Drug Delivery: Science and Technology

Drug Delivery: Science and Technology

Edited by Julian Millar

STATES
ACADEMIC PRESS
www.statesacademicpress.com

States Academic Press,
109 South 5th Street,
Brooklyn, NY 11249, USA

Visit us on the World Wide Web at:
www.statesacademicpress.com

ISBN: 978-1-63989-160-3

Cataloging-in-Publication Data

Drug delivery : science and technology / edited by Julian Millar.
p. cm.
Includes bibliographical references and index.
ISBN 978-1-63989-160-3
1. Drug delivery systems. 2. Pharmaceutical chemistry. 3. Pharmaceutical technology. I. Millar, Julian.
RS199.5 .D78 2022
615.6--dc23

Table of Contents

Preface

Every book is a source of knowledge and this one is no exception. The idea that led to the conceptualization of this book was the fact that the world is advancing rapidly; which makes it crucial to document the progress in every field. I am aware that a lot of data is already available, yet, there is a lot more to learn. Hence, I accepted the responsibility of editing this book and contributing my knowledge to the community.

The various aspects related to the transportation of a pharmaceutical compound to its intended target for the purpose of achieving a specific effect is termed as drug delivery. It consists of different manufacturing techniques, approaches, formulations, storage systems and technologies. The efficiency and safety of a drug are maximized through the application of principles connected to site-specific targeting, route of administration, toxicity, drug preparation and metabolism. Drug delivery focuses on altering the specificity and pharmacokinetics of a drug by formulating it with different excipients, medical devices and drug carriers. Some of the different routes of administration which are considered within this field are sublingual, oral, rectal, inhaled and vaginal. This book discusses the fundamentals as well as modern approaches of drug delivery. Also included herein is a detailed explanation of the science and technology of drug delivery. This book is a vital tool for all researching and studying this field.

While editing this book, I had multiple visions for it. Then I finally narrowed down to make every chapter a sole standing text explaining a particular topic, so that they can be used independently. However, the umbrella subject sinews them into a common theme. This makes the book a unique platform of knowledge.

I would like to give the major credit of this book to the experts from every corner of the world, who took the time to share their expertise with us. Also, I owe the completion of this book to the never-ending support of my family, who supported me throughout the project.

Editor

1

Hybrid Nanocarriers for Potential Drug Delivery

Asadullah Madni, Nayab Tahir, Mubashar Rehman, Ahmed Raza, Muhammad Ahmad Mahmood, Muhammad Imran Khan and Prince Muhammad Kashif

Abstract

Nanocarriers have provided the versatile platform for the delivery of various therapeutic and diagnostic agents. Liposome, niosomes, polymeric and solid lipid nanoparticles are the most promising nanocarriers that have been entered in the clinical trials and become commercially available. However, each system has been associated with some problems that can be minimized by using the combinatorial approach of hybrid nanocarriers. These hybrid systems combine the benefits of different structural components to synergize the outcome of the therapy. In this chapter, the different types of hybrid nanocarriers have been described with particular emphasis on the brief rationale for the development of these hybrid nanocarriers along with different fabrication approaches with greater emphasize on the lipid polymer hybrid nanoparticles. A brief description factors governing the optimized response characteristics and their potential application of these hybrid nanoparticles are also presented.

Keywords: core shell hybrid nanoparticles, drug delivery, hybrid nanoparticles, nanoflowers

1. Introduction

In the recent decades, pharmaceutical nanotechnology has opened a new era for the research in the design and characterization of drug delivery systems (DDS) and biotechnological products. A variety of novel drug delivery systems and strategies emerged for diagnostic and therapeutic applications that explored the different structural components, fabrication methods and mechanisms of drug delivery and targeting [1]. These DDS emphasized on the use of multiple nanomaterials and therapeutic moieties that renovate the current pharmaceutical industry and biomedical sciences toward the better drug therapy [2]. These nanosized particles were utilized for the delivery of various molecules including different drugs, proteins, nucleic acid and other diagnostic agents. Some of these compounds may be encapsulated inside while others were adsorbed on the surface of these nanoparticles. These nanocarriers can amend the pharmacokinetics and pharmacodynamics of drug by enhancing the solubility, permeability and bioavailability in multiple ways. The availability of the encapsulated compound depends upon the nature of formulation components and the other external stimuli which enable the controlled as well as targeted delivery of these encapsulated compounds within the cellular microenvironment [3]. All these parameters ultimately achieve the higher concentration of the encapsulated drug that efficiently reaches the potential target site without affecting the normal tissues. These nanocarriers also aid to implement the concept of rational therapeutics by providing the tunable drug delivery systems based on the patient therapeutic demands.

Despite of excellent in-vitro performance, some drugs demonstrate poor in-vivo results because of low aqueous solubility, poor membrane penetrability, rapid clearance by the reticuloendothelial system, complex pathophysiological states of the disease and uncertain plasma levels leading to drug toxicity, thus, requiring such drug delivery systems that overcome these problems [4]. Latest developments in the material sciences, polymer engineering and nanotechnology have enabled multidisciplinary research to formulate and evaluate different novel drug delivery systems that claimed increased drug solubility, penetration and retention at the targeted site in the body [5].

Among the different nanoparticulate systems, nanoparticles of different composition and lipid based vesicular carriers (liposome, lipid nanocarriers, solid lipid nanoparticles and drug lipid conjugates) have been frequently employed for the medical applications. The nanoparticles may provide versatility in terms of composition. As, these include the polymeric nanocarriers, mesoporous nanoparticles, metal coated (gold, iron and silver), inorganic nanoparticles, quantum dots, carbon nanotubes, dendrimers and magnetic nanoparticles [6, 7]. Furthermore, all these systems were modified to mimic the desired therapeutic properties through different modification method and ligands such as (i) increase in the retention time and stability of the system, (ii) stimuli triggered release, (iii) targeted delivery of various agents and (iv) administration of dual modalities simultaneously [8, 9].

Liposomes and niosomes have been considered as most promising domains among the lipid vesicular carriers. Liposomes are defined as the lipid vesicles having the single or multiple layers of the lipid providing the encapsulation of different therapeutic moieties while niosomes have the same morphology but contain nonionic surfactants instead of phospholipids as major structural components. They provide the better biocompatibility profile, easy surface modification of the vesicles, versatility in the loading of hydrophobic and hydrophilic drugs and improved pharmacokinetic properties [10, 11]. However, drug leakage or fast release from the system, reproducibility, poor physical and chemical stability on storage, higher cost and scale up issues are the major drawbacks associated with the vesicular systems [12, 13].

Nanoparticles (polymeric, organic/inorganic, mesoporous silica, calcium carbonate and different metals, i.e., iron, silver and gold) established the second domain of the nanocarriers. These systems prove superiority in terms of smaller particle size, structural integrity, versatility in the polymeric materials, improved drug loading and release profile. They also provide the targeting capabilities in the case of magnetic iron oxide nanoparticles and better cellular interactions in case of organic and inorganic nanoparticles [14]. Similar to that of vesicular systems, these polymeric nanoparticles have some limitations in term of polymer toxicity, presence of toxic organic solvents, poor entrapment of hydrophilic drugs, polymer degradation and drug leakage before reaching the site of action [15].

The problems associated with the liposomes, polymeric nanoparticles and other carrier systems can be reduced by using a novel combinatorial approach of "hybrid nanoparticles" (HNPs) that utilizes the positive attributes of two different components. These hybrid nanoparticles (HNPs) exploit the benefits of both systems (lipid and polymer/organic and inorganic materials) and the release profile of drug is based on the erosion and degradation of the core material by hydrolysis with in turn determined by water permeation into the outer shell layer and composition of the polymer. The core materials may be protected by the application of multiple layers of the shell materials and the interface of these layer acts as a site for the functionalization of the carrier system for the dual modalities of treatment and diagnosis [16].

Similarly, core shell hybrid nanoparticles using different oils, metal oxides, organic and inorganic components also provide newer system that has multilayered structure having the inner core outer shell with a suitable lipid or oil at the interface to develop a core shell hybrid structure. Recently, use of green approach offer more facile and potentially successful system with the added advantage of solvent-free nanohybrids with greater efficiency.

Such novel system consists of three different structural components as follows:

(i) The inner most core made up of different polymers (poly-lactic-co-glycolic acid [PLGA], polycaprolactone [PCL] and chitosan), lipids (cationic, anionic, zwitterion and neutral phospholipids and nonionic surfactants), inorganic materials (silica, iron oxide) and organic materials (polysaccharides) that encapsulate the therapeutically active moiety.

(ii) The intermediate lipid layer that covers the polymeric/inorganic core and enhance the biocompatibility of that system. It also acts as barrier to minimize the drug leakage and control the rate of polymer/inorganic core degradation by controlling the water permeation into the core.

(iii) The outer most lipid or polymer-conjugate which act as a layer for functionalization of the system by making it target specific through the use of different ligands or increased its circulation and retention time by coating with the PEG. This layer may be modified with a suitably charged moiety to attach the antibodies, aptamer and other such molecules by electrostatic forces [17]. Different types of the hybrid nanocarriers having different morphology and different structural components **Figure 1**.

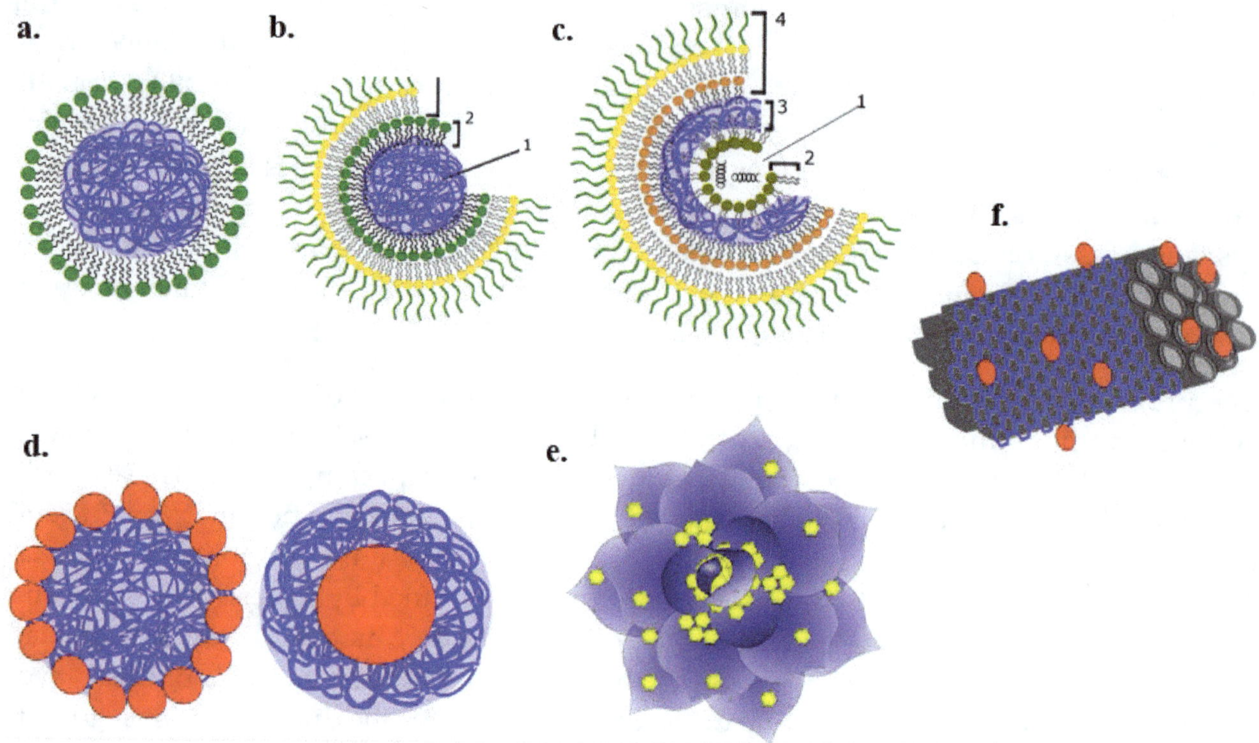

Figure 1. Structure of lipid-polymer hybrid nanoparticles; (a) polymer core-lipid shell hybrid, (b) 3 layers polymer-lipid hybrid nanoparticles consisting of polymeric core (1) and two lipid layers (2,3) shell, (c) 4 layers hollow core lipid-polymer hybrid, consisting of hollow core (1) covered by reverse surfactant layer (2), polymeric shell (3), and outer shells of two lipids (4). (d) organic core-inorganic shell and inorganic core-organic shell hybrid, (e) inorganic (metallic)-protein hybrid nanoflowers, and (f) graphene oxide coated mesoporous silica-inorganic hybrid nanoparticles.

In this chapter, the different types of hybrid nanocarriers have been described with particular emphasis on the brief rationale for the development of these hybrid nanocarriers along with different fabrication approaches with greater emphasize on the lipid polymer hybrid nanoparticles. A brief description factors governing the optimized response characteristics and their potential application of these hybrid nanoparticles are also presented.

2. Method of preparation

Different methods have been employed for the fabrication of hybrid nanocarriers depending upon their chemical composition and applications. The lipid-polymer hybrid, polymer-inorganic hybrid, metal (gold, silver or iron) polymer, silica (SiO_2) based hybrid nanosystems and hybrid polymeric nanocarriers have been most widely investigated [18]. Most of these hybrid carriers utilized two distinctive fabrication approaches. First, a two-step conventional approach process, in which the inner core and outer shell are prepared separately and then are coincubated for the formation of hybrid nanoparticle. The second approach is the single step, in which various state-of-the art techniques of the self-assembling are being incorporated. These processes are further modified with different chemical moieties to obtain versatile hybrid nanoparticles meeting specific need of therapy [19]. In the present chapter, we will focus on the two step conventional as well as single step formulation approaches along with recent innovations have been presented in order to prepare the hybrid nanocarriers with versatile characteristics.

2.1. Conventional two-step method

It was the first technique employed for the fabrication of hybrid nanocarriers. The inner core and outer shell components are prepared in two separate steps employing suitable polymers and chemicals and are then combined to form the hybrid nanoparticle [17]. The foremost type of core shell hybrid nanoparticles contained a core of the polymeric nanoparticles and an outer shell of preformed lipid component such as liposome or lipoparticles in appropriate ratios [20]. Further, the single or multilayered shell is prepared with other techniques such as sonication [21], extrusion or high pressure homogenization and vortexing [22]. The polymeric core is prepared by emulsification-solvent evaporation or solvent diffusion [23], desolvation [24], nanoprecipitation [25, 26], sonication [27] and high pressure homogenization [28] depending upon the hydrophobicity of the loading drugs, their applications [29] and the size of the core.

The single step method is applied when the core materials such as polymers, silica and organic substances are miscible with the drug payload and also are solubilized in the organic solvent [30, 31]. The double emulsification step is employed when the compound is immiscible with the organic solvents and does not form covalent linkage with the core material. As this method requires multiple steps for mixing of different components, relatively larger hybrid nanoparticles are produced [32]. Further, any of the suitable technique such as ultrasonication or extrusion by high pressure homogenization also reduces the particle size as the polymer solution is passed through the nozzle under high pressure. Furthermore, the freeze drying or cooling at normal temperature produced free flowing characteristic particles [33, 34]. Another recent innovation is the application of nanoprecipitation method for the preparation of polymeric core. The polymer is dissolve in the suitable solvent and then precipitated by using the nonsolvent component [26].

The formed polymeric core and lipid vesicles are mixed by vortexing, extrusion, film hydration and ultrasonication techniques in order to formulate the hybrid nanoparticles. The mixing processes provide the energy for the fusion or adsorption of the shell on the inner core material. Additionally, the electrostatic forces among these components also play their role for fabrication of hybrid nanoparticles [35]. It is worth mentioning here that mixing process must be carried out above the phase transition temperature of the lipid component. The formed hybrid nanoparticles are separated by the ultracentrifugation process [36, 37]. Different investigators such as Liang et al. [38] and Zhao et al. [39] prepared the hybrid nanoparticles and nanocells by the emulsification solvent evaporation technique employing the paclitaxel loaded polymeric nanoparticles as core and the PEG or folic acid conjugated octadecyl-quaternary lysine-modified chitosan and cholesterol as lipid shell [38, 39].

2.2. Modified two-step methods

The modifications to the conventional two step method such as spray drying and lithographic molding processes have also been employed for fabrication of hybrid nanoparticles [29]. The inner core is prepared by the spray drying which is dispersed in an appropriate solvent containing the lipid, polymer or any inorganic material. The spray dried lipid coated core shell hybrid nanoparticles were collected after the completion [17].

Freeze or spray dried inhalation hybrid nanoparticles of levofloxacin, ciprofloxacin and isoniazid coated with multiple layers of the lipids were prepared using double emulsion solvent evaporation technique. These hybrid nanoparticles showed better inhalation efficiency, emitted particle size and diameter compared to the conventional two step methods [37, 40]. Another investigations employed nanospray drying for fabrication of hybrid nanoparticles using polyglutamic acid, poly lysine nanoparticles coated with the lipid materials [41]. Recently, Keloglu et al. [42] employed jet spray drying technique for the fabrication of hybrid microfibers-nanoparticles having low density and greater strength using PLGA and poly lactic acid (PLA) [42].

A soft lithography particle molding technique was also utilized for the preparation of hybrid nanocarriers for the delivery of genes to various diseases. De Simon and his coworkers prepared the nanosized particles using the particle replication approach on the silicon wafers. The technique was referred to as Particle Replication in Nonwetting Templates (PRINT) [43]. The process involve the dissolution of the polymer (e.g., PLGA, PLA) in an organic solvents such as dimethyl formamide, methyl acetate and/or dimethyl sulfoxide along with the material to be encapsulated. The PRINT molding device was employed to fabricate the nanoparticles which later were harvested with the help of polyethylene terephthalate sheet [43]. It produces the particles of different shapes and a wide size range depending upon the size of the molding cavities [44].

2.3. Single-step preparation methods

The low encapsulation efficiency due to the leakage of the drugs from the inner core during second step, batch variability and large time consumption are the common problems associated with the conventional two step methods [45]. These constraints can be overcome by designing the simple method that utilized the single step approach and also provide better control on the content uniformity, reproducibility and other characteristics of the system. The method involves the mixing of two different solutions containing the polymer and lipid that self-assembled to form the particles with the core shell hybrid structure [46]. The polymer is dissolved in an appropriate organic solvent while the lipid solution is prepared in the water that may utilize the small fraction of organic solvent as solubilizing agent. The solution containing polymer is added to the lipid phase where the polymer precipitate to formed the nanoparticles and the lipid is self-assembled at the surface to form the hybrid nanoparticles. Single-step preparation is usually achieved by nanoprecipitation, emulsification-solvent evaporation and solvent diffusion methods. These methods and their appropriate modifications are discussed here.

2.3.1. Emulsification solvent evaporation method

Emulsification solvent evaporation method is the most commonly employed single step approach for the fabrication of hybrid nanocarriers. The single emulsification solvent evaporation [47] and double emulsification solvent evaporation (DESE) techniques are employed depending upon the nature and solubility of encapsulating drug. In the ESE method, the oil phase is formed by dissolving the polymer and the drug in the water immiscible organic solvent.

The aqueous solution containing the lipid portion which act as a stabilizer itself during the self-assembling process [48, 49]. The organic phase is then added dropwise into the aqueous phase under the sonication or stirring at the constant speed that results in the formation oil in water emulsion. During the emulsification process, the hydrophobic part of the lipid is adsorbed on the inner core material while the hydrophilic parts arrange themselves toward the aqueous medium forming the lipid coated hybrid nanoparticles [45, 50].

The single ESE method is employed for the encapsulation of hydrophobic drugs with low aqueous solubility [51]. Recently, the folate conjugated lipid polymer hybrid nanoparticles have been prepared by the emulsification solvent diffusion method for the targeted delivery of the doxorubicin using phosphatidylcholine (lecithin 99%) and 1,2-distearoyl-sn-glycero-3-phosphoethanolamine (DPSE)-PEG-COOH as lipid portion and PLGA as a polymeric portion [52]. The ESE method was also employed to formulate duel ligand hybrid nanocarriers for the targeted delivery of docetaxel. The hybrid nanoparticles possessed a uniform monolayer of the lipid over the polymeric core. The cell interaction studies revealed better endocytosis profile with sustained release of the drug by preventing the diffusion of the aqueous medium in the polymeric core. However, the particle were relative larger compared to that prepared by the nanoprecipitation method. This might be attributed to higher drug loading that maintained the therapeutic concentration for the longer period of time [53].

The double emulsification solvent evaporation (DESE) has been employed for the hydrophilic drugs and nucleic acid such as siRNA (small interfering ribonucleic acid) which are not dissolved in different organic solvents along with the other suitable polymers or the core/shell materials [54]. The aqueous solution of desired substance is prepared and is then emulsified in the organic/oil phase containing the lipid and polymer. The resultant primary emulsion is again added to another aqueous solution containing the lipid (lecithin, phosphatidylcholine or DSPE) or surface ligand (PEG, half antibodies, aptamer) and a water-in-oil-in-water (w/o/w) multiple emulsion is prepared. The evaporation of the organic phase results in the formation of hybrid nanoparticles [55]. The particles with hollow core covered with an appropriate shell provide the space for the internalization of hydrophilic and small molecules. The evaporation of the organic solvent provides the multilayered shell which has larger size as compared to the other methods [17].

Su et al. [56] prepared the reduction sensitive hybrid nanoparticles of doxorubicin using chitosan with the sodium dodecyl sulfate employing the double emulsification solvent evaporation method. The amphiphilic chitosan and lipid base micelles core provided a unique nanoconfiguration that is enveloped by the triglycerides which enhanced the loading efficiency and provided the drug release profile up to eight folds [56].

2.3.2. Nanoprecipitation

This method is also known as salting out method. It is a well known method for fabrication of hybrid nanoparticles of size less than 100 nm. This method employs two miscible solvents with different solubilizing capacity for the polymer. First, the polymer core is formed by solubilizing in solvent of greater solubility designated as good solvent which is then added to less soluble solvent designated as poor solvent. The two solutions are mixed by dropwise addition, stirring or sonication. Good solvent being miscible with poor solvent diffuses into later, leaving behind the core nanoparticles due to the precipitation of the polymer [19].

The core forming polymer and lipophilic drug are solubilized in a water-miscible organic solvent like acetone, acetonitrile or ethanol [57]. The lipids, inorganic salts or silica are dispersed in water with moderate heating (~60–75°C) and/or addition of hydroalcoholic mixtures for proper dispersion of the lipids.

The hydrophilic drugs are added to the aqueous phase containing dispersed lipids [58]. The polymer containing organic phase is then added dropwise to lipid dispersion with continuous stirring to precipitate the polymer into nanoparticles. The monodispersed hybrid nanoparticles are collected after suitable application of vortexing, homogenization or ultrasonication [55, 59]. Concurrent to the precipitation process, the self-assembly of lipid molecules around the polymer molecules occurs due to the hydrophobic interactions. The polymer core captures the hydrophobic tails of lipid while the heads are facing toward the aqueous phase [17, 60]. Continuous stirring of dispersion for several hours is helpful in uniform lipid coating of hybrid nanoparticles and to ensure the complete removal of organic solvent [55]. Rotary evaporator may also be helpful for the removal of organic solvents [58].

The literature suggests 10% ethanolic solution is employed for solubilization of lipids and PEG may enhance the stability of hybrid nanoparticles [61]. According to the study of Ling et al. [58], dextran sulfate and lecithin/PEG-PLGA hybrid nanoparticles can entrap higher amounts of hydrophilic moiety, the vincristine.

Wang et al. [62] developed PLGA/TPGS-lecithin hybrid nanoparticles using a modified nanoprecipitation method. The PLGA was dissolved in acetone while lipids were dispersed in either aqueous or 4% ethanolic aqueous solution. An inverse-phase nanoprecipitation method (i.e. aqueous phase was added dropwise into organic phase consisting of acetone, the PLGA and the paclitaxel). Initially, the formation of hybrid nanoparticles was slow due to the higher proportion of organic phase in the mixture. Continuous stirring and addition of water boosted the diffusion which leads to solidification of the hybrid nanoparticles. A stable hybrid nanoparticle formulation with low value of PDI (~0.1) was observed at 5:1 aqueous to organic phase ratio [62].

2.3.3. *Sonication*

Sonication is a fast technique for the fabrication of hybrid nanoparticles which utilizes ultrasonic waves rather than vortexing, solvent evaporation or heating. In this method, the two solutions designated as organic and aqueous phases lead to formation of inner core (polymer) and outer shell or coating materials (lipids), respectively. The sonication has been employed by Fang et al. [63] for the fabrication of hybrid nanoparticles of lecithin-PEG and PLGA by using this approach. The PLGA was dissolved in acetonitrile while the lecithin and the PEG were added in 4% ethanol solution. The former solution was carefully pipetted into the hydro alcoholic solution (aqueous to organic ratio was kept as 10:1). The hybrid nanoparticles were produced as this 'cocktail' mixture was placed in sonicator bath for five minutes at a frequency of 42 kHz and a power of 100 W. The main advantage of this technique is the formation of stable hybrid nanoparticles with short processing time and production rate is 20 times than other processes [63].

The sonication technique has been employed for PLGA and docetaxel hybrid nanoparticles by Liu et al. [64]. In another study, Mandal et al. [65] developed erlotinib loaded hybrid nanoparticles of PCL in which erlotinib and PCL were dissolved in acetone and added to the aqueous phase containing lipids. Hybrid nanoparticles were produced after sonication for 10 minutes at a frequency of 67 kHz and a power of 200 W [65].

A unique method using the combination of modified nanoprecipitation and sonication methods is presented for the fabrication of hybrid nanoparticles. In this method, the lipids melt was mixed with ethanolic solution of Elacridar, a chemosensitizer, and placed in vacuum oven until complete removal of solvents. The doxorubicin being hydrophilic drug was added in water with surfactant (Pluronic-F68) and heated (72–74°C). The drug and surfactant dispersion was mixed with Elacridar-lipid mixture. The whole mixture was stirred for 10 min and then ultrasonicated for two cycles of three minutes. It produced submicron sized lipid emulsion which was dispersed in 4–9 times higher volume of cold water (maintained 4°C) which leads to the formation of hybrid nanoparticles [66, 67].

2.3.4. Green technology for the preparation of hybrid nanocarriers

The use of green technology has revolutionized the synthesis of hybrid nanocarriers due to the ecofriendly procedures that mitigate the threats of toxic impurities and use of the organic solvents. These ecofriendly approaches also provided low operating cost, better stability, compatibility and minimum health hazards [68]. The literature has suggested the successful implementation of solvent free approaches to formulate nanosized systems for the targeted delivery of different therapeutic and diagnostic moieties.

The heat chill method has been employed to prepare micelles using the amphiphilic diblock and triblock copolymers of polycaprolactone (PCL) for the encapsulation of insulin without using any organic solvent and has provide better stability of the entrapped proteins which are liable to denaturation in the presence of different organic solvents [69].

Kumar et al. prepared the green PLGA-oil hybrid nanoparticles of resveratrol employing the acrysol oil (a derivative of castor oil) as nontoxic solvent. The nanoparticles have a smooth outer morphology with improved drug release and stability profile [70].

2.3.5. Preparation of organic/inorganic hybrid nanoparticles

The concept of combining the characteristics of organic and inorganic components is quite old since the time of Egyptian inks. However, the modern organic-inorganic hybrid systems are not prepared by simple mixing these materials but may involve the weak electrostatic linkages (H-bonding or van der Waals forces) or strong chemical bonds, i.e., covalent bonds [71]. Multiple strategies are employed for the preparation of these hybrid particles. These include (i) polymerization of the different monomers, organosilanes and the metal oxides, (ii) self-assembly of different structural components at nanoblock level with different organic and metal components, (iii) the functionalization of preformed nanocarriers with different organic compounds and (iv) making the core with organic materials and coating with the silica and different metallic components [72, 73].

Structural components	Physicochemical properties			Application	References
	Size (nm)	Zeta potential (mV)	Entrapment efficiency (%)		
PLA DPPC PEG-PE	278 ± 16	(+) 20 to 50	N/A	Steric stabilization of hybrid nanoparticles was enhanced at least up to 150 mM NaCl (for more than 1 year at 4°C).	[27]
Paclitaxel PLGA PEGylated octadecyl-quaternized lysine modified chitosan	194 ± 7	22 ± 4	87 ± 2	Folic acid modified polymer core lipid shell hybrid carrier for targeted anti-cancer therapy. Higher internalization up to 14.8 folds was observed in flow cytometry. It also showed higher cytotoxicity than commercial preparation (Taxol®). After 2 hours administration, it showed 3.70 fold higher bio distribution than Paclitaxel injection.	[39]
Levofloxacin Ciprofloxacin Ofloxacin PLGA Phosphatidylcholine (PC), Stearic Acid (SA)	420 260 360	-26 +26 -22	19 4 5	The amount of the polymer and lipid were optimized for highly efficient hybrid system. Hybrid nanoparticles showed higher size and drug encapsulation in comparison to polymeric carriers. Different antibiotics like levofloxacin, ciprofloxacin and ofloxacin were encapsulated. Ciprofloxacin showed less EE due to less lipophilicity. Oppositely charged drug and lipid prevented nanoparticle formation which was remedied by the addition of counter ionic surfactant.	[45]
Doxorubicin PLGA DEPE-PEG Lecithin	118.7 ± 0.75	15.19 ± 3.85	45.76 ± 6.58	Folate receptor mediated drug delivery of anti-cancer agent, doxorubicin, resulted in higher cell internalization and enhanced cell-killing effect toward MCF-7 cells with a significantly lower IC50.	[52]
PLGA DSPE-PEG Poly (β-aminoester) poly-1	280 ± 70	(+) 40 ± 7	N/A	mRNA loaded pH sensitive particles reached cytosol offering low cytotoxicity followed by translation at a frequency of ~30%. Intranasal administration of abovementioned system led to *in vivo* expression of protein as soon as 6 hours after administration.	[57]
Vincristine PLGA Poly ethylene glycol (PEG) Dextran sulfate	121.8–133	-8.5 to -14.6	64.7 to 93.6	Vincristine loaded hybrid nanocarriers resulted in 3.3-fold increase in apparent bioavailability, while its uptake was 12.4-fold higher than plain drug solution.	[58]

Structural components	Physicochemical properties			Application	References
	Size (nm)	Zeta potential (mV)	Entrapment efficiency (%)		
Docetaxel PLGA Lecithin PEG	70–80	-30 to -35	59 ± 4	Docetaxel loaded Hybrid nanoparticle exhibited 20 hourrs as T_{50}. These carriers also exhibited good stability in 10% bovine serum albumin and in 10% plasma solution.	[59]
Paclitaxel PLGA Soybean lecithin D-α-tocopheryl polyethylene glycol 1000 succinate (TPGS)	120–150	-15 to -20	>80	Developed carriers provided sustained release up to 8 days with a high tumor targeting potential through EPR effect. It also showed superior antitumor efficacy by inhibiting 58.8% volume of tumor at day 28.	[62]
PLGA DSPE-PEG	65	-47.7	N/A	A new quick single step preparation method is reported which needs 5 min to get accomplished. This method increased the production rate 20-fold without compromising determinant features of hybrid particles. Particles developed such exhibited good colloidal stability in PBS and serum over 5 days.	[63]
Docetaxel PLGA DEPE-PEG_{2000}	263.6	-20.74	66.88	Folic acid conjugation increased 38.2% for 0.5 hour incubation and 54% increase for 2 hours incubation during cell uptake study. Cell viability studies showed that formulation was 93.65% more effective than commercial preparation Taxotere®.	[64]
Erlotinib DEPE-PEG_{2000} Dipalmitoylphosphatidylcholine (DPPC) N-[1-(2,3-Dioleoyloxy) propyl]-N,N,N-trimethylammonium methyl-sulfate (DOTAP)	161–271	-47	77.18	Erlotinib loaded Core Shell Lipid Polymer Hybrid Nanoparticles demonstrated 170 nm size with 66% Entrapment efficiency and greater uptake and efficiency in A549 cells.	[65]
Doxorubicin Elacridar Pluronic F-68	187–272	-19.7 to -22.9	71.2–89.3	Formulation shows up to 89% encapsulation efficiencies of Dox and GG918 in PLN with more uptake and cytotoxicity of Dox to MDR cells	[67]

Structural components	Physicochemical properties			Application	References
	Size (nm)	Zeta potential (mV)	Entrapment efficiency (%)		
Resveratrol PLGA	375 ± 13	-22 ± 1.6	76 ± 4.2	G-PONHs have higher biocompatibility and stability, but moderate cytotoxicity compared to standard NPs. It also involves the application green synthesis approach for the hybrid nanocarriers	[70]
Paclitaxel Poly-lactic-co-glycolic acid (PLGA) Soybean lecithin 1,2-Distearoyl-sn-glycero-3-phosphoethanolamine (DSPE-PEG)	186.9 ± 8.52	-29.5 ± 2.0	81.34 ± 3.41	More drug reaches target site crossing Blood brain barrier and survival time for mice was PtxR-FPLNs (42 days), Ptx-FPLNs (38 days) compared to PtxR (18 days) and Paclitaxal (14 days)	[76]
Melatonin Poly lactic acid (PLA) Didodecyldimethylammonium bromide (DDAB) Cetyltrimethylammonium bromide (CTAB)	180–218	+15.4 to -36.1	90.35	Coating with cationic lipids provides sustained and prolonged drug release, a pronounced benefit in ophthalmic application	[77]
Docetaxel PLGA DEPE-PEG_{2000} Soybean lecithin	60–70	-40 to -60	~62	The system provides 62% entrapment efficiency and almost 50% drug release in 20 hours. The incorporation of PEG provides stability over 120 hours. TC 50 value ranged between 4.58 and 5.55 mg.	[78]
PLGA DSPE-PEG	50–150	N/A	N/A	Different lipid ratios were evaluated for the entrapment, particle size, stability of the system. The current system provides that pH sensitive release and targeting which aggregate the drug in the acidic tumor microenvironment.	[79]
Poly caprolacton (PCL) Glyceryl tripalmitate	58–2009	-5.82 to -46.31	5.81–60.32	The system indicates biphasic release of the drug in which the burst release id presented in the initial hour. The cellular uptake was 83.3% in L929 cells. It also provides better colloidal stability over 120 hours.	[81]
Human IgG Poloxamer-188	135–799	+16.7 to +17.9	30.3–60	The system was loaded with the SiRNA. Which show the loading capacity of up to 2.04%, entrapment efficiency 60% in the optimized formulation. It provides the targetibility with the antibody and the sustain release was demonstrated by 20% release over the study time.	[82]

Structural components	Physicochemical properties			Application	References
	Size (nm)	Zeta potential (mV)	Entrapment efficiency (%)		
PCL Grape leaf extract Curcumin	~291	-24.3		The resulting drug delivery system improves the antimicrobial efficacy against two bacterial strains in addition to antifungal activity and can be an alternative approach to antibacterial agents.	[83]
Doxorubicin Epoxidized soybean oil Pluronic F68	200–350	-23.1	70 to 80	The system promotes cytotoxicity of DOX against MDR to about eightfolds. Uptake and retention of drug by MDR was also significantly increased.	[84]
Carboxymethyl chitosan Calcium phosphate PEG	102 ± 1.7	-8.25 ± 0.76	78	It gives excellent delivery of siRNA to cancer proximity through EPR effect. Particularly hTERT containing nanoparticles promotes silencing of hTERT expression and induction of cell apoptosis pathways.	[85]
Doxorubicin Sorafenib	126.3 ± 16.4	-21.4 ± 4.6	90.5 ± 3.4 and 70.8 ± 2.8	DOX-SOR combination in iRGD conjugated HNPs produces more apoptotic rates up to 44.7% than 33.4% with plain drug combinations or 37% with HNPs without iRGD.	[86]
Doxorubicin Mitomycin C	~150	~ -25	>90	Co delivery of anticancer agents using HNPs is more effective than simple combination therapy with advantages of high local delivery. It provides the 2–4 fold increase in the cellular uptake of the drug in the cancer cells.	[87]
Lipid modified PEG	24 ± 5	-38 ± 1	N/A	The system describes engineering of functionalized lipid conjugated polymeric nanoparticles with more specific targeting approach and imaging and bio sensing based on fluorescence.	[88]
Doxorubicin Combretastatin A4 PLGA PC DSPE-PEG Cholesterol	180–200	N/A	N/A	The system contains two different therapeutic agents which provide the site targeted release of the anti-angiogenesis agent and the anti-cancer drugs.	[89]
Curcumin PLGA DPPC DSPE-PEG	171.6 ± 8.2	N/A	N/A	By treating the metastatic breast cancer cells with the lipid-polymer hybrid nanoparticles of Curcumin decreased the adhesion onto tumor necrosis factor by 70% in capillary flow.	[90]

Structural components	Physicochemical properties			Application	References
	Size (nm)	Zeta potential (mV)	Entrapment efficiency (%)		
Docetaxel PLA Chitosan	208–255.7	-21.3 to + 52.4	75.9	PLA/chitosan nanoparticles provide rapid initial release of 40% drug in 5 hours and 70% cumulative release in 24 hours.	[91]
Docetaxel Curcumin PLGA	169.6 ± 4.6	-35.7 ± 1.9	89.8 ± 3.1 and 81.9 ±5.6	The drugs loaded hybrid nanoparticles showed enhanced cytotoxicity and tumor growth inhibition.	[92]
Docetaxel DSPE-PEG PLGA	110 ± 13.5	-25.67 ± 1.45	77.65 ± 0.57	The system increases the cellular update of docetaxel 2.5 folds and anti-proliferative activity 2.69–4.23 folds.	[93]
Doxorubicin Chitosan Hyaluronic acid	264 ± 2.2	-12.3 ± 2.0	97.8 ± 1.3	It is used to deliver anticancer drugs which results in enhanced circulation half-life and reduce the elimination of drug	[94]

Table 1. Hybrid nanoparticles with different structural components and their applications.

In conventional sol-gel approach, the hydrolysis process is used to obtain the hybrid system. The reaction involves the organically modified metal oxides which crosslinks with the polymers of multiple functionalities. These components may or may not be present in the organic solvents and possibly trapped within the inorganic material. However, use of self-assembling procedures in last few decades provided new methods for the fabrication. During the process, the inorganic materials (triblocks) were arranged by the use of organic surfactants. The preparation of the mesoporous hybrid with multiple functionalities provide highly porous surface which further modified based on the applications [74].

Shen and Shi [75] reported a method for preparation of the organic/inorganic hybrid based dendrimers. The metal or inorganic nanoparticles were entrapped in the dendrimers template to provide a modified surface morphology which can be tuned by different functional components to provide the biocompatibility and better colloidal stability [75] (**Table 1**).

3. Factors affecting hybrid nanocarriers

Hybrid nanoparticles are trimmed to an acceptable level of particle size, drug carrying capacity and site specificity through incorporation and adjustment of ratios of different chemical components. The variations of structural components of HNPs have an obvious influence on HNPs' characteristics [17, 96]. The principal factors of HNPs' formulation are (i) lipid/polymer ratio, (ii) PEGylation and (iii) polymer nature.

3.1. Lipid/polymer ratio

The lipid covering the polymeric core provides substantial benefits to HNPs and their distinction over nonhybrid nanoparticles. The ratio of two building blocks (lipid-polymer) of hybrid particles have significant role in stabilizing the formulation, monodispersibility and encapsulation efficiency [45, 97].

At a lower L/P ratio, the nanoparticle surfaces are not entirely covered with lipids, which can form bridges with lipid part of other particles causing aggregation and formation of larger particles. At a relative higher lipid concentration, it tends to decrease the production yield as whole amount is not incorporated in particles and free lipids will arrange themselves to form liposomes can affect the homogeneity of formulation. Therefore, the concentration of lipids should be optimized that cover to polymeric core on the basis of particle size and production yield [59, 98]. Chew et al. prepared HNPs with PC and PLGA carrying antibiotics with W_{PC}/W_{PLGA} value <15- up to 90%. At lipid amount below 15% larger particles were formed (800–1000 nm) and a sharp decrease in particle size was observed at an optimum concentration i.e. 30% lipids, an optimum particle size (260–400 nm) and 80% production yield was achieved. The lipid ratio above the optimum concentration i.e. 30% did not reduce particle size but it decreased the yield as the entire lipid was not utilized [45].

An optimum lipid to polymer ratio also provides the colloidal stability of HNPs by providing an optimum surface charge density which is responsible for electrostatic repulsive forces that prevent particle coalescence and stabilizes the formulation. In case where the lipid part is insufficient and the resulting electrostatic repulsive forces are weak, some agents like PEG can be incorporated in the formulations to provide steric repulsion and stabilization of the HNPs [52, 80–98].

The charge on lipid part which is responsible for electrostatic repulsion between particles is shielded when mixture of cationic and zwitterionic lipids is employed. Anionic heads of zwitterionic lipids face outwards which reduces of cationic lipids charge and promotes aggregation of particles. However, the higher cationic lipid concentration may overcome this charge screening and aggregation can be minimized [59, 99]. The zwitterionic lipid such as 1,2-dipalmitoyl-sn-glycero-3-phosphocholine (DPPC) produces less aggregation than a cationic lipid, 1,2-dipalmitoyl-3-trimethylammonium propane (DPTAP). Therefore, it zwitter ionic lipid provides more stability than ionic lipids [55, 59].

The two potential benefits that lipid augments to the HNPs are the encapsulation efficiency and retardant release of the incorporated drugs. The former is achieved by preventing drug leakage during self-assembling process, whereas the latter is due to reduced interaction of lipids with dissolution medium [17, 100]. The charge on the surface of lipids and drugs also affects the entrapment efficiency due to interaction of surface charge of HNPs and the charge of the drug. The loading of ciprofloxacin in the PLGA-PC hybrid system is not successful due to the interaction of cationic drug with the anionic lipids [19, 78].

A significant higher percent encapsulation of docetaxel (59 ± 4) was achieved in HNPs assembled from lecithin, DSPE-PEG and PLGA i.e. compared to PLGA-PEG nanoparticles with 19 ± 3 (mean ± SD). This effect is attributed to the fencing action of lipids which keeps hydrophobic drugs within the core and retards water penetration. The lipid-polymer hybrid formulations also provide a sustained release of drug when compared with nonhybrid formulation due to less water penetration and reduced escape of drug molecules from polymeric core. A consistent 50 % release of docetaxel from lecithin-PLGA hybrid system was observed compared to the PLGA-PEG NPs and PLGA NPs released same amount of drug in 10 hours and 7 hours, respectively. The pH of the dissolution media also affected the encapsulation of drugs, for example, the erlotinib EE % was 77.1%, 28.83% and 18.45% at pH values of 7.4, 5.4 and 3.4, respectively [55, 59, 78, 100].

3.2. PEGylation

The steric stabilization of HNPs systems to withstand salt solutions, buffer actions and uptake by macrophages is provided by the appropriate surface modification by employing PEG. The term is called as PEGylation. PEGs can escalate circulation times of HNPs by preventing particle aggregation, opsonization and adsorption of plasma proteins [27, 78].

Incorporation of PEG-lipid affects the colloidal stability of HNPs by two ways (i) chain length of PEG-lipid and (ii) molar Ratio of PEG-lipid. HNPs coated with PEG-lipid longer chains exhibited more stability than the shorter chain PEG-lipid coated particles. Similarly, at the fixed chain length more PEG-lipid incorporated onto polymer core and thickness of lipid shell increased which lowered the zeta potential and hence stability is enhanced [78, 80].

Yang et al. studied the effect of lipid/polymer ratio and PEGylation on HNPs prepared from PLA/mPEG-PLA polymer and BHEM-Chol cationic lipid. HNPS prepared from mPEG-PLA were smaller and more stable in PBS at the given lipid/polymer ratio than PLA alone [61].

Fang et al. formulated HNPs using 0.10–0.35 lipid-PEG/PLGA ratios without incorporating lecithin. Initially particle reduced with increase in lipid amount and optimized at 0.30 lipid-PEG/PLGA ratio after which further increase in lipids did not affect particle size and PDI. At an optimized (0.30 lipid-PEG/PLGA) ratio, lipid-PEG was replaced with mole equivalents of lecithin. The stable particles of 60 nm were obtained at 50% lipid-PEG replacement. Upon 70% lipid-PEG replacement, the size was increased to 100 nm and at 80% lipid-PEG replacement with lecithin, the unstable particles were obtained. This instability of particles is due to the replacement of higher lipid-PEG content, a major stability component of HNPs [63].

3.3. Nature of polymer

The characteristics such as density and surface charge play an important role in the fabrication of HNPs [35]. The density of polymer also has substantial effect on stability and particle size [59, 78]. HNPs fabricated from high density polymer are less stable toward increasing ionic strength of medium due to the higher sedimentation rate when electrostatic charges are shielded. PLA is 1.18 times denser than poly(styrene); hence, HNPs prepared with PLA core have less colloidal stability toward increasing ionic strength of medium [35]. Zhang et al. evaluated that change in viscosity of PLGA polymer from 0.19 to 0.82 resulted a decrease in particle diameter from 92.7 nm to 66.7 nm [59].

Adsorption of lipid over polymeric particle surface to form lipid shell depends upon curvature and surface charge of particle. Cationic lipids exhibit more adsorption than zwitter ions toward the anionic polymeric core due to the electrostatic attractions polymeric core from anionic polymer PLA has greater affinity for DPTAP cationic lipid than the zwitterionic DPPC. Lipid rearrangement around polymeric core can be quick and complete if the affinity between polymer and lipid is high. Larger size distribution and free lipid structures are observed when lipids cannot rearrange around polymeric core due to weaker affinity. Modification in pH of medium can improve the affinity of polymer for lipid by surface charge variation at different pH levels [35, 101, 102].

4. Applications of hybrid nanocarriers

Hybrid systems combine properties of two or more materials, thus, appear superior to individual material system. Usually, one component of hybrid system is active, whereas other is used to improve biocompatibility, circulation life and targeting. Many new hybrid systems use second material to improve efficiency of first materials. By suitable selection of materials, hybrid systems find wider applications in medical field. Hydrophilic polymers have been widely used to impart stealth property to nanoparticles. However, stealth coating does not improve or impart new functional aspect of nanoparticles. Thus, many researchers do not regard PEG coated as hybrid systems. Similarly, nanoparticles conjugated with targeting ligands cannot be regarded as hybrid system.

4.1. Lipid polymer hybrid nanoparticles (LPHN)

LPHN consists of a drug containing polymeric core which is coated by a lipid shell. In these systems, inner polymer core contains drug and lipid shell is used to enhance penetration through biological membranes and to control drug release. Polymeric core can be made from hydrophilic or hydrophobic polymer. Term lipid-polymer hybrid is also used for systems that contain polymer core with lipid coating. Lipid is preferred carrier material for hydrophobic drugs due to higher encapsulation efficiency and extended release pattern. A polymeric coating is applied over lipid core to impart certain characteristics required for novel biomedical applications.

In addition of polymeric and lipid layers, surface of LPHN may be modified with different materials. In one study, a hydrophobic drug was loaded in a hydrophobic biodegradable polymer to enhance encapsulation efficiency of a hydrophobic drug. Then, a lipid layer is applied to stabilize core and shell, and to prolong drug release. Finally, hydrophilic polymeric layer, consisting of DSPE-PEG (1,2-distearoyl-sn-glycero-3-phosphoethanolamine-N-carboxy (polyethylene glycol)2000) was applied to improve pharmacokinetics of LPHN. The three-layer LPHN showed high encapsulation and sustained release of hydrophilic drug [59]. A hydrophilic polymer monolayer may be applied to LPHN to escape phagocytosis and early removal from body. Generally, polyethylene glycol (PEG) is used to provide this stealth property and enhance circulation time of nanoparticles. PEG will attract water to make an aqueous layer which protect LPHN from attachment of opsonin proteins and let it escape the uptake by reticuloendothelial (RES) system. Hydrophilic polymer layer can also enhance colloidal stability of LPHN due to steric hindrance effect [5]. As stealth layer can also hinder interaction with target cells, PEG can be conjugated with other monomers or polymers to form block copolymers that are specific to certain stimuli. This approach enables long circulating LPHN that can shed stealth layer when come in contact with target cells. The stimuli could be intracellular and extracellular protease enzymes, low pH or reducing agents [103].

Selection of polymeric matrix plays a major role in drug delivery properties of LPHN. LPHN are commonly used for poor water soluble or hydrophobic drugs. A hydrophobic polymer core can encapsulate higher amount of hydrophobic drug and vice versa. Two or more drugs could also be loaded into the core of LPHN. On the other hand, LPHN with hydrophilic and hydrophobic drug could be made to contain one drug in core and the other in shell. Wong et al. [67] prepared LPHN containing lipid core to encapsulate hydrophobic drug Elacridar (GG918) and hydrophilic shell of hydrolyzed polymer of epoxidized soybean oil (HPESO) to encapsulated doxorubicin. They found that both drugs were released in sustained manner for more than 72 hours (**Figure 2**). Simultaneous delivery of chemosensitizer GG918 was able to revert multidrug resistance to anticancer drug doxorubicin. These simultaneously loaded LPHN showed better efficacy than free drug solution or LPHN of any of the two drugs.

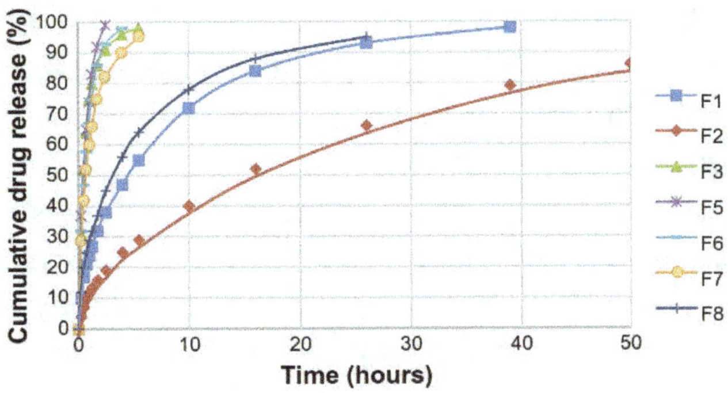

Figure 2. Drug release from gold nanoparticles containing solid lipid nanoparticles. F1 (5mg diacerein) and F2 (10 mg diacerein) show sustained release of drug for 39 and 48 hours. However, F3 had same composition as F2 but drug release was conducted at 40°C. F5 and F6 contained increasing amount of hydrophilic gold nanoparticles with 5 mg diacerein. F7 contained gold nanoparticles same as F6 but 10 mg diacerein. Finally, F8 contained lipophilic gold nanoparticles with 10 mg diacerein. Drug release was faster at higher temperature (F3) as compared to 37°C. Furthermore, hydrophilic gold nanoparticles containing formulations F5, F6 and F7 released drug in less than 5 hours, whereas hydrophobic gold nanoparticles showed prolonged release up to 25 hours.

As a wide variety of polymers and lipids are available, LPHN can be prepared to theoretically load any therapeutic moiety. Nucleic acid based therapeutics i.e. plasmid DNA, antisense oligonucleotide, small interfering RNA and small hairpin RNA, have shown promise to cure many diseases. LPHN have emerged as nonviral carriers for nucleic acid products with low toxicity, immunogenicity and cost of production. Cationic polymers and lipids have been widely investigated for this purpose. Cationic groups can bind negatively charged nucleic acid molecules and deliver to target cells. Zhong et al. [104] prepared LPHN with biodegradable PLGA and two cationic lipids i.e. 1, 2-dioleoyl-3-trimethyammonium-propane (DOTAP) or 3β-[N-(N′,N′-dimethylaminoethane)-carbamyl]cholesterol (DC-Chol). LPHN were prepared by two either with cationic lipid core so that DNA is loaded inside core or with cationic lipid shell so that DNA is loaded on surface. The *in vitro* evaluation was done in human embryonic kidney cells. They found that LPHN with DNA on surface showed higher transfection efficiency than those with DNA inside core. Next, they prepared LPHN with polymer both inside core and on the surface which showed efficiency similar to that of LPHN with DNA on surface. This study concluded that LPHN can show transfection efficiency about 600 times higher than unbound DNA. However, cationic lipids and polymers may have some problems on their own. They may interact with biological components, be nonbiodegradable or toxic after systemic administration. These factors are controlled by hydrophobic chain length, nature of cation group and linkage. To solve these problems, Shi et al. [54] prepared novel LPHN with four distinct layers. First is a hollow core i.e. aqueous droplet containing nucleic acid which is coated by an inner lipid layer of cationic lipid ethylphosphocholine.

The cationic lipid orients itself in such a way that cationic group faces inward and its hydrophobic chain faces outward. Third layer is formed by ester terminated PLGA. It is a hydrophobic polymer that intermingles with protruding chains of cationic lipid. Finally, self-assembled lecithin and DSPE-PEG form outer coating to facilitate transfection and to impart stealth property to LPHN. This LPHN system release loaded siRNA in sustained manner up to 6 days and enhanced gene expression in mice.

A recent trend in drug delivery research has focused on the development of human-like vesicular drug delivery system. This concept emerged when exosome were found to be responsible for cell to cell communication in tumors and regulate tumor microenvironment. It was believed that exosomes isolated from patients may be filled with antitumor drugs and injected back to the patients for personalized treatment. As isolation of exosomes from patients is complicated and very costly, this dream was realized by synthesizing surface antigens of exosomes by genetic engineering and grafting on the surface of drug containing liposomes or other vesicular systems [5]. In addition to this, many bacterial and viral antigens have been used. These antigens are used for the delivery of vaccine and act as immune adjuvant i.e. enhance immune response to vaccine. Moreover, polymeric core produce better adjuvant effects than lipid core. Bershteyn et al. [105] prepared PLGA core and phospholipid bilayer coated LPHN that were stabilized by PEG for simultaneous loading of antigen and adjuvant. The protein adjuvant was covalently bonded on surface and lipophilic adjuvants, such as monophosphoryl lipid A and α-galactosylceramide, which were loaded in lipid bilayer. Immune response was shown at dose as low as 2.5 ng which was detectable after 100 days. It was also found that α-galactosylceramide shows rapid rise in antibody titer whereas monophosphoryl lipid A produced response in sustained manner. Interestingly, coloading of both adjuvants with antigen further increased antigen titer by 12 fold. These results show that LPHN can reduce dose of antigen to reduce cost and side effects.

Term LPHN may also be extended to nanoparticle systems consisting of two or more polymer at least one of which is lipophilic. A hydrophilic shell may be applied to drug containing hydrophobic (or lipophilic) polymeric core to impart mucoadhesion or to make them stealth. For example, PEG or chitosan coating has been widely used to improve circulation life of sustained release solid lipid nanoparticles [106]. On the other hand, a hydrophobic polymer shell may be formed over hydrophilic polymer core to enhance LPHN absorption through biological membranes. This approach is especially useful for oral administration of therapeutic macromolecules [107]. Recently, Liu et al. has synthesized supramolecular vectors for gene delivery. First, adamantyl-terminated polyethyleneimine was admixed with β-cyclodextrin to encapsulate nucleic acid, i.e., DNA or siRNA which was further coated with adamantyl-PEG. The supramolecular vector was stabilized by host-guest interaction. This LPHN system showed low toxicity and high transfection efficiency during in vitro experiments. Graphene is another two-dimensional framework of carbon atoms that is investigated for hybrid applications. When treated with suitable reagents, it can be oxidized, hydroxylated, carboxylated or halogenated. These functional groups can be conjugated with different materials desired for biomedical applications [108].

4.2. Inorganic/organic hybrid nanoparticles (IOHN)

IOHN are synthesized from organic and inorganic materials. Most commonly, core is made of inorganic materials and the shell of an organic material is applied to improve its pharmacokinetic parameters. On the other hand, inorganic shell may be applied to the core of organic materials to impart different properties. IOHN are interesting because they offer properties of both materials. Like organic polymer, they can be functionalized with different groups. Like metallic nanoparticles, inorganic shell provides physical and chemical stability to polymeric core. Generally, the inorganic portion is developed by reduction of metal ions to zerovalent state. Inorganic core is synthesized by mixing metal ions solution with a reducing agent with or without heating. However, inorganic shell may be synthesized either by reduction of metal ions on polymeric core or by deposition of preformed metal colloids on organic core.

Methods for synthesis of organic core and shell have already been discussed in detail in a chapter. We have prepared IOHN consisting of gold core with fatty acid shell. First, gold nanoparticles were synthesized with lecithin bilayer (hydrophilic surface) and lecithin monolayer by acid treatment (hydrophobic surface). The gold nanoparticles were added to molten fatty acids and emulsified with aqueous surfactant solution. Upon cooling, we found that gold nanoparticles with hydrophobic surface are more stable as compared to gold nanoparticles with hydrophilic surface [109]. The presence of gold nanoparticles in core enhanced drug release rate from lipid nanoparticles. This can be attributed to the presence of gold nanoparticles that push drug toward periphery and reduce diffusion path length (**Figure 1**). In another study, we prepared an organic core of lecithin and inorganic shell of gold nanoparticles. First, lecithin nanoparticles were prepared and loaded with drug. Next, preformed gold nanoparticles were adsorbed on its surface. We found that drug release was controlled by both gold nanoparticles. Gold nanoparticles retard release of drug due to physical barrier. Lecithin controlled release of anti-inflammatory drug from core in pH-dependent manner [110]. Gold is also known to possess anti-inflammatory effect. In this study, gold shell was found to synergize anti-inflammatory effect of encapsulated drug diacerein by many folds (**Figure 3**).

Various organic materials have been used to prepare IOHN to improve their performance. The materials that are used to synthesize or stabilize nanoparticles may impart specific function. The most pronounced function is enhanced penetration inside target cells which in turn controls toxicity of IOHN. Freese et al. [47] studied toxicity of gold nanoparticles with different organic coatings with neutral, positive and negative charge. The results showed that IOHN with positive charge coating shows more internalization in cells, and thus, higher toxicity. The cell membrane has a negative charge, whereas the IOHN are positively charged particles. This charge difference triggers the rapid binding to the cell surface and internalization of these IOHNs. As gold can cause toxicity at higher dose, higher internalization in cell will lead to high toxicity [111].

Metallic nanoparticles smaller than 100 nm are usually responsive to different stimuli, a technique that has been widely employed in diagnosis and therapy. IOHN with metallic core can be used for thermotherapy of cancer whereby IOHN produces heat when exposed to external magnetic field. Similarly, metallic moieties, i.e., nanoparticles or tagged polymers, can be bound to core of organic materials. These nanoparticles will be targeted to cancerous tissues and magnetic moieties will produce hyperthermia under external stimuli. When core of organic material is loaded with drug, inorganic part can release the drug by hyperthermia-mediated degradation of core after reaching the target site [5]. In addition to magnetic field, inorganic nanoparticles are also responsive to infrared and ultrasound waves. This makes IOHN interesting candidates for biomedical imaging of targeted tis-

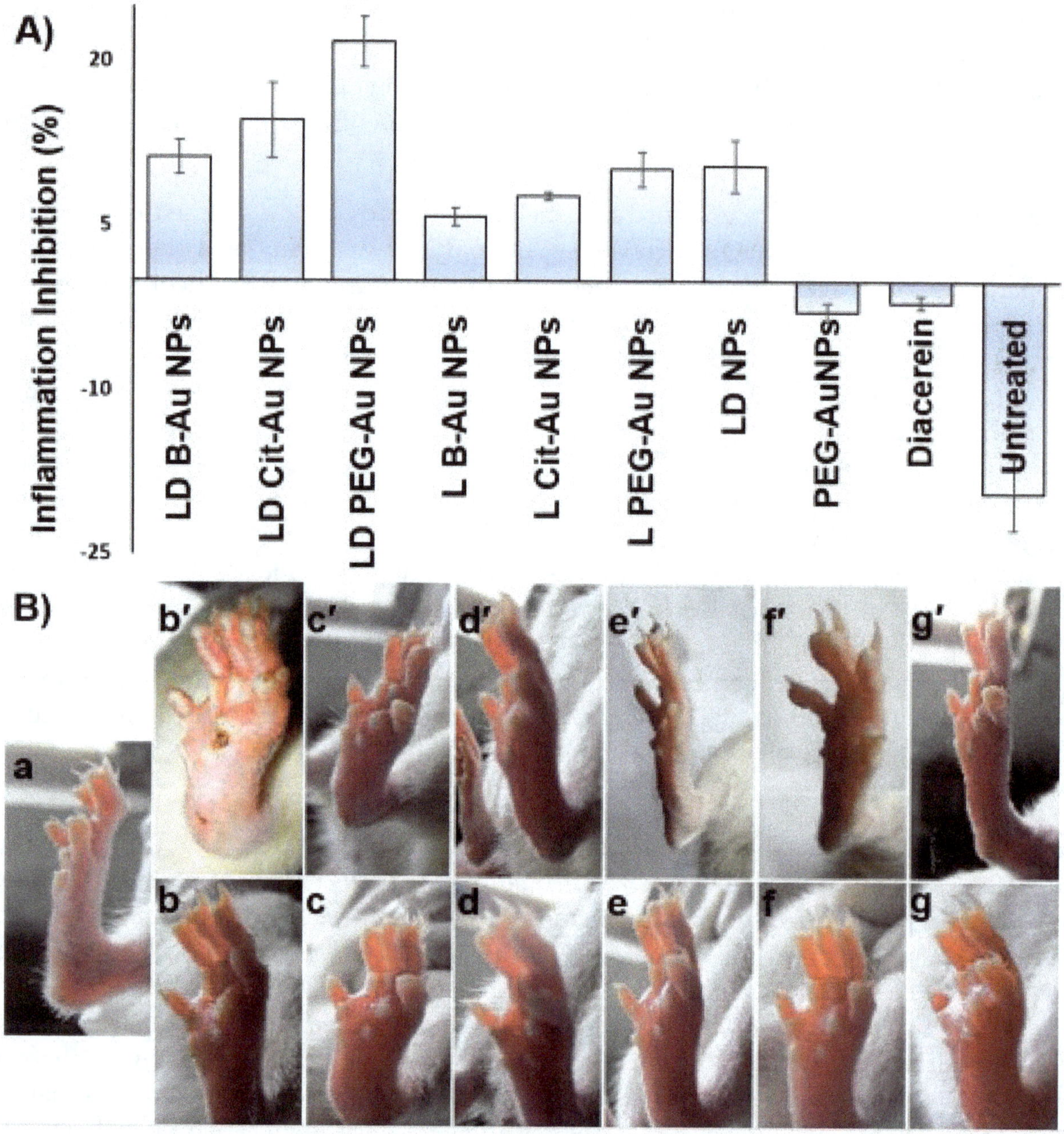

Figure 3. Efficacy of anti-inflammatory drug encapsulated in lecithin core-gold shell hybrid nanoparticles; (A) Anti-inflammatory effect of diacerein is synergized in the presence of gold as compared to pure drug, diacerein. PEG-AuNP = PEG coated gold nanoparticles, LD-NP = diacerein loaded lecithin nano[articles, L PEG-AuNP = Lecithin nanoparticles surface coated with PEG coated gold nanoparticles, L Cit-AuNP = Lecithin nanoparticles surface coated with citrate coated gold nanoparticles, L B-AuNP = Lecithin nanoparticles surface coated with sodium borohydrate coated gold nanoparticles, LD PEG-AuNP = L PEG-AuNP loaded with diacerein, LD Cit-AuNP = L Cit-AuNP loaded with diacerein, LD B-AuNP = L B-AuNP loaded with diacerein. (B) represents decrease in swelling as measured by Vernier caliper before (a, b, c, d, e, f, g) and 3 h after (b′,c′, d′, e′, f′, g′) from untreated (b), diacerein (c), PEG-Au NPs (d), LD PEG-Au NPs (e), LD Cit-Au NPs (f), and LD B-Au NPs (g) treatments groups, while a is normal rat paw.

sues. More recently, multimodal IOHN have ensured imaging and drug release from the same system after systemic administration. This target can be achieved in two ways. First, magnetic field of low frequency or intensity is applied for imaging of IOHN. Once in cancer tissue, intensity or frequency is increased to produce hyperthermia-based cell killing or drug release [112]. Secondly, inorganic materials responsive to more than one stimulus can be used. One stimulus aids in imaging, whereas second stimulus will lead to drug release or thermotherapy [113].

IOHN have also been prepared with hollow core enclosed inside a hybrid shell. Hollow core IOHN can be prepared by many ways. First strategy is to make layer of inorganic or organic material which is then stabilized by other component of IOHN system. Similarly, it can consist of a mixed shell of inorganic and organic materials enclosing hollow core. Metal-tagged polymers with amphiphilic nature self-assemble to form micelles in aqueous solution or after reaching the target microenvironment [114]. Whole virus or virus capsid has been investigated as drug delivery systems by many researchers due to its inherent high penetration in cells.

Portney et al. [115] hybridized virus capsid with quantum dots and single-wall carbon nanotubes to yield hybrid structures that can find various applications. These hybrid structures are very stable to chemical and mechanical stress. IOHN with metallic core and organic shells have been widely investigated for diagnostic application. Although, organic shell usually employed to improve the pharmacokinetics and targeting properties of the metallic nanoparticles but may be beneficial by enhancing the diagnostic efficiency of the system. The most prominent example is nucleic acid-based biosensors with metallic core. When metallic nanoparticles aggregate, they show blue shift due to increase in size. Metallic core is coated with single-stranded DNA (ssDNA) that can identify specific sequence on target DNA and bind it. In bioassay, when metallic nanoparticle conjugated ssDNA start bind target DNA, they come close to each other and test solution color changes from red to blue. This indicates the presence of target DNA as visualized by naked eye or through UV-visible spectrophotometer [116].

4.3. Metalloprotein hybrid nanoflowers (MPHNs)

Although MPHN can be categorized as inorganic-organic hybrid NP, they are discussed here separately due to difference in structure and many fold increased surface area. The flower-like structure of MPHN is due to the presence of proteins that stabilize metallic crystals in the structure. Proteins act as glue and hold metallic crystals in a pattern which mimics flower petals. Unlike inorganic-organic hybrids, synthesis of MPHN occurs in three stages. First stage is the growth stage in which metal ions bond with proteins through amide bond. This acts as nucleation site leading to growth of primary crystals. In the second stage, metalloprotein crystals aggregate to form larger structures bearing primary petals like structures. Finally, anisotropic growth on metalloprotein aggregates leads to formation of complete petals. Generally, their size lies in the range of 2–30 μm which is another reason to differentiate MPHN from OIHN. MPHN is mostly used for bioassay whereby desired enzyme is conjugated with metallic part. Encapsulation efficiency of enzymes in MPHN has been achieved up to 66%. Enzyme loading above or below this limit decreases encapsulation efficiency. Nevertheless, enzyme efficiency of MPHN varies between 85% and 1000%. Enzyme efficiency higher than free enzyme is due to many reasons. MPHN shows high surface area due to petal-like projections. The petals also have hole-like spaces between them that may be up to 100 nm in diameter. It is also observed that immobilized enzyme shows cooperative interaction to enhance enzyme efficiency. Similarly, metal ions, such as copper, calcium and manganese, may also help enzyme in catalysis. Copper (Cu^{2+}) is the most widely used metal with different enzymes. Cu^{2+} and laccase enzyme MPHN have been developed for detection of phenols. The prepared MPHN was adsorbed on filter, and a mixture of phenol and 4-aminoantipyrine was added to it. Laccase-assisted reaction of both compounds produced red antipyrine dyes in 5 minutes. The changes in color will be visible with the naked eye, and UV-visible spectrophotometer can be used for quantitative detection. The MPHN-coated filters are reusable and are much faster than chromatography and mass spectrometry based methods. Likewise, MPHN of Cu^{2+} and horseradish peroxidase was prepared for detection of phenol and hydrogen peroxide. This MPHN was able to detect very low amounts of phenol (1 μM) and hydrogen peroxide (0.5 μM) as change in color was observed with the naked eye. It has been found that hydrogen peroxide induces cell death at concentration higher than 50 μM and the limit of detection of free enzyme is around 20 μM. Thus, these MPHNs will be very efficient to detect slight changes in hydrogen peroxide efficiently even below its threshold level. Cu^{2+} and trypsin MPHN have been used to carry out proteolysis which is an important step in protein identification. The enzyme efficiency of proteolytic MPHN is similar or superior to free enzyme but are fast and reusable.

Another form of nanoflowers is synthesized using deoxyribonucleic acid (DNA) which, like proteins, possesses high number of nitrogen molecules and serves as a template for nanoflowers. In one study, a drug and a dye molecule was bonded to DNA that was used to synthesize nanoflowers. These nanoflowers showed multimodel property of drug delivery and imaging by using FRET technology. More recently, capsular MPHNs have been prepared with improved characteristics. This technique involved coating of MPHN with protamine and silica. Then, metallic core is removed from capsular MPHN system. Capsular nanoflowers show higher enzyme efficiency and improved stability in harsh environmental conditions.

4.4. Mesoporous silica hybrid nanoparticles

Silica has been widely used in drug delivery due to its nontoxic and biocompatible nature. Silica shell has been applied to metallic nanoparticles to reduce their toxicity in various biomedical applications. Mesoporous silica nanoparticles (MSNPs) are silica materials with mesopores of up to 50 nm. They are also termed as hollow mesoporous silica nanoparticles due to the fact that mesopores are hollow. The advantages of MSNP are enhanced surface area and that hollow mesopores can be loaded with therapeutic molecules. First, MSNPs were loaded with drugs. Later, MSNPs were used for the delivery of different dyes and macromolecules such as enzymes. MSNP hybrids have been prepared with both organic and inorganic materials. One problem with the use of MSNP is the leakage of drugs from pores. Sreejith et al. [117] used graphene oxide (GO) coating on MSNP to prevent leakage of drugs. After drug loading, GO coating is applied which acts as blanket to physically block the pores. GO coating also prevents encapsulated drug from environmental degradation. In addition to applications in drug delivery, MSNPs are also used for diagnosis and imaging.

Maji et al. [118] prepared MSNP-GNP (gold nanoparticle) hybrids for detection of hydrogen peroxide. They coated MSNP with graphene oxide, and GNPs were coated on this surface.

The hybrids were first used for electrochemical detection of hydrogen peroxide in the presence of other biological molecules. Later, MSNP-GNPs were successfully used for in vivo imaging in mice. MSNP surface can be modified with different functional groups that provide opportunities to form hybrid with different materials [118].

5. Conclusion and future prospects

Hybrid nanocarriers provide a novel platform that synergizes the effects of therapeutic and diagnostic agents through tunable properties such as particle size, structure, composition, preparatory method and easy surface and charge modifications. Here, we describe the different parameters related to development, optimization as well as characterization to obtain a robust platform for the drug delivery and other biomedical applications. We can still try to focus some unmet challenges of this novel drug delivery system. These challenges include development and optimization of the application of target ligands in appropriate ligand density that will improve the pharmacokinetics as well as pharmacodynamics profiles of all the drugs loaded in these hybrid nanoparticles either single or in combination with other therapeutic and diagnostic agents. Similarly, development of these hybrid nanocarriers at large scale has received less attention. So it is a key parameter to translate the system for large-scale applications by using the different methods mentioned in the section of method of preparation especially the one-step self-assembly method that is likely to improve the production in a facile and economic manner.

Author details

Asadullah Madni*, Nayab Tahir, Mubashar Rehman, Ahmed Raza, Muhammad Ahmad Mahmood, Muhammad Imran Khan and Prince Muhammad Kashif

*Address all correspondence to: asadpharmacist@hotmail.com

Faculty of Pharmacy and Alternative Medicine, The Islamia University of Bahawalpur, Bahawalpur, Pakistan

References

[1] Li M, Luo Z, Zhao Y. Hybrid nanoparticles as drug carriers for controlled chemotherapy of cancer. The Chemical Record. 2016. DOI: 10.1002/tcr.201600029.

[2] Gong J, Chen M, Zheng Y, Wang S, Wang Y. Polymeric micelles drug delivery system in oncology. Journal of Controlled Release. 2012;159(3):312–323. DOI: 10.1016/j.jconrel.2011.12.012.

[3] Mieszawska AJ, Kim Y, Gianella A, van Rooy I, Priem B, Labarre MP, et al. Synthesis of polymer–lipid nanoparticles for image-guided delivery of dual modality therapy. Bioconjugate Chemistry. 2013;24(9):1429–1434. DOI: 10.1021/bc400166j.

[4] Mehnert W, Mäder K. Solid lipid nanoparticles: production, characterization and applications. Advanced Drug Delivery Reviews. 2001;47(2):165–196. DOI: 10.1016/S0169-409X(01)00105-3.

[5] Madni A, Sarfraz M, Rehman M, Ahmad M, Akhtar N, Ahmad S, et al. Liposomal drug delivery: a versatile platform for challenging clinical applications. Journal of Pharmacy & Pharmaceutical Sciences. 2014;17(3):401–426. DOI: http://dx.doi.org/10.18433/J3CP55.

[6] Fan J, Fang G, Wang X, Zeng F, Xiang Y, Wu S. Targeted anticancer prodrug with mesoporous silica nanoparticles as vehicles. Nanotechnology. 2011;22(45):455102.

[7] Prabaharan M, Grailer JJ, Pilla S, Steeber DA, Gong S. Gold nanoparticles with a monolayer of doxorubicin-conjugated amphiphilic block copolymer for tumor-targeted drug delivery. Biomaterials. 2009;30(30):6065–6075. DOI: 10.1016/j.biomaterials.2009.07.048.

[8] Torchilin V. Multifunctional and stimuli-sensitive pharmaceutical nanocarriers. European Journal of Pharmaceutics and Biopharmaceutics. 2009;71(3):431–444. DOI: 10.1016/j.ejpb.2008.09.026.

[9] Krishnamurthy S, Vaiyapuri R, Zhang L, Chan JM. Lipid-coated polymeric nanoparticles for cancer drug delivery. Biomaterials Science. 2015;3(7):923–936. DOI: 10.1039/C4BM00427B

[10] He Y, Zhang L, Song C. Luteinizing hormone-releasing hormone receptor-mediated delivery of mitoxantrone using LHRH analogs modified with PEGylated liposomes. International Journal of Nanomedicine 2010;5:697–705. DOI: 10.2147/IJN.S12129.

[11] Zhang L, Zhu D, Dong X, Sun H, Song C, Wang C, et al. Folate-modified lipid–polymer hybrid nanoparticles for targeted paclitaxel delivery. International Journal of Nanomedicine 2015;10:2101–2114. DOI: 10.2147/IJN.S77667.

[12] Lee S-M, Ahn RW, Chen F, Fought AJ, O'halloran TV, Cryns VL, et al. Biological evaluation of pH-responsive polymer-caged nanobins for breast cancer therapy. ACS Nano. 2010;4(9):4971–4978. DOI: 10.1021/nn100560p.

[13] Montasser I, Shahgaldian P, Perret F, Coleman AW. Solid lipid nanoparticle-based calix [n] arenes and calix-resorcinarenes as building blocks: synthesis, formulation and characterization. International Journal of Molecular Sciences. 2013;14(11):21899–21942. DOI: 10.3390/ijms141121899.

[14] Liechty WB, Kryscio DR, Slaughter BV, Peppas NA. Polymers for drug delivery systems. Annual Review of Chemical and Biomolecular Engineering. 2010;1:149. DOI: 10.1146/annurev-chembioeng-073009-100847.

[15] Reis CP, Neufeld RJ, Ribeiro AJ, Veiga F. Nanoencapsulation I. Methods for preparation of drug-loaded polymeric nanoparticles. Nanomedicine: Nanotechnology, Biology and Medicine. 2006;2(1):8–21. DOI: 10.1016/j.nano.2005.12.003.

[16] Zheng M, Yue C, Ma Y, Gong P, Zhao P, Zheng C, et al. Single-step assembly of DOX/ICG loaded lipid–polymer nanoparticles for highly effective chemo-photothermal combination therapy. ACS Nano. 2013;7(3):2056–2067. DOI: 10.1021/nn400334y.

[17] Hadinoto K, Sundaresan A, Cheow WS. Lipid–polymer hybrid nanoparticles as a new generation therapeutic delivery platform: a review. European Journal of Pharmaceutics and Biopharmaceutics. 2013;85(3):427–443. DOI: 10.1016/j.ejpb.2013.07.002.

[18] Qi D, Cao Z, Ziener U. Recent advances in the preparation of hybrid nanoparticles in miniemulsions. Advances in Colloid and Interface Science. 2014;211:47–62. DOI: 10.1016/j.cis.2014.06.001.

[19] Zhang L, Zhang L. Lipid–polymer hybrid nanoparticles: synthesis, characterization and applications. Nano Life. 2010;1(1):163–173. DOI: 10.1142/S179398441000016X.

[20] Hu C-MJ, Zhang L, Aryal S, Cheung C, Fang RH, Zhang L. Erythrocyte membrane-camouflaged polymeric nanoparticles as a biomimetic delivery platform. Proceedings of the National Academy of Sciences. 2011;108(27):10980–10985. DOI: 10.1073/pnas.1106634108.

[21] Allen TM, Cullis PR. Liposomal drug delivery systems: from concept to clinical applications. Advanced Drug Delivery Reviews. 2013;65(1):36–48. DOI: 10.1016/j.addr.2012.09.037.

[22] Zhang L, Granick S. How to stabilize phospholipid liposomes (using nanoparticles). Nano Letters. 2006;6(4):694–698. DOI: 10.1021/nl052455y.

[23] Mieszawska AJ, Gianella A, Cormode DP, Zhao Y, Meijerink A, Langer R, et al. Engineering of lipid-coated PLGA nanoparticles with a tunable payload of diagnostically active nanocrystals for medical imaging. Chemical Communications. 2012;48(47):5835–5837. DOI: 10.1039/C2CC32149A.

[24] Jain S, Valvi PU, Swarnakar NK, Thanki K. Gelatin coated hybrid lipid nanoparticles for oral delivery of amphotericin B. Molecular Pharmaceutics. 2012;9(9):2542–2553. DOI: 10.1021/mp300320d.

[25] Kamaly N, Xiao Z, Valencia PM, Radovic-Moreno AF, Farokhzad OC. Targeted polymeric therapeutic nanoparticles: design, development and clinical translation. Chemical Society Reviews. 2012;41(7):2971–3010. DOI: 10.1039/C2CS15344K.

[26] Nicolas J, Mura S, Brambilla D, Mackiewicz N, Couvreur P. Design, functionalization strategies and biomedical applications of targeted biodegradable/biocompatible polymer-based nanocarriers for drug delivery. Chemical Society Reviews. 2013; 42(3):1147–1235. DOI: 10.1039/C2CS35265F.

[27] Thevenot J, Troutier A-L, David L, Delair T, Ladavière C. Steric stabilization of lipid/polymer particle assemblies by poly (ethylene glycol)-lipids. Biomacromolecules. 2007;8 (11):3651–3660. DOI: 10.1021/bm700753q.

[28] De Miguel I, Imbertie L, Rieumajou V, Major M, Kravtzoff R, Betbeder D. Proofs of the structure of lipid coated nanoparticles (SMBV™) used as drug carriers. Pharmaceutical Research. 2000;17(7):817–824. DOI: 10.1023/A:1007504124603.

[29] Enlow EM, Luft JC, Napier ME, DeSimone JM. Potent engineered PLGA nanoparticles by virtue of exceptionally high chemotherapeutic loadings. Nano Letters. 2011;11(2): 808–813. DOI: 10.1021/nl104117p.

[30] Chaisri W, Hennink WE, Okonogi S. Preparation and characterization of cephalexin loaded PLGA microspheres. Current Drug Delivery. 2009;6(1):69–75. DOI: 10.2174/156720109787048186.

[31] Cohen-Sela E, Teitlboim S, Chorny M, Koroukhov N, Danenberg HD, Gao J, et al. Single and double emulsion manufacturing techniques of an amphiphilic drug in PLGA nanoparticles: formulations of mithramycin and bioactivity. Journal of Pharmaceutical Sciences. 2009;98(4):1452–1462. DOI: 10.1002/jps.21527.

[32] Kang F, Singh J. Effect of additives on the release of a model protein from PLGA microspheres. AAPS PharmSciTech. 2001;2(4):86–92. DOI: 10.1007/BF02830570.

[33] Dong Y, Feng S-S. Poly(D,L-lactide-co-glycolide)(PLGA) nanoparticles prepared by high pressure homogenization for paclitaxel chemotherapy. International Journal of Pharmaceutics. 2007;342(1):208–214. DOI: 10.1016/j.ijpharm.2007.04.031.

[34] Paillard-Giteau A, Tran V, Thomas O, Garric X, Coudane J, Marchal S, et al. Effect of various additives and polymers on lysozyme release from PLGA microspheres prepared by an s/o/w emulsion technique. European Journal of Pharmaceutics and Biopharmaceutics. 2010;75(2):128–136. DOI: 10.1016/j.ejpb.2010.03.005.

[35] Thevenot J, Troutier A-L, Putaux J-L, Delair T, Ladaviere C. Effect of the polymer nature on the structural organization of lipid/polymer particle assemblies. The Journal of Physical Chemistry B. 2008;112(44):13812–13822. DOI: 10.1021/jp805865r.

[36] Liao Z, Wang H, Wang X, Zhao P, Wang S, Su W, et al. Multifunctional nanoparticles composed of a poly(DL-lactide-coglycolide) core and a paramagnetic liposome shell for simultaneous magnetic resonance imaging and targeted therapeutics. Advanced Functional Materials. 2011;21(6):1179–1186. DOI: 10.1002/adfm.201002314.

[37] Wang H, Zhao P, Su W, Wang S, Liao Z, Niu R, et al. PLGA/polymeric liposome for targeted drug and gene co-delivery. Biomaterials. 2010;31(33):8741–8748. DOI: 10.1016/j.biomaterials.2010.07.082.

[38] Liang XF, Wang HJ, Luo H, Tian H, Zhang BB, Hao LJ, et al. Characterization of novel multifunctional cationic polymeric liposomes formed from octadecyl quaternized carboxymethyl chitosan/cholesterol and drug encapsulation. Langmuir. 2008;24(14):7147–7153. DOI: 10.1021/la703775a.

[39] Zhao P, Wang H, Yu M, Liao Z, Wang X, Zhang F, et al. Paclitaxel loaded folic acid targeted nanoparticles of mixed lipid-shell and polymer-core: in vitro and in vivo evaluation. European Journal of Pharmaceutics and Biopharmaceutics. 2012;81(2):248–256. DOI: 10.1016/j.ejpb.2012.03.004.

[40] Li X, Anton N, Arpagaus C, Belleteix F, Vandamme TF. Nanoparticles by spray drying using innovative new technology: the Büchi Nano Spray Dryer B-90. Journal of Controlled Release. 2010;147(2):304–310. DOI: 10.1016/j.jconrel.2010.07.113.

[41] Hitzman CJ, Elmquist WF, Wattenberg LW, Wiedmann TS. Development of a respirable, sustained release microcarrier for 5-fluorouracil I: in vitro assessment of liposomes, microspheres, and lipid coated nanoparticles. Journal of Pharmaceutical Sciences. 2006;95(5):1114–1126. DOI: 10.1002/jps.20591.

[42] Keloglu N, Verrier B, Trimaille T, Sohier J. Controlled association and delivery of nanoparticles from jet-sprayed hybrid microfibrillar matrices. Colloids and Surfaces B: Biointerfaces. 2016;140:142–149. DOI: 10.1016/j.colsurfb.2015.12.039.

[43] Hasan W, Chu K, Gullapalli A, Dunn SS, Enlow EM, Luft JC, et al. Delivery of multiple siRNAs using lipid-coated PLGA nanoparticles for treatment of prostate cancer. Nano Letters. 2011;12(1):287–292. DOI: 10.1021/nl2035354.

[44] Caldorera-Moore M, Glangchai L, Shi L, Roy K. Step and flash imprint lithography for the fabrication of shape-specific, enzymatically-triggered, drug nanocarriers. UNE. 2016;13:15.

[45] Cheow WS, Hadinoto K. Factors affecting drug encapsulation and stability of lipid–polymer hybrid nanoparticles. Colloids and Surfaces B: Biointerfaces. 2011;85(2):214–220. DOI: 10.1016/j.colsurfb.2011.02.033.

[46] D'Addio SM, Prud'homme RK. Controlling drug nanoparticle formation by rapid precipitation. Advanced Drug Delivery Reviews. 2011;63(6):417–426. DOI: 10.1016/j.addr.2011.04.005.

[47] Freese C, Gibson MI, Klok H-A, Unger RE, Kirkpatrick CJ. Size-and coating-dependent uptake of polymer-coated gold nanoparticles in primary human dermal microvascular endothelial cells. Biomacromolecules. 2012;13(5):1533–1543. DOI: 10.1021/bm300248u.

[48] Chu C-H, Wang Y-C, Huang H-Y, Wu L-C, Yang C-S. Ultrafine PEG-coated poly(lactic-co-glycolic acid) nanoparticles formulated by hydrophobic surfactant-assisted one-pot synthesis for biomedical applications. Nanotechnology. 2011;22(18):185601. DOI: 10.1088/0957-4484/22/18/185601/meta.

[49] Liu Y, Pan J, Feng S-S. Nanoparticles of lipid monolayer shell and biodegradable polymer core for controlled release of paclitaxel: effects of surfactants on particles size, characteristics and in vitro performance. International Journal of Pharmaceutics. 2010;395(1):243–250. DOI: 10.1016/j.ijpharm.2010.05.008.

[50] Bershteyn A, Chaparro J, Yau R, Kim M, Reinherz E, Ferreira-Moita L, et al. Polymer-supported lipid shells, onions, and flowers. Soft Matter. 2008;4(9):1787–1791. DOI: 10.1039/B804933E.

[51] Yang Z, Luo X, Zhang X, Liu J, Jiang Q. Targeted delivery of 10-hydroxycamptothecin to human breast cancers by cyclic RGD-modified lipid-polymer hybrid nanoparticles. Biomedical Materials. 2013;8(2):025012. DOI: 10.1088/1748-6041.

[52] Zheng M, Gong P, Zheng C, Zhao P, Luo Z, Ma Y, et al. Lipid-polymer nanoparticles for folate-receptor targeting delivery of doxorubicin. Journal of Nanoscience and Nanotechnology. 2015;15(7):4792–4798. DOI: 10.1166/jnn.2015.9604.

[53] Yang Z, Tang W, Luo X, Zhang X, Zhang C, Li H, et al. Dual-ligand modified polymer-lipid hybrid nanoparticles for docetaxel targeting delivery to Her2/neu overexpressed human breast cancer cells. Journal of Biomedical Nanotechnology. 2015;11(8):1401–1417. DOI: 10.1166/jbn.2015.2086.

[54] Shi J, Xiao Z, Votruba AR, Vilos C, Farokhzad OC. Differentially charged hollow core/shell lipid–polymer–lipid hybrid nanoparticles for small interfering RNA delivery. Angewandte Chemie. 2011;123(31):7165–7169. DOI: 10.1002/ange.201101554.

[55] Mandal B, Bhattacharjee H, Mittal N, Sah H, Balabathula P, Thoma LA, et al. Core–shell-type lipid–polymer hybrid nanoparticles as a drug delivery platform. Nanomedicine: Nanotechnology, Biology and Medicine. 2013;9(4):474–491. DOI: 10.1016/j.nano.2012.11.010.

[56] Su C-W, Chiang M-Y, Lin Y-L, Tsai N-M, Chen Y-P, Li W-M, et al. Sodium dodecyl sulfate-modified doxorubicin-loaded chitosan-lipid nanocarrier with multi polysaccharide-lecithin nanoarchitecture for augmented bioavailability and stability of oral administration in vitro and in vivo. Journal of Biomedical Nanotechnology. 2016;12(5):962–972. DOI: 10.1166/jbn.2016.2227.

[57] Su X, Fricke J, Kavanagh DG, Irvine DJ. In vitro and in vivo mRNA delivery using lipid-enveloped pH-responsive polymer nanoparticles. Molecular Pharmaceutics. 2011;8(3):774–787. DOI: 10.1021/mp100390w.

[58] Ling G, Zhang P, Zhang W, Sun J, Meng X, Qin Y, et al. Development of novel self-assembled DS-PLGA hybrid nanoparticles for improving oral bioavailability of vincristine sulfate by P-gp inhibition. Journal of Controlled Release. 2010;148(2):241–248. DOI: 10.1016/j.jconrel.2010.08.010.

[59] Zhang L, Chan JM, Gu FX, Rhee J-W, Wang AZ, Radovic-Moreno AF, et al. Self-assembled lipid–polymer hybrid nanoparticles: a robust drug delivery platform. ACS Nano. 2008;2(8):1696–1702. DOI: 10.1021/nn800275r.

[60] He C, Lu J, Lin W. Hybrid nanoparticles for combination therapy of cancer. Journal of Controlled Release. 2015;219:224–236. DOI: 10.1080/17425247.2016.1211637.

[61] Yang X-Z, Dou S, Wang Y-C, Long H-Y, Xiong M-H, Mao C-Q, et al. Single-step assembly of cationic lipid–polymer hybrid nanoparticles for systemic delivery of siRNA. ACS Nano. 2012;6(6):4955–4965. DOI: 10.1021/nn300500u.

[62] Wang G, Yu B, Wu Y, Huang B, Yuan Y, Liu CS. Controlled preparation and antitumor efficacy of vitamin E TPGS-functionalized PLGA nanoparticles for delivery of paclitaxel. International Journal of Pharmaceutics. 2013;446(1):24–33. DOI: 10.1016/j.ijpharm.2013.02.004.

[63] Fang RH, Aryal S, Hu C-MJ, Zhang L. Quick synthesis of lipid–polymer hybrid nanoparticles with low polydispersity using a single-step sonication method. Langmuir. 2010;26(22):16958–16962. DOI: 10.1021/la103576a.

[64] Liu Y, Li K, Pan J, Liu B, Feng S-S. Folic acid conjugated nanoparticles of mixed lipid monolayer shell and biodegradable polymer core for targeted delivery of Docetaxel. Biomaterials. 2010;31(2):330–338. DOI: 10.1016/j.biomaterials.2009.09.036.

[65] Mandal B, Mittal NK, Balabathula P, Thoma LA, Wood GC. Development and in vitro evaluation of core–shell type lipid–polymer hybrid nanoparticles for the delivery of erlotinib in non-small cell lung cancer. European Journal of Pharmaceutical Sciences. 2016;81:162–171. DOI: 10.1016/j.ejps.2015.10.021.

[66] Wong HL, Bendayan R, Rauth AM, Xue HY, Babakhanian K, Wu XY. A mechanistic study of enhanced doxorubicin uptake and retention in multidrug resistant breast cancer cells using a polymer-lipid hybrid nanoparticle system. Journal of Pharmacology and Experimental Therapeutics. 2006;317(3):1372–1381. DOI: 10.1124/jpet.106.101154.

[67] Wong HL, Bendayan R, Rauth AM, Wu XY. Simultaneous delivery of doxorubicin and GG918 (Elacridar) by new polymer-lipid hybrid nanoparticles (PLN) for enhanced treatment of multidrug-resistant breast cancer. Journal of Controlled Release. 2006;116 (3):275–284. DOI: 10.1016/j.jconrel.2006.09.007.

[68] Kumar S, Lather V, Pandita D. Green synthesis of therapeutic nanoparticles: an expanding horizon. Nanomedicine. 2015;10(15):2451–2471. DOI: 10.2217/nnm.15.112.

[69] Payyappilly SS, Panja S, Mandal P, Dhara S, Chattopadhyay S. Organic solvent-free low temperature method of preparation for self assembled amphiphilic poly(ϵ-caprolactone)–poly(ethylene glycol) block copolymer based nanocarriers for protein delivery. Colloids and Surfaces B: Biointerfaces. 2015;135:510–517. DOI: 10.1016/j.colsurfb.2015.07.075.

[70] Kumar S, Lather V, Pandita D. A facile green approach to prepare core-shell hybrid PLGA nanoparticles for resveratrol delivery. International Journal of Biological Macromolecules 2016;84:380–384. DOI: 10.1016/j.ijbiomac.2015.12.036.

[71] Gómez-Romero P, Sanchez C. Hybrid materials, functional applications. An introduction: Wiley-VCH Verlag GmbH & Co. KGaA: Weinheim, Germany; 2004.

[72] Van Bommel KJ, Friggeri A, Shinkai S. Organic templates for the generation of inorganic materials. Angewandte Chemie, International Edition. 2003;42(9):980–999. DOI: 10.1002/anie.200390284.

[73] Sanchez C, Belleville P, Popall M, Nicole L. Applications of advanced hybrid organic–inorganic nanomaterials: from laboratory to market. Chemical Society Reviews. 2011;40(2):696–753. DOI: 10.1039/C0CS00136H.

[74] Corriu RJ, Mehdi A, Reyé C, Thieuleux C. Control of coordination chemistry in both the framework and the pore channels of mesoporous hybrid materials. New Journal of Chemistry. 2003;27(6):905–908. DOI: 10.1039/B302027D.

[75] Shen M, Shi X. Dendrimer-based organic/inorganic hybrid nanoparticles in biomedical applications. Nanoscale. 2010;2(9):1596–1610. DOI: 10.1039/C0NR00072H.

[76] Agrawal U, Chashoo G, Sharma PR, Kumar A, Saxena AK, Vyas SP. Tailored polymer–lipid hybrid nanoparticles for the delivery of drug conjugate: dual strategy for brain targeting. Colloids and Surfaces B: Biointerfaces. 2015;126:414–425. DOI: 10.1016/j.colsurfb.2014.12.045.

[77] Carbone C, Manno D, Serra A, Musumeci T, Pepe V, Tisserand C, et al. Innovative hybrid vs polymeric nanocapsules: the influence of the cationic lipid coating on the "4S". Colloids and Surfaces B: Biointerfaces. 2016;141:450–457. DOI: 10.1016/j.colsurfb.2016.02.002.

[78] Chan JM, Zhang L, Yuet KP, Liao G, Rhee J-W, Langer R, et al. PLGA–lecithin–PEG core–shell nanoparticles for controlled drug delivery. Biomaterials. 2009;30(8):1627–1634. DOI: 10.1016/j.biomaterials.2008.12.013.

[79] Clawson C, Ton L, Aryal S, Fu V, Esener S, Zhang L. Synthesis and characterization of lipid–polymer hybrid nanoparticles with pH-triggered poly(ethylene glycol) shedding. Langmuir. 2011;27(17):10556–10561. DOI: 10.1021/la202123e.

[80] Troutier A-L, Delair T, Pichot C, Ladavière C. Physicochemical and interfacial investigation of lipid/polymer particle assemblies. Langmuir. 2005;21(4):1305–1313. DOI: 10.1021/la047659t.

[81] Devrim B, Kara A, Vural I, Bozkir A. Lysozyme-loaded lipid-polymer hybrid nanoparticles: preparation, characterization and colloidal stability evaluation. Drug Development and Industrial Pharmacy. 2016:1–12. DOI: 10.1080/03639045.2016.1180392.

[82] Dim N, Perepelyuk M, Gomes O, Thangavel C, Liu Y, Den R, et al. Novel targeted siRNA-loaded hybrid nanoparticles: preparation, characterization and in vitro evaluation. Journal of Nanobiotechnology. 2015;13:61. DOI: 10.1186/s12951-015-0124-2.

[83] El-Sherbiny IM, El-Shibiny A, Salih E. Photo-induced green synthesis and antimicrobial efficacy of poly (ε-caprolactone)/curcumin/grape leaf extract-silver hybrid nanoparticles. Journal of Photochemistry and Photobiology B: Biology. 2016;160:355–363.

[84] Wong HL, Rauth AM, Bendayan R, Manias JL, Ramaswamy M, Liu Z, et al. A new polymer–lipid hybrid nanoparticle system increases cytotoxicity of doxorubicin against multidrug-resistant human breast cancer cells. Pharmaceutical Research. 2006;23(7):1574–1585. DOI: 10.1007/s11095-006-0282-x.

[85] Xie Y, Qiao H, Su Z, Chen M, Ping Q, Sun M. PEGylated carboxymethyl chitosan/calcium phosphate hybrid anionic nanoparticles mediated hTERT siRNA delivery for anticancer therapy. Biomaterials. 2014;35(27):7978–7991. DOI: 10.1016/j.biomaterials.2014.05.068.

[86] Zhang J, Hu J, Chan HF, Skibba M, Liang G, Chen M. iRGD decorated lipid-polymer hybrid nanoparticles for targeted co-delivery of doxorubicin and sorafenib to enhance anti-hepatocellular carcinoma efficacy. Nanomedicine. 2016;12(5):1303–1311. DOI: 10.1016/j.nano.2016.01.017.

[87] Zhang RX, Cai P, Zhang T, Chen K, Li J, Cheng J, et al. Polymer–lipid hybrid nanoparticles synchronize pharmacokinetics of co-encapsulated doxorubicin–mitomycin C and enable their spatiotemporal co-delivery and local bioavailability in breast tumor. Nanomedicine: Nanotechnology, Biology and Medicine 2016;12(5):1279–1290. DOI: 10.1016/j.nano.2015.12.383.

[88] Kandel PK, Fernando LP, Ackroyd PC, Christensen KA. Incorporating functionalized polyethylene glycol lipids into reprecipitated conjugated polymer nanoparticles for bioconjugation and targeted labeling of cells. Nanoscale. 2011;3(3):1037–1045. DOI: 10.1039/C0NR00746C.

[89] Sengupta S, Eavarone D, Capila I, Zhao G, Watson N, Kiziltepe T, et al. Temporal targeting of tumour cells and neovasculature with a nanoscale delivery system. Nature. 2005;436(7050):568–572. DOI: 10.1038/nature03794.

[90] Palange AL, Di Mascolo D, Carallo C, Gnasso A, Decuzzi P. Lipid–polymer nanoparticles encapsulating curcumin for modulating the vascular deposition of breast cancer cells. Nanomedicine: Nanotechnology, Biology and Medicine. 2014;10(5):e991-e1002. DOI: 10.1016/j.nano.2014.02.004.

[91] Wang W, Chen S, Zhang L, Wu X, Wang J, Chen J-F, et al. Poly(lactic acid)/chitosan hybrid nanoparticles for controlled release of anticancer drug. Materials Science and Engineering C 2015;46:514–520. DOI: 10.1016/j.msec.2014.10.048.

[92] Yan J, Wang Y, Zhang X, Liu S, Tian C, Wang H. Targeted nanomedicine for prostate cancer therapy: docetaxel and curcumin co-encapsulated lipid-polymer hybrid nanoparticles for the enhanced anti-tumor activity in vitro and in vivo. Drug Delivery. 2016;23(5):1757–1762. DOI: 10.3109/10717544.2015.1069423.

[93] Shi K, Zhou J, Zhang Q, Gao H, Liu Y, Zong T, et al. Arginine-glycine-aspartic acid-modified lipid-polymer hybrid nanoparticles for docetaxel delivery in glioblastoma multiforme. Journal of Biomedical Nanotechnology. 2015;11(3):382–391. DOI: 10.1166/jbn.2015.1965.

[94] Ramasamy T, Tran TH, Choi JY, Cho HJ, Kim JH, Yong CS, et al. Layer-by-layer coated lipid–polymer hybrid nanoparticles designed for use in anticancer drug delivery. Carbohydrate Polymers. 2014;102:653–661. DOI: 10.1016/j.carbpol.2013.11.009.

[95] Wu B, Yu P, Cui C, Wu M, Zhang Y, Liu L, et al. Folate-containing reduction-sensitive lipid-polymer hybrid nanoparticles for targeted delivery of doxorubicin. Biomaterials Science. 2015;3(4):655–664. DOI: 10.1039/C4BM00462K.

[96] Messerschmidt SK, Musyanovych A, Altvater M, Scheurich P, Pfizenmaier K, Landfester K, et al. Targeted lipid-coated nanoparticles: delivery of tumor necrosis factor-functionalized particles to tumor cells. Journal of Controlled Release. 2009;137(1):69–77. DOI: 10.1016/j.jconrel.2009.03.010.

[97] Varthya M, Pawar H, Singh C, Dora CP, Jena SK, Suresh S. Development of novel polymer-lipid hybrid nanoparticles of tamoxifen: in vitro and in vivo evaluation. Journal of Nanoscience and Nanotechnology. 2016;16(1):253–260. DOI: 10.1166/jnn.2016.10651.

[98] Kumar S, Sangwan P, Lather V, Pandita D. Biocompatible PLGA-oil hybrid nanoparticles for high loading and controlled delivery of resveratrol. Journal of Drug Delivery Science and Technology. 2015;30:54–62. DOI: 10.1016/j.jddst.2015.09.016.

[99] Makino K, Yamada T, Kimura M, Oka T, Ohshima H, Kondo T. Temperature-and ionic strength-induced conformational changes in the lipid head group region of liposomes as suggested by zeta potential data. Biophysical Chemistry. 1991;41(2):175–183. DOI: 10.1016/0301-4622(91)80017-L.

[100] Hallan SS, Kaur P, Kaur V, Mishra N, Vaidya B. Lipid polymer hybrid as emerging tool in nanocarriers for oral drug delivery. Artificial Cells, Nanomedicine, and Biotechnology. 2016;44(1):334–349. DOI: 10.3109/21691401.2014.951721.

[101] Mornet S, Lambert O, Duguet E, Brisson A. The formation of supported lipid bilayers on silica nanoparticles revealed by cryoelectron microscopy. Nano Letters. 2005;5(2): 281–285. DOI: 10.1021/nl048153y.

[102] Schmitt J, Danner B, Bayerl TM. Polymer cushions in supported phospholipid bilayers reduce significantly the frictional drag between bilayer and solid surface. Langmuir. 2001;17(1):244–246. DOI: 10.1021/la001275v.

[103] Romberg B, Hennink WE, Storm G. Sheddable coatings for long-circulating nanoparticles. Pharmaceutical Research. 2008;25(1):55–71. DOI: 10.1007/s11095-007-9348-7.

[104] Zhong Q, Chinta DMD, Pamujula S, Wang H, Yao X, Mandal TK, et al. Optimization of DNA delivery by three classes of hybrid nanoparticle/DNA complexes. Journal of Nanobiotechnology. 2010;8(1):1. DOI: 10.1186/1477-3155-8-6.

[105] Bershteyn A, Hanson MC, Crespo MP, Moon JJ, Li AV, Suh H, et al. Robust IgG responses to nanograms of antigen using a biomimetic lipid-coated particle vaccine. Journal of Controlled Release. 2012;157(3):354–365. DOI: 10.1016/j.jconrel.2011.07.029.

[106] Luo Y, Teng Z, Li Y, Wang Q. Solid lipid nanoparticles for oral drug delivery: chitosan coating improves stability, controlled delivery, mucoadhesion and cellular uptake. Carbohydrate Polymers. 2015;122:221–229. DOI: 10.1016/j.carbpol.2014.12.084.

[107] Harde H, Agrawal AK, Jain S. Tetanus toxoids loaded glucomannosylated chitosan based nanohoming vaccine adjuvant with improved oral stability and immunostimulatory response. Pharmaceutical Research. 2015;32(1):122–134. DOI: 10.1007/s11095-014-1449-5.

[108] Badhulika S, Terse-Thakoor T, Villarreal C, Mulchandani A. Graphene hybrids: synthesis strategies and applications in sensors and sensitized solar cells. Frontiers in Chemistry. 2015;3. DOI: 10.3389/fchem.2015.00038.

[109] Rehman M, Asadullah Madni AI, Khan WS, Khan MI, Mahmood MA, Ashfaq M, et al. Solid and liquid lipid-based binary solid lipid nanoparticles of diacerein: in vitro evaluation of sustained release, simultaneous loading of gold nanoparticles, and potential thermoresponsive behavior. International Journal of Nanomedicine. 2015;10:2805. DOI: 10.2147/IJN.S67147.

[110] Javed I, Hussain SZ, Shahzad A, Khan JM, Rehman M, Usman F, et al. Lecithin-gold hybrid nanocarriers as efficient and pH selective vehicles for oral delivery of diacerein—in-vitro and in-vivo study. Colloids and Surfaces B: Biointerfaces. 2016; 141:1–9. DOI: 10.1016/j.colsurfb.2016.01.022.

[111] Umair M, Javed I, Rehman M, Madni A, Javeed A, Ghafoor A, et al. Nanotoxicity of inert materials: the case of gold, silver and iron. Journal of Pharmacy & Pharmaceutical Sciences. 2016;19(2):161–180. DOI: 10.18433/J31021.

[112] McCarthy JR, Weissleder R. Multifunctional magnetic nanoparticles for targeted imaging and therapy. Advanced Drug Delivery Reviews. 2008;60(11):1241–1251. DOI: 10.1016/j.addr.2008.03.014.

[113] Lee N, Yoo D, Ling D, Cho MH, Hyeon T, Cheon J. Iron oxide based nanoparticles for multimodal imaging and magnetoresponsive therapy. Chemical Reviews. 2015;115(19):10637–10689. DOI: 10.1021/acs.chemrev.5b00112.

[114] Shi J, Jiang Y, Wang X, Wu H, Yang D, Pan F, et al. Design and synthesis of organic–inorganic hybrid capsules for biotechnological applications. Chemical Society Reviews. 2014;43(15):5192–5210. DOI: 10.1039/C4CS00108G.

[115] Portney NG, Singh K, Chaudhary S, Destito G, Schneemann A, Manchester M, et al. Organic and inorganic nanoparticle hybrids. Langmuir. 2005;21(6):2098–2103. DOI: 10.1021/la047525f.

[116] Zhou W, Huang P-JJ, Ding J, Liu J. Aptamer-based biosensors for biomedical diagnostics. Analyst. 2014;139(11):2627–2640. DOI: 10.1039/C4AN00132J.

[117] Sreejith S, Ma X, Zhao Y. Graphene oxide wrapping on squaraine-loaded mesoporous silica nanoparticles for bioimaging. Journal of the American Chemical Society. 2012;134(42):17346–17349. DOI: 10.1021/ja305352d.

[118] Maji SK, Mandal AK, Nguyen KT, Borah P, Zhao Y. Cancer cell detection and therapeutics using peroxidase-active nanohybrid of gold nanoparticle-loaded mesoporous silica-coated graphene. ACS Applied Materials & Interfaces. 2015;7(18):9807–9816. DOI: 10.1021/acsami.5b01758.

2

Cellulose-Derivatives-Based Hydrogels as Vehicles for Dermal and Transdermal Drug Delivery

Lavinia Vlaia, Georgeta Coneac, Ioana Olariu,
Vicențiu Vlaia and Dumitru Lupuleasa

Abstract

The use of water-soluble polymers of natural, semisynthetic, and synthetic origin for dermal and transdermal drug delivery systems is manifold. Among the most used biopolymers in the formulation of skin preparations, the cellulose ether derivatives as representatives of semisynthetic polymers distinguish through their specific physicochemical properties, by which the pharmacist can select the appropriate cellulose derivative for a particular purpose. The hydrogels containing cellulose derivatives as gelling agents are widely used as water-soluble ointment bases, because they usually associate the characteristics of both conventional and innovative hydrogels, including especially safety, biocompatibility, biodegradability, and a relatively easy way of preparation and low price. The present chapter describes the following issues: the physicochemical properties of water-soluble cellulose derivatives in relationship with their type and grade; physical and chemical properties of cellulose-derivatives-based hydrogels and their compatibility with other auxiliary substances commonly used in the formulation of pharmaceutical hydrogels; the development and manufacturing of these hydrogels on both small and large scales; the characterization of cellulose derivatives hydrogels as pharmaceutical dosage forms through different compendial and noncompendial methods; and well-recognized and novel applications of cellulose-derivatives-based hydrogels for dermal and transdermal drug delivery.

Keywords: cellulose derivative, hydrogel, dermal, drug delivery, gelation, viscosity

1. Introduction

Over the past decades, the delivery of drugs to and through the skin has gained an increased interest in research and in the pharmaceutical industry, mainly due to the fact that the skin is an easily accessible and painless route for drug administration, which in turn leads to increased patient compliance. Furthermore, dermal and transdermal drug delivery represents an attractive alternative to the conventional oral and parenteral route of administration, as it offers several advantages.

In present-day pharmaceutical and dermatological practice, most of the drug products applied to the skin for either localized or systemic effects are semisolid preparations, such as ointments, creams, and gels. Hydrogels, as conventional semisolid vehicles with hydrophilic properties, are highly valued in dermatology because they are transparent, completely water washable, greaseless, thixotropic, easily spreadable, suitable for the incorporation of lipophilic compounds or insoluble solids, and present good bioadhesive properties. In addition, innovative hydrogel formulations recently developed show other advantageous characteristics, namely biocompatibility, biodegradability, and sensitivity to various external stimuli. Biodegradability is nowadays a preferred and even a required property considering the need for environmentally friendly materials and technologies in different domains.

Hydrogels generally consist of two main components, the gelling agent responsible for the network formation and an aqueous liquid vehicle. Among the gelling agents extensively used in the pharmaceutical compounded and industrialized topical hydrogel formulations are cellulose derivatives (also referred to as cellulosics) such as methylcellulose, carboxymethylcellulose, and hydroxypropylmethylcellulose (HPMC). The cellulose-derivatives-based hydrogels are particularly attractive as ointment bases because they usually associate the characteristics of both conventional and innovative hydrogels. Moreover, the large availability in nature, nontoxicity, and the low cost of cellulose derivatives represent other important features, which recommend these polymers as first choice raw materials for the preparation of pharmaceutical hydrogels.

This chapter focuses on the current design, development, and applications of cellulose-derivatives-based hydrogels as semisolid pharmaceutical dosage forms intended for dermal and transdermal drug delivery.

2. Classification of cellulose derivatives

Cellulose is the most abundant naturally occurring biopolymer, found as the major component of annual plants and natural fibers (e.g., cotton, hardwoods and softwoods, linen, jute, and hemp) and also produced by some bacteria, fungi, and animals [1–5]. This glucose polymer is extensively used in pharmaceutical applications as it fulfills the two essential requirements: biocompatibility and biodegradability [6].

Plant-derived cellulose occurs as fibers, formed of macromolecules that contain hundreds of glucose molecules, determining the variability in chain length and molecular weight. The cellulose molecular weight can reach 1500 Da, each 40–50 glucose units being associated with longitudinal formations, named crystallites, which are oriented parallel to the longitudinal axis of the fiber and have 600–650 nm in length. In cellulose, as a linear polysaccharide polymer, the glucose monomers in pyranose form are linked to unbranched chains by β-1,4-glucosidic bonds, every glucose monomer being flipped related to the next one. Due to this structure, cellulose shows high crystallinity and rigidity and is practically insoluble in water and most organic solvents [7, 8].

In order to alter these disadvantageous properties, which limit its biomedical applications, chemical modification of cellulose, involving reactions of hydroxyl groups such as esterification or etherification, was performed. The extension of these reactions is expressed through the degree of substitution (DS), representing the average number of hydroxyl groups replaced by the substituents; the maximum value of DS is 3. For the cellulose derivatives used in pharmaceutical domain, the DS values correspond to pharmaceutical grades [8, 9].

Cellulose derivatives, named cellulosics, fall within the general class of hydrophilic colloids and have in common that they are hydrophilic, semisynthetic linear macromolecules obtained through chemical modification of cellulose. A more specific classification of cellulose derivatives can be made on the basis of other criteria, namely type of chemical modification of cellulose (etherification or esterification), electrolytic dissociation, and water solubility. Such classifications are useful because they facilitate the discussion of cellulose derivatives properties. Thus, based on the type of chemical modification of cellulose, cellulosics can be divided into two major groups:

- *polymers formed by hydroxyl etherification* with the appropriate alkyl halide of previously alkalinized cellulose. Principal examples of cellulose ethers derivatives used in pharmaceutical applications include methylcellulose (MC), ethylcellulose (EC), benzylcellulose (BC), hydroxyethylcellulose (HEC), hydroxypropylcellulose (HPC), hydroxypropylmethylcellulose (HPMC), hydroxyethylmethylcellulose (HEMC), and sodium carboxymethylcellulose (CMCNa);

- *polymers formed by hydroxyl esterification* with various organic acids, in the presence of a strong acid as catalyst. Some of the most important cellulose esters derivatives used in pharmaceutical domain are: cellulose acetate, cellulose nitrate, cellulose acetate phthalate, hydroxypropylmethylcellulose phthalate, and hydroxypropylmethylcellulose acetate succinate.

Table 1 presents the general chemical structures of cellulose ether derivatives and the formulas of the R groups in these biopolymers, which are further discussed in this chapter.

Cellulose derivatives may also be classified according to their electrolytic dissociation or charge as *nonionic (uncharged) polymers* that do not have an electric charge (i.e., MC, EC, HEC, HPC, HEMC, and HPMC) and *ionic (anionic and cationic) polymers* with electric charge. Among the above-mentioned cellulose derivatives, only NaCMC is an anionic or negatively charged polyelectrolyte at pH values above its isoelectric point, being sensitive to pH and ionic strength variations [9–11].

Cellulose ether derivatives	R groups
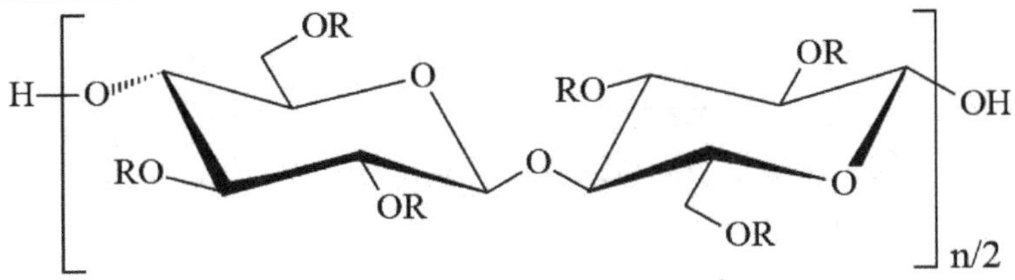	
Methylcellulose	H, CH_3
Ethylcellulose	H, CH_2CH_3
Hydroxyethylcellulose	H, $[CH_2CH_2O]_nH$
Hydroxypropylcellulose	H, $[CH_2CH(CH_3)O]_nH$
Hydroxyethylmethylcellulose	H, CH_3, $[CH_2CH_2O]_nH$
Hydroxypropylmethylcellulose	H, CH_3, $[CH_2CH(CH_3)O]_nH$
Carboxymethylcellulose	H,CH_2COONa

Table 1. Chemical structures of some important cellulose ether and ester derivatives.

In addition, the cellulose derivatives can also be categorized based on their water solubility into two groups: *water-soluble polymers*, including most of the cellulose ethers, and *water-insoluble polymers*, including the cellulose esters and both EC and BC from the group of cellulose ethers. It is to be mentioned that the water-insoluble cellulose derivatives are soluble in various organic solvents.

3. Water-soluble cellulose derivatives

In this section, it will be discussed in detail the physical and chemical properties of several water-soluble cellulose ether derivatives including methylcellulose (MC), hydroxyethylcellulose (HEC), hydroxypropylcellulose (HPC), hydroxypropylmethylcellulose (HPMC), and sodium carboxymethylcellulose (CMCNa), which are widely used as polymeric gelling agents in pharmaceutical hydrogels.

The commercial types of cellulose ethers for pharmaceutical applications are available in various grades, with different molecular weight, structural formula, and distribution of substituent groups and with different degree of substitution. These specific characteristics determine the physicochemical properties of cellulose ethers, such as solubility, viscosity in solution, surface activity and stability to biodegradation, heat, and hydrolytic and oxidative degradation. The solubility and the thermal gelation temperature of aqueous solutions of cellulose ethers are affected by their degree of substitution. But the viscosity of their solutions is directly related to their molecular weight and degree of polymerization. Therefore, the pharmacist has the possibility to select the appropriate cellulose derivative for a particular purpose [12].

3.1. Methylcellulose (MC)

Methylcellulose is included in various pharmacopoeias as *methylcellulose* (i.e., British Pharmacopoeia, BP; Japanese Pharmacopoeia, JP; European Pharmacopoeia, PhEur; United States Pharmacopoeia, USP; and International Pharmacopoeia) and is commercially available as different trade names *Benecel, Methocel, Metolose, Tylose* etc [13].

It is a nonionic, linear, and filiform macromolecule of cellulose, in which approximately 27–32% of the hydroxyl groups are in the form of methyl ether. At present, there are various grades of MC commercially available, having degrees of polymerization in the range of 50–1000, molecular weights (number average) in the range 10,000–220,000 Da, and a degree of substitution in the range 1.64–1.92 [13].

Methylcellulose occurs as a white, fibrous powder or granules, practically odorless and tasteless, and slightly hygroscopic. It swells and disperses slowly in cold water (1–5°C), forming a clear to opalescent, viscous colloidal dispersion, with pH 5.0–8.0. MC is practically insoluble in hot water (70°C), ethanol (95%), and glycerol. This methyl derivative of cellulose has the specific property of forming thermally reversible hydrogels on heating, being classified as a lower critical solution temperature polymer. In addition, other typical physicochemical properties of methylcellulose, which are to be considered for its selection as gelling agent in a pharmaceutical formulation, are presented in **Table 2**.

Specific property	Methylcellulose
Surface tension	MC has an important surface activity, decreasing the surface tension of water from 72.8 dyn/cm to 45–55 dyn/cm for a 0.1% (w/v) solution at 20°C
Stability	Solutions of methylcellulose are stable to alkalis and dilute acids at pH 3–11, at room temperature. At pH less than 3, acid-catalyzed hydrolysis of the glucose-glucose linkages occurs and the viscosity of methylcellulose solutions is reduced
Incompatibilities	MC is incompatible with various drugs (i.e., chlorocresol, mercuric chloride, phenol, resorcinol, tannic acid, silver nitrate, tetracaine), antimicrobial preservatives (i.e., cetylpyridinium chloride, methylparaben, propylparaben and butylparaben), salts of mineral acids, and strong oxidizing agents

Table 2. Several specific properties of methylcellulose important as selection criteria in the formulation stage of a pharmaceutical gel.

3.2. Hydroxyethylcellulose (HEC)

The grades of HEC used in pharmaceutical applications comply with the specifications defined in the *hydroxyethylcellulose* monograph included in different pharmacopoeia (i.e., BP, PhEur, USP, and International Pharmacopoeia). Commercially, HEC is available in different trade names such as *Cellosize HEC, Natrosol, Tylose H* etc.

Hydroxyethylcellulose, a partially substituted poly(hydroxyethyl) ether of cellulose, is a nonionic, hydrophilic polymer, with a linear and filiform chain, having a degree of substitution of minimum 1.5 (three hydroxyls substituted/two units). With a further increase in DS over this minimum, the water solubility of HEC is increased.

There are available several grades of HEC, which differ in viscosity (determined by molecular weight) and in degree of substitution; further, some grades are modified to improve their water dispersibility. Also, HEC may contain a suitable anticaking agent. HEC appears as a white, yellowish-white or grayish-white, odorless and tasteless, and hygroscopic powder. It dissolves readily in either hot or cold water, forming clear, smooth, uniform solutions, with pH 5.0–8.5. HEC is practically insoluble in acetone, ethanol (95% m/v), ether, and most other organic solvents, but it swells or is partially soluble in polar solvents, usually those that are miscible with water such as glycols, dimethyl formamide, dimethyl sulfoxide, and ethanol:water mixtures (70:30, 60:40, 30:70 by weight) [13, 14].

Since the aqueous formulations of HEC are sensitive to biological contamination, a water-soluble antimicrobial preservative should be added for a prolonged storage (i.e., sodium benzoate, sorbic acid, and methyl-propylparaben combinations).

In **Table 3**, other HEC typical properties of interest for its incorporation into a pharmaceutical formulation are presented.

Specific property	Hydroxyethylcellulose
Surface tension	HEC has an insignificant surface activity that lead to a negligible lowering of water surface tension, from 72.8 dyn/cm to 66.8 dyn/cm for a 0.1% (w/v) solution at 20°C
Stability	Although the aqueous solutions of hydroxyethylcellulose are stable over the pH range of 2–12, at room temperature, their greatest stability is achieved in the pH range of 6.5–8.0. The solutions are less stable below pH 3 and under highly alkaline conditions, due to acid hydrolysis and oxidative degradation respectively
Compatibilities	Due to its water solubility and nonionic character, HEC is soluble in many salt solutions that will not dissolve other water-soluble polymers
	For example, HEC dissolves in most 10% salt solutions and many 50% salt solutions, with several exceptions which are mentioned below. Further, HEC is compatible with a wide range of water-soluble materials, including other cellulosic hydrosoluble polymers, natural gums, and surfactants
Incompatibilities	HEC will precipitate in sodium carbonate and sodium sulfate 10% solutions, and in 50% (saturated) solutions of sulfates of bi- and trivalent metals (i.e., magnesium, zinc, and aluminum), di- and trisodium phosphate, ferric chloride, sodium nitrate, sodium sulfite. HEC is also incompatible with some quaternary disinfectants and partially compatible with the following water-soluble compounds: casein, gelatin, methylcellulose, polyvinylalcohol, and starch
Safety	Generally, HEC is considered as an essentially nontoxic and nonirritant material, being mainly used in ophthalmic and cutaneous pharmaceutical formulations

Table 3. Some specific properties of hydroxyethylcellulose as gelling agent.

3.3. Hydroxypropylcellulose (HPC)

According to Ph. Eur. and USP-NF, hydroxypropylcellulose intended for pharmaceutical use, is a partially substituted poly(hydroxypropyl) ether of cellulose, which may contain no more than 0.6% of silica or another suitable anticaking agent. HPC, also known as hyprolose and oxypropylated cellulose, is made by the Aqualon Division of Hercules Inc. and Nippon Soda Co., Ltd. (NISSO) under the brand names Klucel and NISSO HPC, respectively. The pharmaceutical grades of HPC are commercially available in several different viscosity types with molecular weight in the range of 50,000–1,250,000, depending on the degree of polymerization.

This ether of cellulose is a hydrophilic, nonionic, linear thread-like polymer where some of the hydroxyl groups of the cellulose have been hydroxypropylated, forming $-OCH_2CH(OH)CH_3$ groups. Moreover, the added hydroxypropyl groups can also be etherified during HPC preparation, leading to a value of moles of substitution (the number of moles of hydroxypropyl group per glucose ring) higher than 3. Hence, HPC with good water solubility must have a DS value of 2.5 and an MS value of approximately 4.

Hydroxypropylcellulose occurs as a white to slightly yellow-colored, odorless and tasteless powder. It feature a remarkable combination of properties: solubility in cold or hot polar organic solvents such as methanol (1:2), ethanol 95% (1:2.5), isopropyl alcohol (1:5), propyleneglycol (1:5); water solubility (1:2) below 38°C, forming a smooth, clear, colloidal solution; surface activity; aqueous thickening and stabilizing properties. HPC is insoluble in hot water, precipitates as a highly swollen floc in the temperature range 40–45°C, but this precipitation is completely reversible; thus, the gelation of HPC occurs on heating and yields to thermally reversible gels, similar to MC. It is also practically insoluble in aliphatic and aromatic hydrocarbons, glycerin, and oils [13, 15, 16].

In addition, other physical and chemical properties of pharmaceutical grades hydroxypropylcellulose are indicated in **Table 4**.

Specific property	Hydroxypropylcellulose
Surface tension	HPC is a surface active cellulose polymer, lowering the surface tension of water, from 72.8 dyn/cm to 46.3 dyn/cm for a 1% (w/v) solution, at 20°C
Stability	Aqueous solutions of hydroxypropylcellulose are stable in the pH range of 6–8, at room temperature. However, under highly acid or alkaline conditions, the degradation of polymer can occur, due to acid hydrolysis or alkaline oxidation
Compatibilities	The compatibility of hydroxypropylcellulose with inorganic salts varies according to the salt and its concentration
	For example, HPC dissolves in most 2–3% salt solutions and few 10% salt solutions. Further, HEC is compatible with a wide range of organic materials, including water-soluble as well as solvent-soluble resins, polymers (i.e., natural gums, semisynthetic, and synthetic polymers), surfactants, and organic liquids
Incompatibilities	In aqueous solutions, HPC will precipitate in the presence of 10% aluminum, ammonium or sodium sulfates, disodium phosphate, sodium acetate, carbonate, chloride, and thiosulfate. This polymer tends to be salted out in the presence of high concentrations of other dissolved compounds
Safety	Generally, HPC is considered as an essentially nontoxic and nonirritant material, being widely used as excipient in oral and topical pharmaceutical formulations. It does not exhibit skin irritation or skin sensitization. It is GRAS listed and is included in the FDA Inactive Ingredients Database (for oral solid dosage forms such as capsules and tablets, and also for topical and transdermal preparations)

Table 4. Some typical properties of hydroxypropylcellulose used in pharmaceutical applications.

3.4. Hydroxypropylmethylcellulose (HPMC)

It is also known as hypromellose, a nonproprietary name under which this cellulose derivative is found in different pharmacopoeias (BP, JP, PhEur, and USP) or their current editions. In addition, hydroxypropylmethylcellulose intended for use in pharmaceutical applications is produced by different manufacturers and commercialized under several trade names such as *Benecel MHPC, Methocel, Metolose, Pharmacoat, Tylopur, Tylose MO* [17–21].

Hypromellose is the propyleneglycol ether of methylcellulose, described by the PhEur as a partly *O*-methylated and *O*-(2-hydroxypropylated) cellulose. This nonionic, water-soluble polymer is available in several grades that differ in viscosity and extent of substitution. Different viscosity grades of HPMC are identified by an attached number indicating the apparent viscosity, in mPa s, of a 2% (w/w) aqueous solution at 20°C. The substitution type of hypromellose is specified in the pharmacopoeias as a four-digit number following the nonproprietary name, e.g., hypromellose 2208. The first two digits indicate the approximate percentage content of the methoxy group (OCH_3) and the second two digits indicate the approximate percentage content of the hydroxypropoxy group ($OCH_2CH(OH)CH_3$), calculated on a dried basis.

Methocel and *Metolose* grades	Compendial (JP, PhEur, USP) substitution type	Nominal viscosity (mPa s)
Methocel K3 Premium LV	2208	3
Methocel K100 Premium LVEP	2208	100
Methocel K4M Premium	2208	4000
Methocel K15M Premium	2208	15,000
Methocel K100M Premium	2208	100,000
Methocel E3 Premium LV	2910	3
Methocel E5 Premium LV	2910	5
Methocel E6 Premium LV	2910	6
Methocel E15 Premium LV	2910	15
Methocel E50 Premium LV	2910	50
Methocel E4M Premium	2910	4000
Methocel F50 Premium	2906	50
Methocel F4M Premium	2906	4000
Metolose 60S	2910	50, 4000, 10,000
Metolose 65SH	2906	50, 400, 1500, 4000
Metolose 90SH	2208	100, 400, 4000, 15,000

Table 5. The substitution type and typical viscosity values for 2% (w/v) aqueous solutions of Methocel (Dow Wolff Cellulosics) and Metolose (Shin-Etsu Chemical Co. Ltd.). Viscosities measured at 20°C [13, 17, 20, 21].

In the case of *Methocel* products of Dow Wolff Cellulosics, the substitution type is incorporated into the product name as an initial letter "*E*", "*F*," and "*K*," the number that follows stands for the viscosity (in mPa s) of that product measured at 2% concentration in water at 20°C; further, in referring the viscosity, the letter "*C*" is frequently used to represent 100 and the letter "*M*" is used to represent 1000 (**Table 5**). Also, several suffixes are used to identify special products: "*P*" denotes Methocel Premium grade products which means they are compliant with the USP, PhEur, and JP; "*LV*" stands for Low Viscosity products; "*CR*" refers to a Premium, Controlled Release grade (**Table 5**). On the other hand, the *Metolose SH* types of Shin-Etsu Chemical Co. Ltd. may be distinguished based on the degree of substitution by a number preceding the initial letters "*SH*" which identify the hypromellose products (**Table 5**) [13, 17, 20, 21].

The percentage content of methoxy and hydroxypropoxy groups affects both the molecular weight that is approximately 10,000–1,500,000, and the physicochemical properties of HPMC, such as solubility, surface activity, and thermal gelation [13]. HPMC appears as a white or creamy-white fibrous or granular powder, which is odorless and tasteless. It is soluble in cold water, forming a transparent, viscous, and surface active colloidal solution (the surface tension range from 42 dyn/cm to 64 dyn/cm). Certain types and grades of hypromellose are also soluble in various binary cosolvent systems such as ethanol/water, isopropanol/water, ethanol/dichloromethane, isopropanol/dichloromethane, providing a unique combination of solubility in organic solvents and water. However, hypromellose is practically insoluble in hot water, chloroform, ethanol (95%), and ether.

Another interesting characteristic of HPMC is the thermoreversible gelation behavior in aqueous media, which can be explained as follows: the aqueous solutions of hypromellose, obtained at room temperature, turn into gels when heated to their specific gel temperature (50–90°C); the resulting gels are completely reversible and liquefy upon cooling to room temperature, returning to their solution form. The thermoreversible gelation of hypromellose is particularly affected by several factors, such as its concentration in solvent media and the nature of additives. Thus, the additives that impart a solubilizing effect (i.e., ethanol, propyleneglycol, PEG 400) raise the gel point of HPMC, whereas the additives that exhibit a coagulant effect (i.e., glycerol, sorbitol, and most electrolytes) lower the gel temperature. In the past decade, numerous studies on thermoreversible gelation behavior of HPMC solutions have been carried out [22–26].

In addition, hypromellose possesses several other physicochemical characteristics, which are generally, similar to those of the above described cellulose ether derivatives of pharmaceutical grade. Some of these properties are presented below: HPMC in powder form is a stable material, although it is hygroscopic; aqueous solutions of HPMC are predisposed to microbial spoilage and require the addition of an antimicrobial preservative; in solution, hypromellose is stable in a wide pH range (3–11); HPMC is incompatible with some oxidizing agents, but exhibits a higher tolerance for salts in solution than MC; it is generally regarded as nontoxic an nonirritating excipient, being extensively used in topical pharmaceutical formulations and cosmetics; also, it is GRAS listed [13].

3.5. Carboxymethylcellulosesodium (CMCNa)

Among the two salt forms of carboxymethylcellulose (calcium and sodium) available for industrial use, sodium carboxymethylcellulose is commonly used for pharmaceutical preparations, including hydrogels. This cellulose ether derivative, also known as carmellose sodium, must comply with the compendial requirements of *carmellose sodium* or *carboxymethylcellulose sodium* monographs listed in BP, PhEur, JP, and respectively USP, which describe it as the sodium salt of polycarboxymethyl ether of cellulose, with a 6.6–10.8% sodium content. It is commercially available as various trade names such as *Akucell, Aqualon CMC, Aquasorb, Blanose, Tylose CB,* and *Walocel C.*

CMCNa is a hydrophilic, anionic polymer, with a linear, filiform chain, prepared by partial substitution of the two, three, and six hydroxyl groups of cellulose by carboxymethyl groups. The carmellose sodium pharmaceutical grades are available in a wide variety of types with regard to the degree of substitution, viscosity, and particle size. The value of DS varies in the range 0.6–1, affecting some of the polymer physicochemical properties. Hence, as the DS value is higher, the solubility in water and sodium content of CMCNa increase and a better polymer tolerance for other components in solution is achieved. The viscosity of different types of carmellose sodium depends on their polymerization degrees and molecular weights which are of 100–2000 and 90,000–700,000, respectively. Particle size has a pronounced effect on the ease of dispersing and dissolving CMCNa.

Sodium carmellose occurs as granular or fibrous, white to slightly off white, odorless, tasteless, and hygroscopic powder. It is slightly soluble in water at all temperatures, forming clear, viscous colloidal solutions, but is practically insoluble in most organic solvents such as ethanol (95%), methanol, acetone, ether, and toluene. However, it can be dissolved in aqueous mixtures if the content in water-miscible solvent is less than 40% (by weight). The powder of CMCNa presents a high chemical and microbiological purity and stability, and is not surface active. The aqueous solutions of carboxymethylcellulose sodium exhibit maximum viscosity and stability at pH 7–9, although they are stable over a broad pH range (2–10); at pH < 2, precipitation of CMC acid can occur, and at pH > 10 the viscosity of solutions decreases rapidly. Similar to HPMC, sodium carmellose exhibits thermoreversible gelation behavior in aqueous media. Also, its aqueous solutions are sensitive to microbiological attack and should contain a preservative for prolonged storage [13, 27, 28, 29].

Being a polyelectrolyte, CMCNa is sensible to pH and ionic strength variations. Therefore, its compatibility in solution with other components (**Table 6**) is another critical characteristic for the formulation of a pharmaceutical hydrogel.

In the past decade, cross-linked networks of CMC have been obtained and reported by applying chemically and physically cross-linking technologies. The chemically cross-linking method involves the use of bifunctional cross linkers such as epichlorhydrin [30], multifunctional carboxylic acids [31–34], ethyleneglycol diglycidyl ether [32], and polyethyleneglycol diglycidyl ether [35]. However, some of these reagents such as epichlorhydrin and ethyleneglycol diglycidyl ether produce large amounts of toxic byproducts under the cross-linking conditions, requiring their elimination through extensive washing, thus affecting the biocompatibility of the resulted hydrogel and the environmental safety of the production process. Considering these environmental and health safety risks, a physical cross-linking method, namely the radiation technology based on γ or electron-beam irradiation under relatively mild conditions, has attracted increased interest [36, 37]. This method presents some advantages: the addition of chemical reagents is not required, the side products are not present, and the simultaneously sterilization of the final hydrogel is possible.

Common excipients compatible with CMCNa in solution	Common excipients incompatible with CMCNa in solution
Most hydrophilic nonionic and anionic polymers and gums	Xanthan gum
	Gelatin, pectin and collagen forming complexes
Most 10% and 50% inorganic salts of monovalent cations, which form soluble salts of carboxymethylcellulose, with a prerequisite condition: the polymer should be dissolved in water before adding the salt	Most inorganic salts of bivalent (Ca^{2+}, Ba^{2+}, Mg^{2+}, Co^{2+}, Fe^{2+}, Mn^{2+}, and Zn^{2+}) and trivalent cations (Al^{3+}, Fe^{3+}), and also trace amounts of heavy metals cations (Ag^{+}, Cu^{2+}, Pb^{2+}, Zr^{2+}), which form precipitates

Table 6. Compatibility of carboxymethylcellulose sodium with other components in solution.

Although cross-linked CMC is a water-insoluble biopolymer, it is capable to absorb large amounts of water and swells to form superabsorbent hydrogels that exhibit superior mechanical properties and viscoelasticity compared with conventional sodium CMC-based hydrogels [38]. Due to this characteristic, the cross-linked CMC-based hydrogels were recently studied as potential wound dressing materials, as well as dermal and transdermal drug delivery systems [35, 38, 39].

Similar to the others cellulose ether derivatives, sodium carmellose is a safe excipient, being regarded as nontoxic and nonirritant. It is GRAS listed and included in different databases of inactive ingredients. Consequently, this polymer is extensively used in oral, topical, and some parenteral formulations, in cosmetics, toiletries, and food products [13].

4. Colloidal dissolution and gelation as processes involved in the formation of cellulose-derivatives-based hydrogels

To obtain a topical semisolid drug product, such as a medicated hydrogel, which meets the specific requirements, one of the major objectives of its formulation is the excipients selection and preparation of the base (hydrogel base) with semisolid consistency, jelly-like structure, and bioadhesive properties. Further, the hydrogel base must be stable, formed of compatible components, and therapeutically acceptable. Due to the specific jelly-like structure, hydrogels preserve their shape during the stockage, spread evenly, and adhere to the skin surface. In order to achieve this goal of hydrogel formulation, the knowledge of processes involved in the formation of hydrogels, such as colloidal dissolution and gelation of hydrophilic polymers, are of great importance as they are closely related with the physical and chemical properties of the gelling agent.

Based on the jelly-like structure, cellulose derivatives hydrogels are categorized as single-phase, reversible (or physical) gels composed of a network of organic macromolecules dissolved in water, without the existence of definite boundaries between the two components. However, due to the large size of the dissolved molecules, cellulose derivatives hydrogels are considered, on the microlevel, as biphasic colloidal systems, consisting of colloidal polymer and a liquid phase (water) [16, 40].

According to the formation mechanism of hydrogel, all cellulose derivatives described in the previous section are biopolymers that form hydrogels independently of pH, but in the case of MC, HPC, and HPMC the hydrogel formation is temperature dependent. Usually, the water-soluble cellulose derivatives form hydrogels in the concentrations of 1–10% (by weight), depending on the polymerization degree. The gelation of cellulose ether derivatives has been extensively studied for decades and numerous of these studies have been reviewed in several scientific journals and books [24, 39–47].

It is generally accepted that the gelation of water soluble cellulose ether derivatives is due to some physical processes such as molecular entanglements, hydrophobic associations between macromolecules and hydrogen bonding. The filiform macromolecules chains connect at both ends by forming some intermolecular bonds as a result of interaction between the existing functional groups. Also, entanglements develop from the interpenetration of random-coil flexible chains of polymers. Thus, they form a continuous three-dimensional network that occupies the entire system and entraps the entire amount of water. The formation of cellulose-derivatives-based hydrogels occurs in three stages. The first stage, identified as the diffusion of water molecules into the polymer network, is attributed to hydrogen bonding between the water molecules and the hydrophilic functional groups of macromolecules including carboxyl and hydroxyl groups. So, the solvent molecules will be oriented along the polymer chain, increasing the rigidity of the dispersed system. The second stage, correspond to relaxation of the polymer chains by hydration, when large amounts of water permeated into the polymer network are spontaneously absorbed by the macromolecules that swell and therefore greatly enhance the gel volume. In this stage of hydrogel formation, the interactions between polymer and water molecules through coordinate bonds lead to the formation of very stable complexes of hydration. Also, wetting determines the enhancement of macromolecule chains permeability and their stretching, accompanied by a more or less linear arrangement. The third stage, namely the polymer network expansion displayed through the increase of the gel volume, is due to water absorption and swelling of macromolecules. The stronger macromolecules hydration is the lower mobility of water molecules and the higher stability of the cross-linked gel network [9, 11, 16, 48].

The two main processes, namely colloidal dissolution and gelation, involved in the formation of cellulose-derivatives-based hydrogels, depend on several physicochemical factors (i.e., properties of cellulose-based polymers determined by chemical structure, macromolecular chain configuration, molecular weight, degree of substitution and also by the composition of the aqueous media, the pH, and the temperature) and thus influence to a great extent the formulation of a suitable pharmaceutical hydrogel. In general, lower temperature, higher concentration, and higher molecular weight of polymer promote gelation of cellulose ether derivatives, leading to firmer hydrogels. In most cases, the gelation of polymer is affected in the presence of relatively high concentrations of electrolytes, surfactants, sugar, or some natural gums, which reduce the polymer hydration and consequently the gelation temperature by the "salting out" phenomenon; the magnitude of this effect depends not only on the nature and concentration of the other dissolved components, but also on the substitution degree of the polymer. Generally, the cellulose ether derivatives with lower substitution degrees tend to exhibit a higher tolerance for the other dissolved components in the system. Due to the stability of aqueous solutions of water-soluble cellulose derivatives in a wide range of pH values (3–11), the gel formation is affected only under highly acid or alkaline conditions [9, 11, 16, 48].

Among the water soluble cellulose derivatives, MC, HPC, and HPMC are lower critical solution temperature polymers (**Table 7**) that form thermoreversible hydrogels [49, 50].

In order to understand and clarify the thermal gelation of these biopolymers, in the past two decades a large number of studies have been performed using different techniques. However, it was not reached a consensus in all cases, due the complexity of this process involving several different phenomena which can occur during the sol-gel transition.

Cellulose derivative	Trade name and type	Methoxy, DS	Methoxy, wt%	Hydroxypropoxy, MS	Hydroxypropoxy, wt%	Gelation temperature (°C)
MC	Benecel™ A	1.8	27.1–31.5	–	–	56
	Methocel A	1.8	30	–	–	50
	Metolose SM	1.8	Not specified	–	–	50–55
HPC	Klucel™ HPC	–	–	3.4–4.4	Not specified	40–45
	Nisso HPC	–	–	Not specified	53.4–77.5	40–45
HPMC	Benecel™K	Not specified	20.0–24.0	Not specified	7.0–12.0	80
	Benecel™E	Not specified	28.0–30.0	Not specified	7.0–12.0	63
	Methocel E	1.9	29.0	0.23	8.5	63
	Methocel F	1.8	28.0	0.13	5.0	63
	Methocel J	1.3	18.0	0.82	27	62
	Methocel K	1.4	22.0	0.21	8.1	85
	Metolose 60SH	1.9	28.0–30.0	0.25	7.0–12.0	65–66
	Metolose 65SH	1.8	27.0–30.0	0.15	4.0–7.5	61–65
	Metolose 90SH	1.4	19.0–24.0	0.20	4.0–12.0	75

Table 7. Thermal gelation temperatures of various grades and types of methyl- and/or hydroxypropyl-derivatives of cellulose.

In the case of the above-mentioned three cellulose derivatives (MC, HPC, and HPMC) is generally accepted that the formation of thermoreversible hydrogels occurs in two stages: (1) the formation of water clusters around the methyl or hydroxypropyl substituents of the polymer chains (the hydrophobic portions), which will be isolated one from another at low temperatures (below 50°C); (2) the phase separation accompanied by gelation at high temperatures (above 50°C).

For methylcellulose, the sol-gel transition is currently defined as the transformation from a clear solution to a turbid strong gel. Although the gelation of MC has been extensively studied by various analytical techniques (NMR, differential scanning calorimetry, IR attenuated total reflectance spectroscopy, small-angle neutron scattering, static and dynamic light scattering, and rheology) and the researchers have proposed different gelation mechanisms, the specific molecular interactions that govern this process is still unclear. However, the results of various studies, which were in good agreement one with another, indicated several factors and/or phenomena which play an important role in the gelation of MC [24, 51–64]:

- the first stage (pregel state) is mainly governed by hydrophobic interactions between highly methylated glucose regions, but also by bundles of residual native cellulose crystals, liquid crystal phases, and intermolecular bonding between unsubstituted hydroxyl groups along the polymer chains;

- the second stage (gel state), when the phase separation and gelation occur almost simultaneously, results from micellar interactions, formation of crystallites of trimethylated glucose rings, hydrophobic polymer-polymer interactions, and entangled physical cross links between chains leading to a three-dimensional network.

Recently, it was confirmed experimentally by rheological measurements that a nucleation and growth mechanism is also involved in the gelation of MC, as the gelation temperature depends on the heating rate [65].

The same group of researchers has also demonstrated by cryogenic transmission electron microscopy and small-angle neutron scattering that MC hydrogels have a heterogeneous fibrillar structure that is responsible for their turbidity [66, 67].

For HPMC, the formation of thermoreversible hydrogels is, similar to MC, a two-stage process. Conventionally, it is considered that the mechanism of HPMC gelation involves polymer reptation and dissociation of cellulosic bundles followed by exclusion of water (syneresis) from heavily methoxylated regions of the macromolecule. This syneresis allows hydrophobic interactions between the respective macromolecules accompanied with the formation of polymer clusters, which further associate in a three-dimensional network. This specific mechanism of gelation is supported by the results obtained from several experimental techniques including: differential scanning calorimetry, IR attenuated total reflectance spectroscopy, UV/VIS and fluorescence spectroscopy, polarized light microscopy, and oscillatory rheometry [22, 26, 68–71].

However, several studies have indicated some differences between MC and HPMC regarding thermal gelation properties and gel network structure. Generally, these differences are generated by the presence of hydroxypropyl substituents along the HPMC polymeric chains that hinder the gelation process by inhibiting intermolecular association. This observation is supported by the fact that HPMC has a higher gelation temperature and forms weaker thermosensitive gels compared to MC. Also, as the temperature rise to ca. 55°C, hydroxypropyl derivative of MC precipitates and causes only clouding of the solution, but no gelation, unlike MC [53, 72–74].

On the other hand, hydroxypropylcellulose being soluble in water at room temperature undergoes the gelation in these conditions. Increasing the temperature above the cloud point (40–45°C), the resulted hydrogel suddenly becomes opaque, loses its gel-like characteristics (evidenced by a marked reduction in/rapid decrease in viscosity) and exhibits a sudden shrinking in volume. These effects are due to separation of the polymer as a highly swollen precipitate at the above-mentioned temperature that corresponds to its phase transition temperature (or lower critical solution temperature). However, the polymer precipitation is reversible, because upon cooling the system below 40°C, redissolution of polymer and restoring of original viscosity take place [13, 15].

In contrast to MC and HPMC, only a few studies have investigated the gelation mechanism of HPC by NMR spectroscopy and thermal analysis [75, 76].

As the results from all these studies fitted well one with another, it was proposed the following plausible explanation of the HPC gelation mechanism. At room temperature, due to its high DS and uniform distribution of substituents along the polymeric chains, the HPC backbone has a little hydrophilic character that promotes a hydrophobic effect with water in solution, being extended, and mobilized. At elevated temperature, this hydrophobic structure breakdown and the cellulose backbones of the polymer chains coil into supramolecular helical structure. Although the cellulose backbones of the polymer chains are immobilized in this way, the hydroxypropyl substituents remain solvated projecting outward from the coiled backbone into the solvent and exhibiting a cilia-type motion. These cilia keep adjacent coils apart, leading to a highly dispersed solid phase (precipitate), with no gel-like properties.

Finally, the only one "smart" cellulose derivative, namely sodium carboxymethylcellulose, does not form thermoreversible hydrogels and is soluble in either hot or cold water, because it is an anionic polyelectrolyte. Consequently, the three-stage process of hydrogel formation, described above, is mainly determined in the presence of electrostatic charges attached to the polymer network, which enhance the polymer swelling capability in water by two mechanisms: (1) due to the electrostatic repulsion between the electric charges of the same sign, the macromolecule chains are forced to get more elongated than in a neutral network; (2) enhanced water penetration in the polymer network, due to the presence in the hydrogel of counterions to ensure the electrical neutrality [39]. Nevertheless, the gelation of sodium carboxymethylcellulose is influenced by pH and ionic strength variations (due to the presence of different inorganic salts). In addition, it is generally accepted that the firmness of NaCMC hydrogels increases with the increase in carboxymethyl substitution, molecular weight and polymer concentration [13, 28, 29].

5. Physical and chemical properties of cellulose derivatives hydrogels

Cellulose derivatives hydrogels are interesting as water-soluble ointment bases and topical drug delivery systems, because they present several advantageous characteristics: transparency (especially HPMC- and NaCMC-based hydrogels); high water content (80–95%), which is responsible for their favorable cooling effect and washability; nongreasy, being practically free from fats or fatty substances; porosity; nonocclusive; safety, as they are nontoxic and nonallergenic; are well tolerated by skin and different mucosa (oral, buccal, ophthalmic, nasal, auricular, vaginal, and rectal); are mucoadhesive and bioadhesive materials, adhering well to skin, mucosa and suppurative wounds, and providing intimate contact between the drug and the site of action; can be safely sterilized. They also may be formulated to ensure excellent spreading properties or to optimize drug delivery. Other important advantages of cellulose derivatives hydrogels include biocompatibility, biodegradability, smart stimuli-responsive behavior (in the case of NaCMC), compatibility with most active substances and auxiliary pharmaceutical components (excepting NaCMC which is an anionic polyelectrolyte). Also, the availability in nature and the low cost of cellulose derivatives make them more attractive as gelling agents [16, 45, 39, 77–81]. It is noteworthy that the cellulose derivatives hydrogels are considered biocompatible because they are similar to living tissues, with regard to physical properties, based on their water content, soft consistency, and low interfacial tension with water or biological fluids [39, 82].

The physical properties of cellulose derivatives hydrogels can be divided into two groups: transitional properties (including swelling behavior, sol-gel transition or gel point, and physical aging) and rheological properties (including rigidity, yield point, and rupture strength). These properties of cellulose derivatives hydrogels are directly related to their structure through their polymeric composition, because the selected cellulose derivative decisively influences the network structure as well as the final hydrogel properties [80].

5.1. Transitional properties

5.1.1. Swelling behavior

The capacity to absorb water or aqueous solutions and the permeability (the rate at which the liquid is absorbed into the hydrogel structure) are the most important features characterizing hydrogels, including those based on cellulose derivatives. Generally, the amount of the aqueous medium incorporated in a hydrogel is determined gravimetrically and is expressed as fractional hydration (W) or as swelling ratio (r):

$$W = (w_1 - w_0)/w_1 \text{ or } r = (w_1 - w_0)/w_0$$

where w_1 andw_0 are the weights of the swollen and dry gels, respectively. Also, the amount of water absorbed by a polymer can be described by the equilibrium swelling as the maximum degree of the polymer swelling.

Hydrogels of cellulose derivatives are considered highly swollen gels (containing large percentages of water), because of the high solubility of these polymers in water, high flexibility of the polymeric chains and a large free volume available between polymeric chains [40, 83–85].

However, the water content at the swelling equilibrium of cellulose derivatives hydrogels is influenced basically by the nature of the monomer that makes them up, by the type and density of the cross link (entanglements) and also, by other factors including temperature, pH, and the composition of the hydration medium (the presence of salts and nonsolvents). So, dynamic and equilibrium studies carried out by the Peppas group on hydrogel discs of HEC, HPC, HPMC K4M, and HPMC K100M [44] showed that the volume-swelling ratio and the swelling time (the time when hydrogel discs reached the equilibrium state, namely the gel thickness became essentially constant) of the polymer were dependent on their hydrophilicity and number of junctions or entanglements per original chain. Thus, the equilibrium state for HEC was reached after 240 h, for HPC and HPMC K100M after 260 h, and for HPMC K4M after 170 h, whereas the obtained volume-swelling ratios up to 190 h of swelling ranked the polymers as follows: HPC < HPMC K4M < HPMC K100M < HEC. The swelling kinetics of the studied HPMC polymers in the dynamic state was accurately described by the equation used to calculate the volume-swelling ratio, Q:

$$Q = V_s / V_d$$

where V_s is the volume of the swollen gel and V_d is the initial volume of the dry disc. At equilibrium, the swelling kinetics of HPMC polymers correlated well with the Flory-Rehner equation, describing the average molecular weight between two consecutive entanglements, $\overline{M_e}$:

$$\frac{1}{\overline{M_e}} = \frac{2}{\overline{M_n}} - \frac{\left(\frac{v}{V_1}\right)\left[ln\left(1 - v_{2,s}\right) + v_{2,s} + x_1 v_{2,s}^2\right]}{\left(v_{2,s}^{1/3} - \frac{v_{2,s}}{2}\right)}$$

where $\overline{M_n}$ is the number average molecular weight of the cellulose ether tested, v is its specific volume, V_1 is the molar volume of water, $v_{2,s}$ is the polymer fraction in the swollen gel at equilibrium ($v_{2,s} = 1/Q$), and x_1 is the Flory or polymer-water interaction parameter [44]. From detailed explanation given in this paper, further references are made only for HEC and HPC. In the swollen state, HEC formed the thicker hydrogel layer, signifying that the largest amount of water is physically and chemically trapped in the HEC hydrogel structure. This entrapment was attributed to the relatively high number of entanglements which holds the network structure together at equilibrium. In contrast, HPC formed the thinnest hydrogel layer, meaning that the interactions between the HPC chains are very strong and that water molecules occupy a smaller volume than in the case of HEC. This behavior is supported by the higher number of entanglements and the relatively high molar substitution for HPC, and also by the large volume occupied by hydroxypropyl substituents in the network structure of the HPC hydrogel [44].

As in the case of other hydrogels, the equilibrium degree of swelling influences different properties of cellulose derivatives hydrogels, including permeability, surface properties and surface mobility, optical properties, mechanical properties, and solute diffusion coefficient through these hydrogels. Consequently, the knowledge of the swelling characteristics of cellulose derivatives is of great importance in their pharmaceutical applications [80, 83].

5.1.2. Sol-gel transition (gel point)

Sol-gel transition is an essential property of most cellulose derivatives hydrogels as they are thermoreversible and is dependent on several factors, including polymer concentration and temperature.

The critical gelling concentration is the concentration below which the polymer and the solvent form a sol rather than a macroscopic gel, under the current experimental conditions [86]. For thermoreversible hydrogels of cellulose derivatives (MC, HPC, and HPMC), the critical gelling concentration obviously depends on temperature because, above the melting temperature, this concentration is nominally infinite, requiring a maximum gelation temperature and a critical gelation time [87]. The critical gelling concentration of cellulose derivatives depends on the polymer-polymer and polymer-solvent interactions, their hydrophilic-lipophilic character and molecular weight, and the flexibility of the chain [16, 88, 89]. Moreover, certain additives such as electrolytes, sorbitol, sucrose, and solvents (glycerin, ethanol, propyleneglycol, and polyethyleneglycol 400) can have different effects on the gel point and critical gelling concentration of cellulose derivatives [23]. Thus, it was demonstrated that most electrolytes, as well as sorbitol, sucrose and glycerin depress the gel point, whereas other cosolvents (ethanol, propyleneglycol, and polyethyleneglycol 400) raise the gel point of various grades of methylcellulose [90]. In **Table 8**, the minimal concentration domains for the most used cellulose derivatives as gelling agents in pharmaceutical hydrogels are listed.

Cellulose derivative	Gelling concentrations (wt %)	Required additives
Carboxymethylcellulose	4–6	Na^+
	10–25	Na^+
Methylcellulose	2–4	
Hydroxypropylcellulose	8–10	
Hydroxypropylmethylcellulose	2–10	

Table 8. Gelling concentrations of cellulose derivatives commonly used in topical hydrogels [18].

5.1.3. Physical aging

As the structure of cellulose derivatives hydrogels have not reached the equilibrium, these gels physically age as they move toward respective equilibrium. It is important to consider this physical aging of cellulose derivatives hydrogels, because it is accompanied by changes in gels microstructure where noncovalent cross links are breaking and reforming [16].

5.2. Rheological properties

The mechanical properties of cellulose derivatives hydrogels as water-soluble ointment bases must be considered during the development of a topical medicated hydrogel, as they are very important not only for the establishment of the topical drug formulation and the manufacturing method, but also for packaging, storage, and application.

Due to their semisolid consistency, cellulose derivatives hydrogels are viscoelastic, semistiff gels that exhibit a pseudoplastic flow [91]. These rheological properties are strongly related to the concentration and average molecular weight of the polymer, the gel structure and interchain interactions, and entanglements. So, the hydrogels of methylcellulose and hydroxypropylcellulose of 3–6% concentration exhibit a pseudoplastic character, while those of sodium carboxymethylcellulose types of high molecular weight and low substitution, with a concentration of 5–6% exhibit thixotropy, in addition to pseudoplastic flow. The apparent viscosity or gel strength of cellulose derivative hydrogels increases with an increase in their effective cross-link density or in the concentration and molecular weight of the polymer. Also, a rise in temperature decrease the apparent viscosity of these hydrogels, but under normal conditions, this effect is reversible. In addition, as it was discussed in the previous section, changes in apparent viscosity and consequently in other rheological properties of cellulose derivatives hydrogels can occur when different components such as salts, surfactants, solvents or nonsolvents, and other compatible polymers are added in the formulation. The effects of these additives have been extensively studied in the past decades and are presented in each cellulose derivative technical book [15, 17, 28, 29, 92–94].

6. Preparation of cellulose-derivatives-based hydrogels as pharmaceutical dosage forms

Cellulose-derivative-based hydrogels are relatively easy to prepare. In pharmaceutical applications, these hydrogels can be formulated with or without a drug substance. Medicated dermal gels can contain, in addition to the cellulose derivative as gelling agent and active substances, antimicrobial preservatives (i.e., methylparaben and propylparaben, or chlorhexidinegluconate), stabilizers (i.e., edetate disodium), dispersing agents (i.e., alcohol and/or glycerol, propyleneglycol, sorbitol), and permeation enhancers [95–98]. Minimum gel-forming concentrations of cellulose derivatives are different, based on the type and the molecular weights of these derivatives, but the medium range is about 4–6% (w/v), as mentioned before (**Table 8**). The most widely used hydrophilic external phase, in the preparation of these gels, is purified water. If the addition of cosolvents as dispersing agents is necessary, care should be taken to avoid their evaporation or degradation during gel preparation.

In manufacturing of dermal pharmaceutical cellulose derivatives hydrogels on a small scale (as in extemporaneous compounding), but also on a large scale (industry), the obtaining of an uniform preparation depends in a great extent on several factors including order of mixing, processing conditions, duration of swelling, and removal of entrapped air.

Mixing the above-mentioned components with the gelling agent should be made considering their influence on the gelling process. If the rate and extent of swelling of the gelling agent is affected by these ingredients, they are mixed after the gel formation. If such interference does not occur, the drug and the other additives are mixed prior to the swelling process; in this case, the effects of swelling duration, mixing temperature, and other processing conditions on the physicochemical stability of the drug and additives are also to consider. In general, the following order of mixing is recommended: (1) the drug substances are dissolved or suspended in the hydrophilic phase necessary for the gel preparation; (2) the other additives are dissolved in the obtained solution or in a small amount of the hydrophilic phase respectively; (3) if necessary, the drug dispersion is mixed with the additives solution; (4) the powder of the gelling agent is added under light stirring in the obtained solution/dispersion and allowed to swell.

In the preparation of cellulose derivatives hydrogels, the temperature and pH of the dispersion are critical parameters, as the gelation mechanism of these polymers is temperature dependent and their optimum stability depends on pH. Thus, the macromolecules dispersion is recommended to be heated either before, or after the polymer swelling. In case of MC and HPMC, the heating is indicated before the swelling occurs, but in case of HPC, HEC, and NaCMC, which dissolve better in hot water, the heating of their molecular dispersions is performed after de particle swelling. Practically, the general preparation method of most cellulose derivatives hydrogels involve the dispersion of polymer powder in cold water by using mechanical mixing to form uniform lump-free dispersion, followed by heating to about 60–80°C of the obtained dispersion, which is then gradually cooled to room temperature to form a gel. Also, there are differences regarding the pH values of dispersion medium favorable for gel formation: NaCMC, MC, and HPMC form gels over a wide pH range (4–10), whereas HPC and HEC form gels at a pH of 6–8 and respectively at alkaline pH condition. Another critical parameter in the preparation of cellulose derivatives hydrogels is the duration of polymer swelling. Generally, a swelling duration of about 24–48 h helps in obtaining homogeneous gels, as the cellulose polymers require about 48 h for complete hydration.

Finally, removal of the entrapped air is also an important issue to consider in the manufacturing of cellulose derivatives hydrogels, because the presence of air bubbles in the gel, which is inevitable, affects their transparency. The incorporation of air bubbles into the gel can be minimized by positioning the propeller at the bottom of the mixing container. Further removal of air bubbles by different methods including long - term standing, low -temperature storage, sonication, or inclusion of silicon antifoaming agents is commonly used. In addition, in large scale production vacuum vessel deaerators are used to remove the entrapped air [95, 97–99].

Figure 1 shows the flow chart of the fabrication process of a cellulose derivative hydrogel.

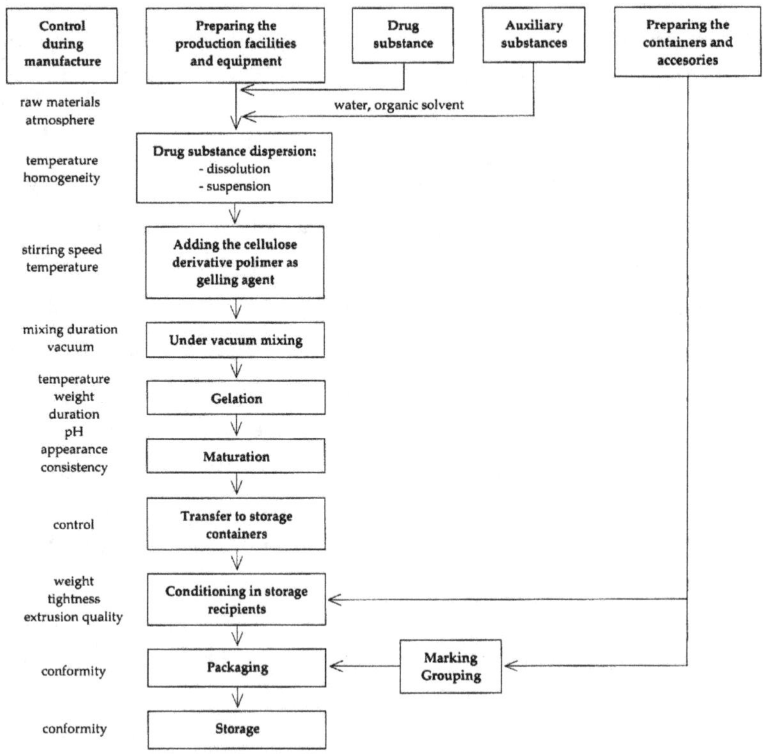

Figure 1. Flow chart of the manufacturing processes of a cellulose derivative hydrogel.

In small scale, the preparation of hydrogels by dispersing of polymer by hand or mechanically, in hot/cold water or in a nonsolvent, is carried out using simple equipment and utensils existing in the pharmacy laboratory, such as: mortars and pestles of porcelain or glass, beakers, magnetic stirrers, and different propeller mixers. In large scale production of pharmaceutical cellulose derivatives hydrogels, different mills, separators, mixers, deaerators, and shifters are used. **Figure 2** present two different processing machines for the hydrogels preparation: a single mixing kettle equipment with slow agitation to avoid air entrapment (a) and "one bowl" vacuum processing machine (b) which is designed to control the processing temperature, and to mix (using a counterrotating mixing system), homogenize (using a high-shear rotor/stator system) and remove the entrapped air (during the product recirculation) [95, 98].

7. Characterization of cellulose derivatives hydrogels as dermal pharmaceutical dosage forms

The physicochemical, microbial and biological characteristics of cellulose-derivatives-based hydrogels are evaluated by a variety of pharmacopoeial and nonpharmacopoeial tests that are carried out to assess the quality and performance of hydrogel formulations and to minimize the batch-to-batch variations. Generally, the US, European, Japanese, and many other pharmacopoeias recommend the following tests: appearance (transparency or clarity), homogeneity, particle size analysis, pH, minimum fill, rheological measurements (viscosity, consistency), stability, microbial screening, *in vitro* drug release testing and assay. Consequently, a range of experimental techniques are used, more often in tandem, to characterize these hydrogels, providing appropriate evidences for their quality and performance.

The transparency or "clarity" of hydrogels is determined by visual methods or is measured as light transmittance by spectroscopy. Their homogeneity is usually assessed by visual examination and the surface morphology by scanning electron microscopy, which analyze under an electron microscope the lyophilized hydrogel gold sputter coated [99, 100]. Optical microscopy, dynamic light scattering and laser diffraction are currently used to determine the size, shape and granulometric distribution of particles of the suspended active substances, as these particles characteristics can influence several properties of a medicated hydrogel such as the rheological properties, stability, and therapeutic activity. Since these properties of cellulose derivatives hydrogel may be also affected by their pH, this parameter must be considered in their quality control. The pH is measured by potentiometry, using either special pH electrodes designed for viscous gels, or conventional pH electrodes for water diluted gels [101]. The content uniformity assessment of hydrogel product can be supported by the minimum-fill test that is performed to compare the weight of product filled into each container labeled with their weight.

Rheological analysis of cellulose derivatives hydrogels is very important for their characterization and quality control, providing valuable information for their formulation, manufacturing, use, and therapeutic activity. Rheological properties of cellulose derivatives hydrogels are determined by mechanical techniques using more often small-deformation and penetrometric measurements. Small-deformation measurements can be performed under both continuous shear and dynamic oscillatory conditions, being used to determine the viscoelastic properties of these gels. Continuous shear instruments (i.e., rotational viscosimeter, cone-

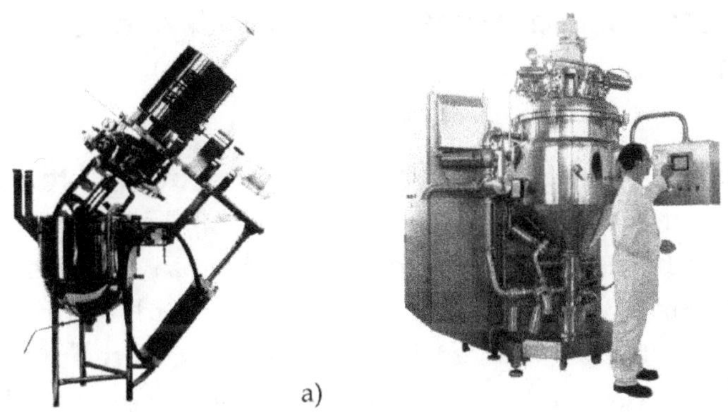

a) b)

Figure 2. Processing machines for the hydrogels preparation: (a) Stainless steel jacketed kettle with agitator (courtesy of Lee Industries, Inc., Philipsburg, Pennsylvania); (b) vacuum processing machine used for the preparation of gels (courtesy of Fryma Koruma, Rheinfelden, Switzerland).

and-plate viscosimeter) measures the apparent viscosity, yield stress, and shear modulus G(or modulus of rigidity), and generates a complete rheogram for a particular hydrogel, allowing to identify its flow behavior. Unlike continuous shear measurements, dynamic oscillatory testing, using rheometers, does not modify the hydrogel microstructure and measures another two important parameters, namely the storage modulus G' and the loss modulus G'', reflecting the hydrogel viscoelasticity [23, 102–105]. The consistency determination is a specific test for semisolids, including the hydrogels and is performed by penetrometry, according to pharmacopoeial specifications [101]. This compendial method measures the hardness of hydrogels, but the other rheological characters of these systems reflected by consistency (i.e., rigidity, spreadability, elasticity, and adhesiveness) can be also measured by different noncompedial techniques, using modern instruments such as texture analyzers [106]. Further, as it was mentioned in Section 5, rheological measurements are powerful experimental techniques for probing both the sol-gel transition and swelling behavior of cellulose derivatives hydrogels.

Due to their high water content, cellulose derivatives hydrogels are susceptible to physical, chemical, and microbial stability alterations. Syneresis, a commonly observed phenomenon of physical instability of these hydrogels, can be determined by water loss from the gel network after a heating-cooling cycle. In the case of medicated cellulose derivatives hydrogels, the chemical stability of active substances into the gel is evaluated by accelerated aging studies, which use different analytical methods to evidence the possible drug degradation in the hydrogel, under extreme conditions of temperature, moisture and light [95].

Although is a noncompendial test, *in vitro* drug release testing is of high interest as it can reflect the combined effects of several formulation parameters (i.e., the type of cellulose derivative as gelling agent, the drug concentration, the pH, and viscosity of hydrogel) on the *in vitro* drug release and permeation parameters. In the last decade, continuous efforts in international harmonization have been made to standardize the methodology and the study protocols of *in vitro* drug release from dermal products [107, 108].

8. Applications of cellulose-derivatives-based hydrogels for dermal and transdermal drug delivery

Cellulose-derivatives-based hydrogels, as pharmaceutical dosage forms, have been developed with their end use mainly in topical drug delivery [109]. These hydrogels are widely used as water-soluble ointment bases usually for dermal and, in a lesser extent, for transdermal delivery of various categories of drugs including nonsteroidal anti-inflammatory agents, antifungals, antibiotics, anesthetics, analgesics, antiallergics, antiseptics, keratolytics, revulsive agents, β-blockers etc. From the formulations intended for dermal delivery, the drug has to pass through the *stratum corneum*, the outermost layer of the skin to reach the subjacent skin layers. Therefore, medicated dermal formulations ensure the drug localization in the skin layers. Instead, from transdermal formulations the drug is transported in the skin dermis and then enters into the systemic circulation [110]. However, the excellent barrier properties of the *stratum corneum* limit the drugs penetration through the skin in both dermal and transdermal drug delivery. Therefore, several strategies have been used to enhance and control the drug transport across the skin, and to increase the number of the delivered drugs. These strategies involve both chemical methods, based on the use of penetration enhancers that temporarily increase the skin permeability, and physical methods, in which a driving force is provided to act on the drug [110].

8.1. Dermal drug delivery

Dermal medicated hydrogels based on cellulose derivatives are intended to treat different acute or chronic, mild or moderate skin conditions (i.e., eczema, dermatitis, psoriasis, acne, warts, inflammations, and allergies).

Medicated gel formulations based on cellulose derivatives were obtained by dispersing the drug directly into the hydrogel vehicle or by entrapping the drug in colloidal carriers (micro- and nanoemulsions, liposomes, niosomes etc.) acting as percutaneous enhancers. In the past decades, the favorable effect of cellulose derivatives hydrogels on dermal drug delivery has been demonstrated by a large number of published original scientific papers, academic reviews, monographs and books focused on preparation, characterization and applications of cellulose derivative hydrogels [85, 89, 111–117].

Due to their specific properties, some of gel-forming cellulose derivatives, such as NaCMC and MC are used for the development of wound dressings, usually in combination with other hydrophilic polymers and propyleneglycol, which act as humectant and preservative. These hydrogels proved to be effective as treatment for burned tissues and nonhealing diabetic ulcers [16, 39, 118, 119].

In **Table 9** are included the main studies that have been conducted in the past decade on cellulose-derivatives-based hydrogels as vehicles for dermal delivery of different drugs.

This section provides a survey of the relevant results of the recent reports published in the last decade.

Kouchak and Handali [121] studied the effect of some skin penetration enhancers, including sodium tauroglycocholate, lauric acid, and ethanol on the *in vitro* permeation of aminophylline from 3% HPMC-based hydrogels through snake skin. Sodium tauroglycholate and ethanol at concentration of 100 μg/ml and 60%, respectively, produced a 6-fold increase of the permeation parameters (flux and permeation coefficient), being the optimum enhancers for aminophylline, intended to be used as anticellulitic agent.

From the class of antifungal agents, clotrimazole, bifonazole, and fluconazole were selected as model drugs that were solubilized in emulsion or microemulsion systems, which were then loaded in a cellulose derivative-based hydrogel in order to improve the viscosity of the emulsion/microemulsion and make it suitable for cutaneous application. Shahin et al. [125] studied several jojoba oil-based emulgel formulations as potential clotrimazole delivery vehicles. Jojoba oil was used as lipophilic phase, Span 60 and Brij 35 were used as surfactants, propyleneglycol was selected as humectant and for its aesthetic benefits, and hydroxypropylmethylcellulose and/or Carbopol 934P were chosen as gelling agents; triethanolamine was used to neutralize the formula containing carbomer to the pH range 5.5–6.5. It was found that the concentration and type of the gelling agent significantly influenced the viscosity and the consistency of the examined systems. Also, the *in vitro* clotrimazole release data showed an inverse correlation between the concentration of the gelling agent and the extent of the released drug. The formulation containing the combination of two gelling agents, HPMC and Carbopol 934P, in concentrations of 1% and 0.2%, respectively, showed stable rheological properties (shear thinning behavior with little thixotropy), high extent of drug release and superior antifungal activity in comparison to a commercially available preparation [125].

Drug	Cellulose derivative as gelling agent	Pharmaceutical dosage form	References
Alaptide	HEC, HPC, MC	Hydrogel	[120]
Aminophylline	HPMC	Hydrogel	[121]
Bifonazole	HPMC	Microemulsion-loaded hydrogel	[122]
Clarithromycin	HPMC	Emulgel	[123]
Chlorphenesin	HPMC	Emulgel	[124]
Clotrimazole	HPMC	Emulgel	[125]
Diclofenac sodium	CMCNa	Hydrogel	[126]
Etoricoxib	HPMC	Hydrogel	[127]
Fluconazole	CMC	Emulgel, microemulsion-loaded hydrogel	[128]
	HPMC	Hydrogel	[129]
Ketorolac tromethamine	HPMC	Hydrogel	[130]
Lidocaine	HPC	Hydrogel	[131]
Lidocaine hydrochloride			
Meloxicam	HPC	Hydrogel	[132, 133]
Mepivacaine		Hydrogel	[134]
Piroxicam	HPMC	Emulgel	[135]
	MC, HPMC, CMC	Microemulsion-loaded hydrogel	[136]
Propranolol hydrochloride	HPMC	Hydrogel	[137]

Table 9. Overview of cellulose-derivatives-based hydrogels as vehicles for cutaneous delivery of drugs.

In order to improve the solubility and skin permeability of bifonazole, Sabale et al. [122] investigated several oil-in-water microemulsion-loaded hydrogels composed of bifonazole (1%) water, oleic acid as oil, Tween 80/isopropyl alcohol as surfactant/cosurfactant mixture, and two grades of HPMC (K15M and K100M) in concentrations of 1, 1.5, and 2%. After optimization of the microemulsion formulation by 3^2 factorial design and of the polymer concentration for preparation of microemulsion-loaded hydrogel based on viscosity, the composition of the optimized microemulsion-loaded hydrogel was bifonazole (1%), oleic acid (6.25%), Tween 80/isopropyl alcohol (55%, 3:1), water (38.75%), and HPMC K100M (2%).

The results of the *ex vivo* permeation study through excised rat skin indicated that bifonazole presented a permeability of 84% within 10 h and a sustained release from the optimized formulation, due to the presence of the gelling agent; the drug release was accurately described by the zero order model. Also, the developed preparation exhibited a good stability over a period of 3 months, no skin irritancy and an antifungal activity comparable with a marketed bifonazole cream [122].

Salerno et al. [128] studied the *in vitro* fluconazole release from different topical dosage forms, aiming to determine a formulation with the capacity to deliver the whole active compound and maintain it within the skin, in order to be considered as a useful formulation, either for topical mycosis treatment or as adjuvant in a combined therapy for Cutaneous Leishmaniasis. Sodium carboxymethylcellulose was used for emulgels and microemulsion-loaded hydrogels as gelling agent, and propyleneglycol and diethyleneglycol monoethyl ether (Transcutol P®) were used for each dosage form as solvent for the drug and also as penetration enhancers. The microemulsion-loaded hydrogel containing Transcutol P® delivered the whole applied dose of fluconazole, and showed the highest ability to penetrate pig skin (a four times greater of total amount drug released than that from lipogels) and an important ability to keep the drug within the skin layers; also this formulation proved to be the most effective in regard of the *in vitro* antifungal activity. Further, the authors concluded that in the case of CMCNa-based dosage forms (emulgels and microemulsion-loaded hydrogels), the viscosity was not the main parameter governing the fluconazole release, as these systems showed similar viscosity, but different rates of the released drug [128]. Other study investigated the *in vitro* release of fluconazole from different hydrophilic gels, containing HPMC, chitosan or poloxamer 407 as gelling agents, propyleneglycol as cosolvent and various penetration enhancers (glycerol, PEG 400, Tween 80, and cetrimide). Among the studied hydrogels, those based on HPMC produced the higher percentages of fluconazole released after 6 h, either in the presence or absence of glycerol (66.66 and 71.65%, respectively), glycerol was found to be the most effective release enhancer [129].

Nonsteroidal anti-inflammatory agents, such as diclofenac sodium, oxicams (piroxicam, meloxicam), and ethoricoxib, were used as model drugs in several studies investigating the effects of the structure and the components of the vehicle on drug release and penetration from cellulose-derivative-based hydrogels [126, 127, 130, 132, 133, 135, 136]. A base-gel formulation consisting of 2.5% hydroxypropylcellulose (Klucel), propyleneglycol, ethanol, and water (1:1:1) was selected to investigate the effect of four penetration enhancers (dimethylsulfoxide, Tween 20, oleic acid, and menthol) on *in vitro* permeability of meloxicam through IPM-saturated cellulose membranes and human cadaver skin [132]. Permeation studies through human cadaver skin showed that the highest flux value (2.43 ± 0.47 $\mu g/cm^2/h$), with a corresponding enhancement ratio of 27.5, was obtained from HPC-based hydrogel containing 5% menthol as penetration enhancer. According to the authors, the developed meloxicam gel formulation consisting of 2.5% Klucel® gel, 0.3% meloxicam, 5% menthol, and the mixture of propyleneglycol, ethanol, and water (1:1:1) offers the possibility to deliver through the skin therapeutically effective amounts of meloxicam [132]. The potential of 2.5% hydroxypropylcellulose hydrogel, containing a combination of enhancers, to produce a required flux of meloxicam to maintain therapeutic concentration, was confirmed by another study performed by Chang et al. [133]. The effects of a combination of four penetration enhancers (ethanol, propyleneglycol, menthol, and azone) acting by different mechanisms, on the penetration of meloxicam sodium from HPC-based hydrogels through rat skin, was investigated by the response surface methodology. Also, the uniform design technique was applied to prepare systematical model formulations, which were composed of four formulation factors (the content of ethanol, propyleneglycol, menthol and azone); the penetration rate (flux) was chosen as the response. The obtained results demonstrated, on one hand, that the optimal meloxicam sodium hydrogel formulation can be designed using this response surface methodology, and on the other hand, that menthol influenced, in the greatest extent, the skin permeation of meloxicam sodium, followed by azone, ethanol, and propyleneglycol respectively. The optimal transdermal formulation, containing 1% meloxicam, 2.5% HPC, 37.1% ethanol, 15.4% propyleneglycol, 2.9% menthol, 4.3% azone, and water, had appropriate flux value (467.6 ± 89.3 μg/cm^2/h) which met the required flux value of meloxicam (400 μg/h) for maintaining a therapeutic concentration. Further, the *in vivo* absorption study showed that meloxicam could be determined at 1 h after 2.3 cm^2 topical administration and reached steady-state concentration in about 12 h; the bioavailability of the optimal meloxicam sodium gel was about 50.1% [133]. In another study, aiming to determine the optimal base that promote the *in vitro* release of piroxicam, several gel bases consisting of different polymers in various concentrations (3% MC, 2% CMC, 3% HPMC, 0.5% Carbopols 934 and 940, and 20% Pluronic F-127) were evaluated [136]. In each of these gel bases, piroxicam (0.5%) was incorporated as such and in the form of a microemulsion, consisting of oleic acid as oil, Tween 80 as surfactant and propyleneglycol as cosurfactant. The developed gel formulations were evaluated for their rheological properties, stability and *in vitro* piroxicam release through an artificial membrane. Comparison of the *in vitro* release results showed that the 3% MC and 3% HPMC gel bases loaded with piroxicam-microemulsion released the higher amounts of drug after 180 min (97% and 94%, respectively). However, considering also the rheological properties and shelf life, the above mentioned HPMC gel-base loaded with microemulsion was proposed as the most suitable vehicle for topical delivery of piroxicam [136].

Prakash et al. studied the *in vitro* release of ethoricoxib through rat epidermis and human cadaver skin from several hydroethanolic gels based on different polymers as gelling agents (Carbopol, HPMC K4M, MC, and HPC) in the presence of various permeation enhancers such as DMSO, lemongrass oil, menthe oil, and oleic acid [127]. The results of *ex vivo* permeation study revealed that hydroethanolic gel containing 2% HPMC with 2% lemongrass oil produced the highest cumulative amounts of ethoricoxib permeated at 6 h (99.28%), similarly as the studied marketed product (99.89%). Also, this formulation showed comparable anti-inflammatory activity with the marketed product.

In our research work, a hydroethanolic gel based on 2% HPMC and 60% ethanol was used as vehicle for a hydrophilic model drug (propranolol hydrochloride) in the presence of some terpenes as penetration enhancers (menthol, camphor, eucalyptol, thymol, and α-bisabolol) at 5% concentration [137]. The results of our *in vitro* permeation study through pig ear skin, indicated that eucalyptol and α-bisabolol were the most effective terpenes in enhancing the skin transport of propranolol hydrochloride from HPMC-based hydroethanolic gels. Thus, we considered that the gel formulations consisting of 3% propranolol hydrochloride, 2% HPMC, 60% ethanol, and 5% terpene (eucalyptol or α-bisabolol) should be an alternative to oral dosage forms of this drug, recently reported as an effective treatment for infantile haemangioma [137].

These studies, but also many other, showed that the release properties of topical formulations and consequently of the base, are mainly controlled by the drug thermodynamic activity, particle size and diffusion through the preparation. Generally, the diffusion coefficient of a solute in a base is inversely related to the viscosity of the continuous phase. Consequently, the drug release decreases with the increase of viscosity, which is due to the increase in gelling agent concentration. Also, it was suggested that high polymer concentrations increase the resistance to diffusion in a greater extent than expected, because the drug particles are trapped by the polymer macromolecules and they are much closed to the respective entities. Moreover, at high polymer concentrations the density of chain structures increases, thus limiting the drug movement area. Therefore, in the case of gels, including those based on cellulose derivatives, it is considered more appropriate to relate the diffusion coefficient of drug particles in solution to the gel microviscosity, which controls the movement of the particles [138, 139].

8.2. Transdermal drug delivery

Nowadays, transdermal drug delivery is considered an attractive alternative to the conventional drug delivery methods (oral administration and injection) used for the systemic delivery of drugs. Hydrogels, including cellulose-derivatives-based hydrogels, were proposed and studied as transdermal drug delivery systems due to their several benefits including ease of application and delivery, sustained and controlled drug release, reduced systemic side effects, bypass of hepatic first pass effects and potential to provide a better feeling for the skin compared with conventional ointments and patches [140]. A recent research paper evidenced that a 1% HPMC-based hydrogel formulation produced higher permeation rates of diltiazem hydrochloride through rabbit skin (1569.5 $\mu g/cm^2$) than other studied gel formulations (organogels and bigels). Moreover, *in vivo* study of diltiazem hydrochloride as transdermally applied antihypertensive agent revealed that the HPMC-based hydrogel formulation produced a faster and sustained antihypertensive effect compared with other studied gels. The superiority of diltiazem hydrochloride hydrogel based on 1% HPMC in terms of drug permeation through the skin was attributed to high water content that facilitates the release of the hydrophilic drug from the gel-base and increases epidermal cell hydration, thus enhancing the drug diffusion across *stratum corneum* [141].

However, numerous drugs such as hydrophilic, high molecular weight, and charged active substances are not able to penetrate the skin, because of their structure and physicochemical properties. Therefore, in the recent past, physical penetration enhancement techniques including ionophoresis, sonophoresis, electroporation, and laser irradiation gained attention in transdermal drug delivery research. The therapeutic effects of above-mentioned electrically assisted techniques, used alone as well in combination or further, in conjunction with chemical enhancers, for transdermal drug delivery were intensively investigated [110, 142–147]. Furthermore, hydrogels proved to be suitable formulations for assisted transdermal delivery by ionophoresis, sonophoresis, and electroporation due to their advantageous characteristics such as ease of loading into the device, suitability with the electrode design, good flexibility and fitting with the skin contour, strength, transparency, stability, and high electrical conductivity, which is attributed to their high water content [116, 148, 149].

A number of studies reported the successfully transdermal delivery of different drugs from cellulose-derivatives-based hydrogels using ionophoresis alone and combined with other enhancement physical or chemical techniques. Tavakoli et al. [150] investigated the transdermal iontophoretic delivery of celecoxib from several gel formulations, containing different gelling agents (sodium alginate, sodium carboxymethyl cellulose, hydroxypropyl methylcellulose, and Carbopol 934P). Among the studied gel-bases, the hydrogel containing 4% HPMC K4M was considered the optimal formulation for the iontophoretic studies, as it showed higher spreadability and ability to retain on the skin, and released the highest percent of celecoxib after 5 h (41.5%). The findings of the *ex vivo* studies showed that iontophoretic transport of celecoxib from HPMC K4M-based hydrogels through rat skin was 2-fold higher than the passive flux [150].

Recently, the feasibility of using a 2% HEC-based hydrogel as gel-base for successful iontophoretic transdermal delivery of the E-selectin antagonist CGP69669A, a sialyl Lewisx-glycomimetic with potential activity against inflammatory skin diseases was reported. Although the *in vitro* drug permeation through porcine and human skin from the hydrogel formulation was lower than from aqueous solution, the skin deposition (more relevant for the local treatment of dermatological conditions) was 3-fold higher, which was attributed to the occlusive effect of the gel layer on the skin surface, increasing the degree of dermal hydration and consequently promoting the permeation of the hydrophilic CGP69669A [151].

Nandy et al. studied the efficacy of iontophoresis used alone and in combination with chemical enhancers (L-menthol and Tween 20) on transdermal delivery of atenolol from an aqueous solution and several hydrogel formulations based on 3% sodium carboxymethly cellulose or 3% methylcellulose, through excised abdominal rat skin. The obtained results demonstrated that cellulose-derivatives-based hydrogels were more suitable than a solution as transdermal iontophoretic delivery systems, ensuring a sustained release of atenolol. Also, compared with passive delivery, iontophoresis increased the atenolol transport from all studied gel formulations through rat skin. Moreover, the synergistic effects of iontophoresis and chemical enhancers were revealed. Considering this and the superiority of L-menthol as penetration enhancer compared to Tween 20, the NaCMC- and MC-based hydrogel formulations, containing 1.5% atenolol and 2% L-menthol combined with iontophoresis were considered as the best drug delivery systems to achieve the desired drug level [152]. The advantageous combination of iontophoresis and penetration enhancers for transdermal delivery was also recently evidenced in the case of diclofenac sodium formulated as hydroxyethylcellulose-based hydrogels containing different terpenes. The diclofenac sodium hydrogel containing geraniol produced an iontophoretic flux 5.16-fold higher than the passive control, being considered as optimal formulation [153]. Another research report revealed the feasibility of using carboxymethylcellulose-based hydrogels for transdermal delivery of buprenorphine under the application of iontophoresis or electroporation, separately or together [154].

8.3. Commercial products

A list of examples of pharmaceutical gel products, based on cellulose derivatives with their corresponding therapeutic activity, is shown in **Table 10**. The pharmaceutical gel products containing HPC offer the advantage of the polymer compatibility with high percentages of alcohol.

Commercial gel and manufacturer	Cellulose derivative	Drug and therapeutic activity
Persa-Gel 10 (Otho Derm)	Hydroxypropyl methylcellulose	Benzoyl peroxide; antibacterial
Diclac gel (Hexal AG)	Hydroxypropyl methylcellulose	Diclofenac sodium; antiinflammatory, analgesic
Xylocaine jelly (Astra)	Hydroxypropyl methylcellulose	Lidocaine HCl; anesthetic
ArthriCare triple-medicated gel (Commerce)	Hydroxypropyl methylcellulose	Methyl salicylate, menthol; analgesic, revulsive
Erygel (Herbert)	Hydroxypropylcellulose	Erythromycin; antibiotic for acnee
Retin-A gel (Ortho)	Hydroxypropylcellulose	Retinoic acid; antiacne
Compound W gel (Whitehall)	Hydroxypropylcellulose	Salicylic acid; keratolytic
DuoPlant gel (Schering-Plough)	Hydroxypropylcellulose	Salicylic acid; keratolytic
Hydrisalic gel (Pedinol)	Hydroxypropylcellulose	Salicylic acid; keratolytic
Keralyt gel (Summers)	Hydroxypropylcellulose	Salicylic acid; keratolytic
Fungicure-Tolnaftate gel (Alva-Amco Pharmacal Companies, Inc.)	Hydroxypropylcellulose	Tolnaftate; antifungal
Naftin (Merz Pharmaceuticals, LLC)	Hydroxyethylcellulose	Naftifine; antifungal
Nurofen gel (Reckitt Benckiser Healthcare Int. Ltd.)	Hydroxyethylcellulose	Ibuprofen; antiinflammatory, analgesic
IntraSite™ Gel (Smith and Nephew)	Sodium carboxymethyl cellulose	Wound dressing
GranuGel™ (ConvaTec)	Sodium carboxymethyl cellulose	Wound dressing
Purilon Gel™ (ColoPlast)	Sodium carboxymethyl cellulose	Wound dressing
Aquacel Ag™ (ConvaTec)	Sodium carboxymethyl cellulose	Silver ions; wound dressing

Commercial gel and manufacturer	Cellulose derivative	Drug and therapeutic activity
Silvercel™ (Johnson & Johnson)	Sodium carboxymethyl cellulose	Silver ions; wound dressing

Table 10. Some commercially available gels containing cellulose derivatives.

9. Conclusion

Due to their typical properties, several water-soluble cellulose derivatives, namely methylcellulose, hydroxyethylcellulose, hydroxypropylcellulose, hydroxypropylmethylcellulose, and sodium carboxymethylcellulose, have gained increasing interest for pharmaceutical applications, being currently used as gelling agents in the development of topical drug delivery systems. Among the specific properties, which support the extensively use of water-soluble cellulose derivatives as thickening agents in dermal gel formulations, it can be mentioned the diversity of cellulose derivatives, with broad compatibility with many active substances and wide range of viscosities correlated with variable polymer concentrations. In the presence of water, these hydrophilic cellulose derivatives form reversible hydrogels composed of networks of dissolved macromolecules, which possess specific properties in terms of swelling behavior, gel point and sensitivity to external stimuli. The cellulose-derivatives-based hydrogels are widely used as water-soluble ointment bases for dermal and transdermal drug delivery, due to their unique characteristics such as transparency, high water content, spreadability, good skin tolerability, bioadhesiveness, availability, and also biocompatibility and biodegradability, which make them similar with living tissues. In addition, these hydrogels with or without drug substances are relatively easy to prepare either on a small scale (as in extemporaneous compounding) and on a large scale (industry). Although numerous medicated and nonmedicated hydrogels based on cellulose derivatives have been developed, studied and even patented, only few have reach the pharmaceutical market. Therefore, more studies on this topic are expected so as to fully explore the potential of cellulose derivatives hydrogels as dermal and transdermal drug delivery systems.

Author details

Lavinia Vlaia[1*], Georgeta Coneac[1], Ioana Olariu[1], Vicenţiu Vlaia[1] and Dumitru Lupuleasa[2]

*Address all correspondence to: vlaia.lavinia@umft.ro

1 Faculty of Pharmacy, "Victor Babeş" University of Medicine and Pharmacy, Timişoara, Romania

2 Faculty of Pharmacy, "Carol Davila" University of Medicine and Pharmacy, Bucureşti, Romania

References

[1] Nevell TP, Zeronian SH. Cellulose Chemistry and Its Applications. New York: Halsted Press, John Wiley; 1985. p. 22–26.

[2] Kimura S, Itoh T. Evidence for the role of the glomerulocyte in cellulose synthesis in the tunicate, Metandrocarpauedai. Protoplasma. 1995;186:24–33.

[3] Lin CC, Aronson JM. Chitin and cellulose in cell walls of oomycete, *Apodachlya* sp. Arch Mikrobiol. 1970; 72:111–114.

[4] Römling U. Molecular biology of cellulose production in bacteria. Res Microbiol. 2002; 153:205–212.

[5] Somerville C. Cellulose synthesis in higher plants. Annu Rev Cell Dev Biol. 2006;22:53–78.

[6] Prabhu DM, Li WJ. The most abundant and natural source: cellulose and its derivatives and their applications. In: Mondal IH, editor. Cellulose and Cellulose Derivatives: Synthesis, Modification and Applications. New York: Nova Science Publishers Inc.; 2015. p. 3–16.

[7] Varshney VK, Naithani S. Chemical functionalization of cellulose derived from nonconventional sources. In: Kalia S, editor. Cellulose Fibers: Bio- and Nano-Polymer Composites. Heidelberg: Springer-Verlag Berlin; 2011. p. 43–60.

[8] Kamel S, Ali N, Jahangir K, Shah SM, El-Gendy AA. Pharmaceutical significance of cellulose: a review. eXPRESS Polym Lett. 2008;2(11):758–778.

[9] Popovici I. Dispersii liofile. Dispersii hidrofile. In: Popovici I, Lupuleasa D, editors. Tehnologie Farmaceutică, vol. 2. Iaşi: Polirom; 2008. p. 43–89.

[10] Tosh B. Esterification and etherification of cellulose: synthesis and application of cellulose derivatives. In: Mondal IH, editor. Cellulose and Cellulose Derivatives: Synthesis, Modification and Applications. New York: Nova Science Publishers Inc.; 2015. p. 259–298.

[11] Bowman BJ, Ofner III CM, Schott H. Colloidal dispersions. In: Troy D, editor. Remington: The Science and Practice of Pharmacy, 21st ed. Philadelphia: Lippincott Williams & Wilkins; 2005. p. 293–318.

[12] Bajerová M, Gajdziok J, Dvořáčková K, Masteiková R, Kollár P. Semisynthetic cellulose derivatives as the base of hydrophilic gel systems. Čes Slov Farm. 2008; 57(2):63–69.

[13] Rowe RC, Sheskey PJ, Quinn ME, editors. Handbook of Pharmaceutical Excipients. London: Pharmaceutical Press; 2009. p. 118–121, 311–314, 317–322; 438–441.

[14] Aqualon, NATROSOL®Hydroxyethylcellulose A Nonionic Water-Soluble Polymer. Physical and Chemical Properties. Wilmington; Ashland Aqualon Functional Ingredients. Technical literature; 1999.

[15] Ashland Aqualon Functional Ingredients. Technical literature: Klucel Hydroxypropylcellulose Physical and Chemical Properties; 2012.

[16] Ofner III CM, Klech-Gelotte CM. Gels and Jellies.In: Swarbrick J, editors. Encyclopedia of Pharmaceutical Technology, 3rd ed. vol. 3. New York: Informa Healthcare; 2007. p. 1875–1890; 1885–1886.

[17] Dow Chemical Company. Methocel Cellulose Ethers Technical Book. USA; 2002.

[18] Dow Chemical Company. Using METHOCEL Cellulose Ethers for Controlled Release of Drugs in Hydrophilic Matrix Systems. USA; 2000.

[19] Grover JA. Methylcellulose and derivatives. In: Whistler RL, BeMiller JN, editors. Industrial Gums: Polysaccharides and Their Derivatives, 3rd ed. California: Academic Press Inc.; 1993. p. 475–500.

[20] ShinEtsu: Metolose. Water-Soluble Cellulose Ethers. Japan; 2005

[21] Thakur VK, Thakur MK. Handbook of Polymers for Pharmaceutical Technologies, Structure and Chemistry. Beverly: Scrivener Publishing LLC; 2015.

[22] Silva SM, Pinto FV, Antunes FE, Miguel MG, Sousa JJ, Pais AA. Aggregation and gelation in hydroxypropylmethyl cellulose aqueous solutions. J Colloid Interface Sci. 2008;327(2):333–340.

[23] Joshi SC. Sol-gel behavior of hydroxypropyl methylcellulose (HPMC) in ionic media including drug release. Materials. 2011;4:1861–1905.

[24] Banks SR, Sammon C, Melia CD, Timmins P. Monitoring the thermal gelation of cellulose ethers in situ using attenuated total reflectance Fourier transform infrared spectroscopy. Appl Spectrosc. 2005;59(4):452–459.

[25] Acevedo A, Takhistov P, de la Rosa CP, Florián V. Thermalgelation of aqueous hydroxypropylmethylcellulose solutions with SDS and hydrophobic drug particles. Carbohydr Polym. 2014;102:74–90.

[26] Yoo YJ, Um IC. Examination of thermo-gelation behavior of HPMC and HEMC aqueous solutions using rheology. Korea-Australia Rheol J. 2013;25(2):67–75.

[27] Dow Chemical Company. Pharma & Food Solutions. WALOCEL™ C. USP/EP Carboxymethyl Cellulose Sodium for Pharmaceutical Applications; 2014.

[28] Aqualon Division of Hercules Inc. Booklet 250-10H. Aqualon® Sodium carboxymethylcellulose. Physical and Chemical Properties. Wilmington; 1999.

[29] Hennink WE, Van Nostrum CF. Novel crosslinking methods to design hydrogels. Adv Drug Deliv Rev. 2002;54(1):13–36.

[30] Chang C, Duan B, Cai J, Zhang L. Superabsorbent hydrogels based on cellulose for smart swelling and controllable delivery. Eur Polym J. 2010;46:92–100.

[31] Kono H, Onishi K, Nakamura T. Characterization and bisphenol A adsorption capacity of cyclodextrin-carboxymethylcellulose-based hydrogels. Carbohydr Polym. 2013;98:784–792.

[32] Lin OH, Kumar RN, Rozman HD, Noor MAM. Grafting of sodium carboxymethyl cellulose (CMC) with glycidylmethacrylate and development of UV curable coatings from CMC-g-GMA induced by cationic photoinitiators. Carbohydr Polym. 2005;69:57–69.

[33] Demitri C, Del Sole R, Scalera F, Sannino A, Vasapollo G, Maffezzoli A, Ambrosio L, Nicolais L. Novel superabsorbent cellulose-based hydrogels crosslinked with citric acid. J App Polym Sci. 2008;110:2453–2460.

[34] Akar E, Antinis KA, Seki Y. Preparation of pH and ionic-strength responsive biodegradable fumaric acid crosslinked carboxymethylcellulose. Carbohydr Polym. 2012;90:1634–1641.

[35] Kono H. Characterization and properties of carboxymethyl cellulose hydrogels crosslinked by polyethyleneglycol. Carbohydr Polym. 2014;106:84–93.

[36] Wach RA, Rokita B, Bartoszek N, Katsumura Y, Ulanski P, Rosiak JM. Hydroxyl radical-induced crosslinking and radiation-initiated hydrogel formation in dilute aqueous solutions of carboxymethylcellulose. Carbohydr Polym. 2014;112:412–415.

[37] Wach RA, Mitomo H, Nagasawa N, Yoshii F. Radiation crosslinking of carboxymethylcellulose of various degree of substitution at high concentration in aqueous solutions of natural pH. Radiat Phys Chem. 2003;68:771–779.

[38] Barbucci L, Leone G, Vecchiullo A. Novel carboxymethylcellulose-based microporous hydrogels suitable for drug delivery. J Biomater Sci Polym Ed. 2004;15(5):607–619.

[39] Sannino A, Demitri C, Madaghiele M. Biodegradable cellulose-based hydrogels: design and applications. Materials. 2009;2:353–373.

[40] Gulrez SKH, Al-Assaf S, Phillips GO. Hydrogels: methods of preparation, characterization and applications. In: Carpi A, editor. Progress in Molecular and Environmental Bioengineering – From Analysis and Modeling to Technology Applications. Rijeka: InTech; 2011. p. 117–150.

[41] Desbrières J, Hirrien M, Rinaudo M. A calorimetric study of methylcellulose gelation. Carbohydr Polym. 1998;37(2):145–152.

[42] Hirrien M, Chevillard C, Desbrières J, Axelos MAV, Rinaudo M. Thermogelation of methylcelluloses: new evidence for understanding the gelation mechanism. Polymer. 1998;39(25):6251–6259.

[43] Burchard W. Solubility and solution structure of cellulose derivatives. Cellulose. 2003;10(3):213–225.

[44] Baumgartner S, Kristl J, Peppas NA. Network structure of cellulose ethers used in pharmaceutical applications during swelling and at equilibrium. Pharm Res. 2002;19(8):1084–1090.

[45] Augustine R, Rajendran R, Cvelbar U, Mozetic M, George A. Biopolymers for health, food and cosmetic applications. In: Thomas S, Durand D, Chassenieux C, Jyotishkumar P, editors. Handbook of Biopolymer-Based Materials: From Blends and Composites to Gels and Complex Networks. Weinheim: Wiley-VCH; 2013. p. 801–819.

[46] Omidian H, Park K. Hydrogels. In: Siepman J, Siegel R, Rathbone M, editors. Fundamentals and Applications of Controlled Release Drug Delivery. New York: Springer; 2012. p. 75–106.

[47] Hatakeyama H, Hatakeyama T. Interaction between cellulosic polysaccharides and water. In: Nishinari K, editor. Hydrocolloids. Part I. Philadelphia: Elsevier Science BV; 2000. p. 261–270.

[48] Durand A, Hervé M, Hourdet D. Thermogelation in aqueous polymer solutions. In: McCormick CL, editor. Stimuli-Responsive Water Soluble and Amphiphilic Polymers. ACS Symposium Series, vol. 780. Washington, DC: American Chemical Society; 2009. p. 181–207.

[49] Yokota S, Matsuyama K, Kitaoka T, Wariishi H. Thermally responsive wettability of self-assembled methylcellulose nanolayers. Appl Surf Sci. 2007;253:5149–5154.

[50] Jain S, Sandhu S, Malvi R, Gupta B. Cellulose derivatives as thermoresponsive polymers: an overview. J Appl Pharm Sci. 2013;3(12):139–144.

[51] Kometani N, Tanabe M, Su L, Yang K, Nishinari K. In situ observations of thermoreversible gelation and phase separation of agarose and methylcellulose solutions under high pressure. J Phys Chem B. 2015;119(22):6878–6883.

[52] Budslov DK, Sushko NI, Tretinnikov ON. Study on thermal gelation of methylcellulose in water using FTIR-ATR spectroscopy. Appl Spectrosc. 2008;75(4):514–518.

[53] Haque A, Morris ER. Thermogelation of mehylcellulose. Part I: molecular structures and processes. Carbohydr Polym. 1993;22:161–173.

[54] Takahasi M, Shimazaki M, Yamamoto J. Thermoreversible gelation and phase separation in aqueous methylcellulose solutions. J Polym Sci B. 2001;39:91–100.

[55] Li L. Thermal gelation of methylcellulose in water: scaling and thermoreversibility. Macromolecules. 2002;35:5990–5998.

[56] Li L, Thangamathesvaran PM, Yue CY, Tam KC, Hu X, Lam Y C. Gel Network structure of methylcellulose in water. Langmuir. 2001;17(26):8062–8068.

[57] Sarkar NJ. Thermal gelation properties of methyl and hydroxypropyl methylcellulose. Appl Polym Sci. 1979;24:1073–1087.

[58] Joshi SC, Su JC, Liang CM, Lam YC. Gelation of methylcellulose hydrogels under isothermal conditions. J Appl Polym Sci. 2008;107(4): 2101–2108.

[59] Kato T, Yokoyama M, Takahashi A. Melting temperatures of thermally reversible gels. Colloid Polym Sci. 1978;256:15–21.

[60] Kobayashi K, Huang C, Lodge TP. Thermoreversible gelation of aqueous methylcellulose solutions. Macromolecules. 1999;32:7070–7077.

[61] Sekiguchi Y, Sawatari C, Kondo T. A gelation mechanism depending on hydrogen bonding formation in regioselectively substituted O-methylcelluloses. Carbohydr Polym. 2003;53:145–153.

[62] Chatterjee T, Nakatani AI, Adden R, Brackhagen M, Redwine D, Shen H, Li Y, Wilson T, Sammler RL. Structure and properties of aqueous methylcellulose gels by small-angle neutron scattering. Biomacromolecules. 2012;13(10):3355–3369.

[63] Thirumala S, Gimble JM, Devireddy RV. Methylcellulose based thermally reversible hydrogel system for tissue engineering applications. Cells. 2013;3:460–475.

[64] Balaghi S, Edelby Y, Senge B. Evaluation of thermal gelation behavior of different cellulose ether polymers by rheology. AIP Conf Proc. 2014;1593:755–761

[65] Arvidson SA, Lott JR, McAllister JW, Zhang J, Bates FS, Lodge TP, Sammler RL, Li Y, Brackhagen M. Interplay of phase separation and thermoreversible gelation in aqueous methylcellulose solutions. Macromolecules. 2013;46(1):300–309.

[66] Lott JR, McAllister JW, Arvidson SA, Bates FS, Lodge TP. Fibrillar structure of methylcellulose hydrogels. Biomacromolecules. 2013;14:2484–2488.

[67] Lott JR, McAllister JW, Wasbrough M, Sammler RL, Bates FS, Lodge TP. Fibrillar structure in aqueous methylcellulose solutions and gels. Macromolecules. 2013; 46(24): 9760–9771.

[68] Ford JL. Thermal analysis of hydroxypropylmethylcellulose and methylcellulose: powders, gels and matrix tablets. Int J Pharm. 1999;179:209–228.

[69] Sarkar N. Kinetics of thermal gelation of methylcellulose and hydroxypropylmethylcellulose in aqueous solutions. Carbohydr Polym. 1995;26(3):195–203.

[70] Xu XM, Song YM, Ping Q., Wang Y, Liu XYJ. Effect of ionic strength on the temperature-dependent behavior of hydroxypropyl methylcellulose solution and matrix tablet behavior. Appl Polym Sci. 2006;102 (4):4066–4074.

[71] Sammon C, Bajwa G, Timmins P, Melia CD. The application of attenuated total reflectance Fourier transform infrared spectroscopy to monitor the concentration and state of water in solutions of a thermally responsive cellulose ether during gelation. Polymer. 2006;47:577–584.

[72] Haque A, Richardson RK, Morris ER, Gidley MJ, Caswell DC. Thermogelation of methylcellulose. Part II: Effect of hydroxypropyl substituents. Carbohydr Polym. 1993;22:175–186.

[73] Fairclough JPA, Yu HAO, Kelly O, Ryan AJ, Sammler RL, Radler M. The interplay between gelation and phase separation in aqueous solutions of methylcellulose and hydroxypropyl methylcellulose. Langmuir. 2012;28(28):10551–10557.

[74] Bodvik R, Dedinaite A, Karlson L, Bergström M, Bäverbäck P, Pedersen J.S, Edwards K, Karlsson G, Varga I, Claesson PM. Aggregation and network formation of aqueous methylcellulose and hydroxypropulmethylcellulose solutions. Colloid Surf A: Physicochem Eng Aspects. 2010;354:162–171.

[75] Robitaille L, Turcotte N, Fortin S, Charlet G. Calorimetric study of aqueous solutions of hydroxypropyl cellulose. Macromolecules. 1991;24(9):2413–2418.

[76] Ibbett RN, Philp K, Price DM. ^{13}C NMR studies of the thermal behavior of aqueous solutions of cellulose ethers. Polymer. 1992;33(19):4087–4094.

[77] Fernandes EM. Bionanocomposites from lignocellulosic resources: properties, applications and future trends for their use in the biomedical field. Prog Polym Sci. 2013;38(10–11):1415–1441.

[78] Hoare TR, Kohane DS. Hydrogels in drug delivery: progress and challenges. Polymer. 2008;49:1993–2007.

[79] Patel A, Mequanint K. Hydrogel biomaterials. In: Fazel-Rezai R, editor. Biomedical Engineering – Frontiers and Challenges. New York: InTech; 2011. p. 275–296.

[80] Blanco MD, Olmo RM, Teijón JM. Hydrogels In: Swarbrick J, editor. Encyclopedia of Pharmaceutical Technology, 3rd ed., vol. 3. New York: Informa Healthcare;2007. p. 2021–2039.

[81] Ahmed EM. Hydrogel: preparation, characterization, and applications. A review. J Adv Res. 2015;6(2):105–121.

[82] Miyamoto T, Takahashi S, Ito H, Inagachi H, Nioshiki Y. Tissue biocompatibility of cellulose and its derivatives. J Biomed Mater Res. 1989;23(1):125–133.

[83] Peppas N. Hydrogels. In: Ratner BD, Hoffman AS, Schoen FJ, Lemons JE, editors. Biomaterial Science. An Introduction to Materials in Medicine. 2nd ed. New York: Elsevier Academic Press; 2004. p. 100–107.

[84] Peppas NA, Mikos AG. Preparation methods and structure of hydrogels. In: Peppas NA, editor. Hydrogels in Medicine and Pharmacy, vol. 1. Boca Raton: CRC Press; 1986. p. 1–27.

[85] Hoffman AS. Hydrogels for biomedical applications. Adv Drug Deliv Rev. 2002;43: 3–12.

[86] Clark AH, Ross-Murphy SB. Structural and mechanical properties of biopolymer gels. Adv Polym Sci. 1987;83:57–192.

[87] Nijenhius K. Thermoreversible networks. Viscoelastic properties and structure of gels. Adv Polym Sci. 1997;130:169–193.

[88] Florence AT, Attwood D. Physicochemical Principles of Pharmacy. 5th ed. London: Pharmaceutical Press; 2011. p. 292–294.

[89] Peppas NA, Bures P, Leobandung W, Ichikawa H. Hydrogels in pharmaceutical formulations. Eur J Pharm Biopharm. 2000;50:27–46.

[90] Levy G, Schwarz TW. The effect of certain additives on the gel point of methylcellulose. J Am Pharm Assoc. 1958;47(1):44–46.

[91] Vennat B, Lardy F, Arvouet-Grand A, Pourrat A. Comparative texturometric analysis of hydrogels based on cellulose derivatives, carraghenates, and alginates: evaluation of adhesiveness. Drug Dev Ind Pharm. 1998;24(1):27–35.

[92] Michailova V, Titeva St, Kotsilkova R, Krusteva E, Minkov E. Influence of aqueous medium on viscoelastic properties of carboxymethylcellulose sodium, hydroxypropylmethyl cellulose, and thermally pre-gelatinized starch gels. Colloids Surf A. 1999;149(1–3):515–520.

[93] Mata J, Patel J, Jain M, Ghosh G, Bahadur P. Interaction of cationic surfactants with carboxymethylcellulose in aqueous media. J Colloid Interf Sci. 2006;297:797–804.

[94] Kolodziejska J. The effect of saccharic alcohols on rheological parameters of dental anti-inflammatory gels and on pharmaceutical availability of sodium ibuprofen. Acta Pol Pharm. 2006;63(2):127–133.

[95] Mahalingam R, Li X, Jasti BR. Semisolid dosages: ointments, creams, and gels. In: Gad SC, editor. Pharmaceutical Manufacturing Handbook. Production and Processes. New Jersey: Wiley-Interscience, John Wiley & Sons Inc.; 2008. p. 291–306.

[96] Betageri G, Prabhu S. Semisolid preparations. In: Swarbrick J, editor. Encyclopedia of Pharmaceutical Technology, 3rd ed., vol. 3. New York: Informa Healthcare;. 2007. p. 3257–3274.

[97] Popa EA, Popovici I, Braha SL. Forme farmaceutice bioadezive. In: Popovici I, Lupuleasa D, editors. Tehnologie Farmaceutică, vol. 2. Iaşi: Polirom; 2008. p. 715–791.

[98] Allen LV Jr, Ansel HC. Ointments, creams, and gels. Semisolid dosage forms and transdermal delivery systems. In: Ansel's Pharmaceutical Dosage Forms and Drug Delivery Systems. 10th ed. Philadelphia: Wolters Kluwer Health; 2014. p. 316–342.

[99] El Fray M, Pilaszkiewicz A, Swieszkowski W, Kurzydlowski KJ. Morphology assessment of chemically modified cryostructured poly(vinyl alcohol) hydrogel. Eur Polym J. 2007;43:2035–2040.

[100] Aouada FA, de Moura MR, Fernandes PRG, Rubira AF, Muniz EC. Optical and morphological characterization of polyacrylamide hydrogel and liquid crystal systems. Eur Polym J. 2005;41:2134–2141.

[101] Directorate for the Quality of Medicines of the Council of Europe. European Pharmacopoeia. 8th ed. Strasbourg Cedex: Council of Europe; 2014. p. 24, 28, 299–301.

[102] Lin SY, Amidon GL, Weiner ND, Goldberg AH. Viscoelasticity of cellulose polymers and mucociliary transport on frog palates. Int J Pharm. 1993;95:57–65.

[103] Rudraraju VS, Wyandt CM. Rheological characterization of microcrystalline cellulose/ sodium carboxymethyl cellulose hydrogels using a controlled stress rheometer: part I. Int J Pharm. 2005;292(1–2):53–61.

[104] Dolz-Panas M, Roldan-Garcia C, Herraez-Dominiquez JV, Belda-Maximino R. Thixotropy of different concentrations of microcrystalline cellulose:sodium carboxymethyl cellulose gels. J Pharm Sci. 1991;80:75–79.

[105] Hoare T, Zuralowski D, Langer R, Kohane DS. Rheological blends for drug delivery. I. Characterization in vitro. J Biomed Mater Res A. 2010;92:575–585.

[106] Jones DS, Woolfson AD, Djokic J. Texture profile analysis of bioadhesive polymeric semisolids: mechanical characterization and investigation of interactions between formulation components. J Appl Polym Sci. 1996:61(12):2229–2234.

[107] OECD Guidance document for the conduct of skin absorption studies. OECD series on testing and assessment. No. 28. Paris: Environment Directorate;, 2004. p. 12–24.

[108] FDA Guidance for Industry SUPAC-SS. Nonsterile Semisolid Dosage Forms, Scale-Up and Postapproval Changes: Chemistry, Manufacturing, and Controls. In Vitro Release Testing and In Vivo Bioequivalence Documentation. U.S. Department of Health and Human Services, Food and Drug Administration, Center for Drug Evaluation and Research; June 1997.

[109] Shokri J, Adibkia K. Application of cellulose and cellulose derivatives in pharmaceutical industries. In: van de Ven T, Godbout L, editors. Cellulose – Medical, Pharmaceutical and Electronic Applications. Rijeka: InTech; 2013. p. 47–66.

[110] Trommer H, Neubert RHH. Overcoming the stratum corneum: the modulation of skin penetration. Skin Pharmacol Physiol. 2006;19:106–121.

[111] Ibrahim MM, Hafez SA, Mahdy MM. Organogels, hydrogels and bigels as transdermal delivery systems for diltiazem hydrochloride. Asian J Pharm Sci. 2013;8(1):48–57.

[112] Vlaia L, Olariu I, Coneac G, Vlaia V, Popoiu C, Stanciulescu C, Mut AM, Szabadai Z, Lupuleasa D. Percutaneous penetration enhancement of propranolol hydrochloride

from HPMC-based hydroethanolic gels containing terpenes. Farmacia. 2014;62(5):991–1008.

[113] Pillai AB, Nair JV, Gupta NK, Gupta S. Microemulsion-loaded hydrogel formulation of butenafine hydrochloride for improved topical delivery. Arch Dermatol Res. 2015;307(7):625–633.

[114] Csóka G, Pásztor E, Marton S, Zelkó R, Antal I, Klebovich I. Formulation of thermoresponsive transdermal therapeutic systems using cellulose derivatives. Acta Pharm Hung. 2007;77(2):102–107.

[115] Valenta C, Auner BG. The use of polymers for dermal and transdermal delivery. Eur J Pharm Biopharm. 2004;58(2):279–289.

[116] Caló E, Khutoryanskiy VV. Biomedical applications of hydrogels: a review of patents and commercial products. Eur Polym J. 2015;65:252–267.

[117] Trombino S, Cassano R. Cellulose and its derivatives for pharmaceutical and biomedical applications. In: Mondal IH, editor. Cellulose and Cellulose Derivatives: Synthesis, Modification and Applications. NewYork: Nova Science Publishers; 2015. p. 405–419.

[118] Zheng WJ, Gao J, Wei Z, Zhou J, Chen YM. Facile fabrication of self-healing carboxymethylcellulose hydrogels. Eur Polym J. 2015;72:514–522.

[119] Aly FU. Preparation and evaluation of novel topical gel preparations for wound healing in diabetics. Int J Pharm Pharm Sci. 2012;4(4):76–77.

[120] Sklenář Z, Vitková Z, Herdová P, Horáčková K, Šimunková V. Formulation and release of alaptide from cellulose-based hydrogels. Acta Vet Brno. 2012;81:301–306.

[121] Kouchak M, Handali S. Effects of various penetration enhancers on penetration of aminophylline through shed snake skin. Jundishapur J Nat Pharm Prod. 2014;9(1):24–29.

[122] Sabale V, Vora S. Formulation and evaluation of microemulsion-based hydrogel for topical delivery. Int J Pharm Invest. 2012;2(3):140–149.

[123] Baibhav J, Singh G, Rana AC, Saini S. Development and characterization of clarithromycin emulgel for topical delivery. Int J Drug Dev Res. 2012;4(3):310–323.

[124] Mohamed MI. Optimization of chlorphenesin emulgel formulation. AAPS J. 2004;6(3):81–87.

[125] Shahin M, Hady SA, Hammad M, Mortada N. Novel jojoba oil-based emulsion gel formulations for clotrimazole delivery. AAPS PharmSciTech. 2011;12(1):239–247.

[126] Gupta A, Mishra AK, Singh AK, Gupta V, Bansal P. Formulation and evaluation of topical gel of diclofenac sodium using different polymers. Drug Invent Today. 2010;2(5):250–253.

[127] Prakash PR, Rao NGR, Soujanya C. Formulation, evaluation and antiinflammatory activity of topical etoricoxib gel. Asian J Pharm Clin Res. 2010;3(2):126–129.

[128] Salerno C, Carlucci AM, Bregni C. Study of in vitro drug release and percutaneous absorption of fluconazole from topical dosage forms. AAPS PharmSciTech. 2010;11(2): 986–993.

[129] Abdel-Mottaleb MMA, Mortada ND, Elshamy AA, Awad GAS. Preparation and evaluation of fluconazole gels. Egypt J Biomed. Sci. 2007;23:35–41.

[130] Hosny KM, Tayeb MM, Fallatah OM, Mahmoud AA, Mandoura MS, Al-Sawahli MM. Preparation and evaluation of ketorolac tromethamine hydrogel. Int J Pharm Sci Rev Res. 2013;20(2):269–274.

[131] Sawant PD, Luu D, Ye R, Buchta R. Drug release from hydroethanolic gels. Effect of drug's lipophilicity (log *P*), polymer-drug interactions and solvent lipophilicity. Int J Pharm. 2010;396(1–2):45–52.

[132] Jantharaprapap R, Stagni G. Effects of penetration enhancers on *in vitro* permeability of meloxicam gels. Int J Pharm. 2007;343:26–33.

[133] Chang JS, Huang YB, Hou SS, Wang RJ, Wu PC, Tsai YH. Formulation optimization of meloxicam sodium gel using response surface methodology. Int J Pharm. 2007;338:48–54.

[134] Cho CW, Choi JS, Shin SC. Enhanced local anesthetic action of mepivacaine from the bioadhesive gels. Pak J Pharm Sci. 2011;24(1):87–93.

[135] Shokri J, Azarmi Sh, Fasihi Z, Hallaj-Nezhadi S, Nokhodchi A, Javadzadeh Y. Effects of various penetration enhancers on percutaneous absorption of piroxicam from emulgels. Res Pharm Sci. 2012;7(4): 225–234.

[136] Abd-Allah FI, Dawaba HM, Ahmed AMS. Preparation, characterization, and stability studies of piroxicam loaded microemulsions in topical formulations. Drug Discov Ther. 2010;4(4):267–275.

[137] Vlaia L, Olariu I, Coneac G, Vlaia V, Popoiu C, Stănciulescu C, Muţ AM, Szabadai Z, Lupuleasa D. Percutaneous penetration enhancement of propranolol hydrochloride from HPMC-based hydroethanolic gels containing terpenes. Farmacia. 2014;62(5):991–1008.

[138] Al-Khamis KI, Davis SS, Hadgraft J. Microviscosity and drug release from topical gel formulations. Pharm Res. 1986;3(4):214–217.

[139] Davis SS, Khanderia M. The influence of the rheological properties of the vehicle on the release of drugs from semi-solid ointments. Proceedings 1st International Conference on Pharmaceutica Technology, APGI, Paris; 1977. p. I: 30–47.

[140] Simões S, Figueiras A, Veiga F. Modular hydrogels for drug delivery. J Biomater Nanobiotechnol. 2012;3:185–199.

[141] Ibrahim MM, Hafez SA, Mahdy MM. Organogels, hydrogels and bigels as transdermal delivery systems for diltiazem hydrochloride. AJPS. 2013;8:48–57.

[142] Prausnitz MR, Langer R. Transdermal drug delivery. Nat Biotechnol. 2008;26(11):1261–1268.

[143] Azagury A, Khoury L, Enden G, Kost J. Ultrasound mediated transdermal drug delivery. Adv Drug Deliv Rev. 2014;72:127–43.

[144] Wang Y, Thakur R, Fan Q, Michniak B. Transdermal iontophoresis: combination strategies to improve transdermal iontophoretic drug delivery. Eur J Pharm Biopharm. 2005;60(2):179–191.

[145] Charoo NA, Rahman Z, Repka MA, Murthy SN. Electroporation: an avenue for transdermal drug delivery. Curr Drug Deliv. 2010;7(2):125–136.

[146] Khan A, Yasir M, Asif M, Chauhan I, Singh AP, Sharma R, Singh P, Rai S. Iontophoretic drug delivery: history and applications. JAPS. 2011;1(3):11–24.

[147] Escobar-Chávez JJ, Bonilla-Martínez D, Villegas-González MA, Rodríguez-Cruz IM, Domínguez-Delgado CL. The use of sonophoresis in the administration of drugs throughout the skin. J Pharm Pharm Sci. 2009;12(1):88–115.

[148] Vikram K, Kiran B, Rahul T. Enhancement of iontophoretic transport of diphenhydramine hydrochloride thermosensitive gel by optimization of pH, polymer concentration, electrode design and pulse rate. Pharm Sci Tech. 2007;8:E1–E6.

[149] Stamatialis DF, Rolevink HH, Gironès M, Nymeijer DC, Koops GH. *In vitro* evaluation of a hydroxypropyl cellulose gel system for transdermal delivery of timolol. Curr Drug Deliv. 2004;1:313–319.

[150] Tavakoli N, Minaiyan M, Heshmatipour M, Musavinasab R. Transdermal iontophoretic delivery of celecoxib from gel formulation. Res Pharm Sci. 2015;10(5):419–428.

[151] Gratieri T, Wagner B, Kalaria D, Ernst B, Yogeshvar N, Kalia YN. Cutaneous iontophoretic delivery of CGP69669A, a sialyl Lewisx-mimetic, *in vitro*. Exp Dermatol. 2012;21:226–228.

[152] Nandy BC, Gupta RN, Rai VK, Das S, Tyagi LK, Roy S, Meena KC. Transdermal iontophoretic delivery of atenolol in combination with penetration enhancers: optimization and evaluation on solution and gels. Int J Pharm Sci Drug Res. 2009;1(2):91–99.

[153] Arunkumar S, Shivakumar HN, Desai BG, Ashok P. Effect of gel properties on transdermal iontophoretic delivery of diclofenac sodium. e-Polymers. 2016;16(1):25–32.

[154] Fang JY, Sung KC, Wang JJ, Chu CC, Chen KT. The effects of iontophoresis and electroporation on transdermal delivery of buprenorphine from solutions and hydrogels. J Pharm Pharmacol. 2002;54(10):1329–1337.

3

Lipid-Based Nano-Delivery for Oral Administration of Poorly Water Soluble Drugs (PWSDs): Design, Optimization and *in vitro* Assessment

Mohsin Kazi

Abstract

Currently, more than 90% of compounds identified are water insoluble and or poorly water soluble, which is a bottle neck in the development of many new drug candidates. These poorly soluble drug molecules are difficult to formulate using conventional approaches and are associated with numerous formulation-related performance issues. Formulating these compounds using lipid-based systems is one of the rapidly growing interests and suitable drug delivery strategies. Lipid formulations such as self-emulsifying/microemulsifying/nanoemulsifying drug delivery systems (SEDDS/SMEDDS/SNEDDS) have been attempted in many researches to improve the bioavailability and dissolution rate for their better dispersion properties. One of the greatest advantages of incorporating the poorly soluble drug into such formulation products is their spontaneous emulsion and or microemulsion/nanoemulsion formation in aqueous media. The performance and ongoing advances in manufacturing technologies have rapidly introduced lipid-based drug formulations as commercial products into the marketplace with several others in clinical development. The current chapter aims to present the characteristics feature, development and utilization of oral lipid-based nanoformulations within the drug delivery regime. The content of the chapter also provides an insight into the *in vitro* evaluation of lipid-based nanosystems and their limitations.

Keywords: lipid-based formulation, self-nanoemulsifying drug delivery systems (SNEDDS), poorly water soluble drugs (PWSDs), lipid formulation classification systems (LFCS), solubility enhancement

1. Introduction

Due to the continuous rise in the number of low solubility drug molecules and lack of more targeted drug therapies, the drug development has become more complex and challenging job within the industry. In fact, up to 90% of today's drug candidates are suffering from low aqueous solubility, which is commonly associated with low bioavailability, high intra- and inter-subject variability and lack of dose suitability [1, 2]. In keeping these challenges in mind, drug formulators must seek new techniques and innovative formulation approaches to overcome such hurdles and ensure effective treatments for the patients in need.

It is more than a decade, when lipid-based formulations have been considered as a well-established strategy for improving oral bioavailability and minimizing variable food effect of poorly soluble compounds. Lipids have been used as carriers in various delivery systems for drug administration, including solutions, suspensions, emulsions, and more attractively self-emulsifying/microemulsifying/nanoemulsifying drug delivery systems (SEDDS/SMEDDS/SNEDDS) that are designed to increase solubility and bioavailability of drugs belonging to the BCS Class II–IV [3]. Among several approaches, which are currently available to incorporate active pharmaceutical drugs into lipid vehicles in a variety of dosage forms, SEDDS, SMEDDS and or SNEDDS have proved to be the most successful approaches in improving the bioavailability [4]. The initial key achievement of these formulation systems (SEDDS/SMEDDS/SNEDDS) is to increase the solubilization of the poorly water soluble drugs (PWSDs) by the formation of emulsions and or micellar systems (colloidal solutions).

These systems advantageously present the drug in solubilized form, and their relatively smaller droplet sizes provide a large interfacial area enhancing the activity of pancreatic lipase to hydrolyze triglycerides and thereby promoting faster drug release containing mixed micelles of bile salts. The development of Neoral® (cyclosporin A) as a commercial product exhibits an excellent example of the utilization of these systems [5].

Nanotechnology has become a buzzword for scientific experts, and efforts are ongoing to extend its applications in various medical and pharmaceutical aspects. The nanoscale technologies can be generally categorized into: lipid-based nanocarriers, polymeric nanocarriers, inorganic nanocarriers, and drug nanoparticles or nanosuspensions [6]. Within the lipid-based nanocarriers category, there has been a resurgence of interest in nanoemulsions since low energy emulsification methods, such as spontaneous or self-nanoemulsification, have been developed. SNEDDS are anhydrous homogenous liquid mixtures, composing oil, surfactant, drug and/or cosolvents, which spontaneously form transparent nanoemulsion (20–250 nm droplet size) upon aqueous dilution with mild agitation [6, 7].

Being nanosized, SNEDDS offer a strong alternative to the more conventional oral formulations of lipophilic compounds. SNEDDS introduce the drug in solution within nanosized oil droplets. These fine droplets are emptied rapidly from the stomach resulting in faster drug release all over the gastrointestinal (GI) tract. An additional advantage of SNEDDS over simple oily solutions is granting much larger interfacial area for partitioning of the drug between oil and water leading to ease of dispersibility [8]. In contrast to oily solutions, SNEDDS does not depend on the action of bile salts, enzymes and/or other effects related to the (fed/fasted) state of the stomach [9]. Thus, SNEDDS can reduce the variability in rate and extent of absorption and grant more reproducible plasma concentration levels [10].

Compared with conventional nanoemulsions, SNEDDS can offer the advantages of improved physical and/or chemical stability of the formulation and ability to fill them into unit dosage forms, such as soft/hard capsules, which improve their commercial viability, patient compliance/tolerability and reduce palatability-related concerns [6]. A key feature of a successful SNEDDS formulation is its capability to hold the drug in solution, throughout the GIT, for sufficient time to allow for absorption [11]. Many PWSDs have high solubility in SNEDDS formulations but could make a risk of precipitation after aqueous dispersion of the formulation or during its digestion in the intestine [12].

The current chapter will provide all the information to probe factors which influence the selection of successful lipid nanoformulations and affect the fate of the PWSDs after oral administration. The investigational research presented in this chapter will also provide additional information regarding current practice of lipid formulations with a particular emphasis on self-nanoemulsifying drug delivery systems (SNEDDS), the trends and perspectives and the fate of PWSDs formulated in SNEDDS.

2. Lipid nanoformulations: design approach

Lipid excipients are comprised of a large group of physically and chemically diverse glycerides, which may be used in simple (single oil solutions of the drug substance) or in more complex nanocarriers (SMEDDS/SNEDDS, drug dissolved in the mixture of glyceride, surfactant and or cosolvent), with considerable flexibility in formulation design [12].

Simple oil formulations are generally composed of mono-, di-, or triglycerides or their derivatives and differ on the content of medium- (C_6-C_{10} in chain length) or long-chain (C_{12}-C_{24} in chain length) fatty acids. Glyceride esters are water immiscible, and their solvent capacities for drug substances vary according to the fatty acid chain length. Many lipid excipients (oils, surfactants), which are regarded as acceptable food grade materials, expected to be well tolerated by the body [13], even as parenteral emulsion dosage form [14]. These excipients have a history of use in a wide variety of pharmaceuticals.

In simple terms, lipid nanoformulations can be distinguished according to their dispersion and digestion in the aqueous content of the gut [15, 16]. Emulsion droplet size has been considered to be an important part in the performance of self-nanoemulsifying systems since particle size can determine the rate and extent of drug release *in vitro* [17]. However, the relative digestion rate would be expected to vary if the formulation is modified, and the critical factor is the fate of the drug after digestion of the formulation, in particular whether or not the drug remains in a solubilized state.

Function	Composition and description	Commercial name	Supplier
Oil	**Medium-chain triglycerides (C_8-C_{10})**: Fractionated coconut oil and palm seed oil, triglycerides of caprylic/capric acid	Miglyol 812, 810, Capmul MCM, Captex 355, etc.	Gattefosse corporation, France; Abitec Corp., Janesville, USA; Sasol GmbH, Witten, Germany; Nikko Chemicals Co., Tokyo, Japan; **Cremer Oleo GmbH & Co. KG,** Hamburg, Germany; Lipoid, Germany; BASF Co., Germany
	Long-chain triglycerides (C_{14}-C_{22}): Vegetable oils are glyceride esters of mixed unsaturated long-chain fatty acids, commonly known as long-chain triglycerides	Soybean oil, sesame oil, corn oil, olive oil, peanut oil, cottonseed oil, rapeseed oil, etc.	
	Mixed mono-, di- and triglycerides: Novel semisynthetic medium- and long-chain derivatives. Esters of propylene glycol and mixture of mono- and diglycerides of caprylic/capric acid	Imwitor 988, Imwitor 308, Maisene 35-1, etc.	
	Polar oil: Some excipients which are traditionally thought of as hydrophobic surfactants, such as sorbitan fatty acid esters	Span 80, 85, etc.	
Nonionic surfactant	**Water insoluble:** Oleate esters, such as polyoxyethylene (20) sorbitan trioleate, PEG-6-sorbitan oleate and polyoxyethylene (25) glyceryl trioleate are commonly used in the pharmaceutical industries	Polysorbate 85 (Tween 85), TO-106 V, Tagat TO, etc.	
	Water soluble: The popular castor oil derivatives with saturated alkyl chains resulting from hydrogenation of materials derived from a vegetable oil. Other derivatives include polysorbate 80 which are predominantly ether ethoxylates and phospholipids	Cremophor RH40, Cremophor EL, HCO30, Tween 20, 80, poloxamer 407, various Labrasols, Labrafac Labrafils, Gelucires, Soy phosphatidylcholine, etc.	
Cosolvent	The most popular water soluble cosolvents are propylene glycol, polyethylene glycol, ethanol and glycerol. Others are diethylene glycol monoethyl ether, propylene carbonate, tetrahydrofurfuryl alcohol, polyethylene glycol ether	PG, PEG 300, PEG 400, 600, transcutol, glycofurol, etc.	
Other excipient	Many oil-soluble antioxidants	α-Tocopherol, β-carotene, butylated hydroxytoluene (BHT), butylated hydroxyanisole (BHA), propyl gallate, ascorbyl palmitate, etc.	

Table 1. Common excipients for designing self-nanoemulsifying formulations and the list of their suppliers.

2.1. Excipients used to design lipid-based nanoformulations

Excipients play a key role in designing successful nanoformulations with a sound control strategy and influence business-critical and clinically significant drug product performance outcomes such as stability, bioavailability and manufacturability. The design of lipid-based nanoformulations, particularly SNEDDS, is comparatively simple as the drug need to be incorporated into a suitable oil-surfactant mixture, which could be filled in a soft or hard gelatin capsules. Various choices of lipid excipients are available in the market. Numerous lipids are amphiphilic in nature, which contain both hydrophilic and lipophilic portions (fatty acid) [18]. The morphology of the lipids should be assessed as melting point increases when the length of fatty acid chain increases, but it decreases when unsaturation of the fatty acid increases [19]. Choice of excipients for successfully designed lipid-based nanocarriers is determined based on factors, such as miscibility; solvent capacity; self-dispersibility; digestibility; irritancy; toxicity; purity; chemical stability; compatibility with capsule; melting point; and cost. Since these excipients can affect the drugs bioavailability, it is necessary to identify the characteristics of these excipients. Details of the lipids (oils, nonionic surfactants, cosolvents), their compositions and list of suppliers are given in **Table 1**.

3. Lipid nanocarriers and recent advancements in oral drug delivery

Lipid-based nanoformulations as drug delivery vehicles signify a promising strategy that incorporates or encapsulates the drug molecules and are biodegradable or biocompatible. They are containing nanosized droplets typically ranging from 0 to 250 nm [20]. The entrapped drug molecules can be taken intact and protected against degradation by gastrointestinal (GI) fluids, while drug absorption through the GI epithelium or lymphatic transport can be enhanced. Possible mechanisms of transport of these nanocarriers across GI mucosa are introduced later in the chapter. These focus on effects of size and surface properties of the nanocarriers on the nonspecific or targeted uptake by enterocytes and/or M cells. Applications of various oral nanocarrier formulations, such as lipid nanoparticles and SMEDDS/SNEDDS, are reviewed in several recent publications [4, 21, 22]. **Figure 1** shows an encapsulated SNEDDS designed for oral administration, which are the most efficient formulations for improving the apparent aqueous solubility of PWSDs.

Within the scope of the current chapter, the most advanced SNEDDS and/or SMEDDS systems have been explored as potential nanocarriers, which are much more stable kinetically and thermodynamically and showed great potential for improving the bioavailability of orally administered drugs. In a pure drug nanoparticle formulation, submicron size particles of drugs are stabilized in aqueous medium with generally regarded as safe (GRAS) listed excipients blend. Such formulation can be used for drugs with poor solubility in water and oil, high melting point, high log *P* and high dose.

When saquinavir (HIV protease inhibitor) in 1995 was marketed for the first time as mesylate salt formulation in a hard gelatin capsule (Invirase®), its bioavailability was only 4% and highly variable [23]. Later on, after 2 years, a self-nanoemulsifying formulation of saquinavir (Fortovase®) containing medium-chain mono- and diglycerides, povidone and α-tocopherol was able to increase bioavailability threefold higher than Invirase® in humans [23, 24]. Several other published [10, 25, 26] and unpublished case studies are also available that established the significance of rational approach in designing SMEDDS/SNEDDS which can improve the *in vivo* absorption of the PWSDs. The commercial product such as amprenavir (agenerase), ciprofloxacin (cipro), fenofibrate (fenogal), liponavir/ritonavir (kaletra, norvir), etc., have been formulated using suitable SMEDDS/SNEDDS [24, 27].

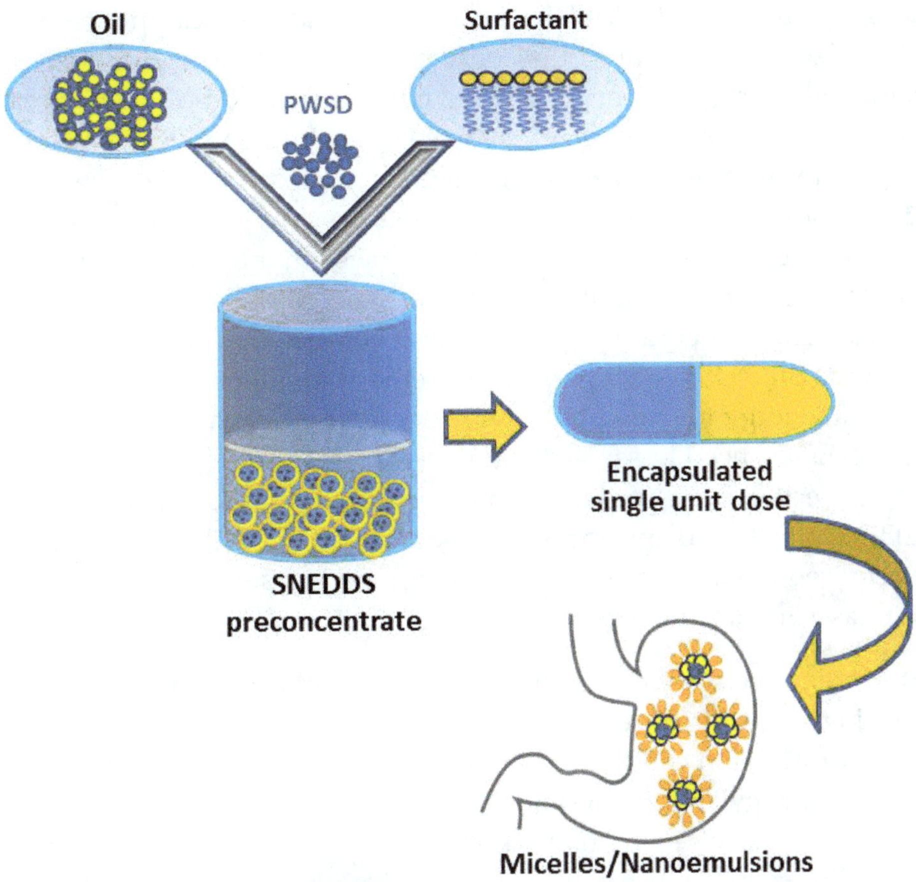

Figure 1. The encapsulated SNEDDS designed for oral administration of PWSDs. *Adapted with permission from Ref. [21].

4. Concept of nanoemulsions within lipid-based formulation

The potentiality of nanoemulsions within lipid-based drug delivery systems was explored almost four decades ago. In simple term, nanoemulsions are the emulsions comprising nanosized droplets and they are well dispersed, transparent and kinetically stable for several months. Their physical stability can be improved by careful selection of surfactants and the ratio of oil/water/surfactant and also the efficiency of equipment used to reduce droplet sizes.

Not only for oral delivery, nanoemulsions are used as greater transmucosal and transdermal drug delivery vehicles due to their remarkable wetting, spreading and penetration abilities.

4.1. SMEDDS vs SNEDDS

SMEDDS and SNEDDS are almost similar lipid dosage form which can be prepared from same materials comprising a simple mixture of oils, surfactants and possibly cosolvents. SMEDDS have the ability to form fine oil in water (O/W) microemulsion, and SNEDDS produce nanoemulsion upon mild agitation in the presence of an aqueous (preferably intestinal) media [28]. The structure provides both SMEDDS and SNEDDS as good candidates for oral delivery of PWSDs with adequate solubility in oil only or oil/surfactant blends and establishes the desired reproducible pharmacokinetic profile. Upon dilution, SMEDDS form transparent microemulsions, with a droplet size of <50 nm [11], while SNEDDS produce transparent dispersions of oil and water stabilized by surfactants, with droplet sizes between 20 and 250 nm and kinetically but not thermodynamically stable systems [29]. These two systems are the most famous colloidal dispersions within lipid-based systems but physicochemically different. Structures and properties of nanoemulsion can be changed on long-term storage but not for microemulsions at same temperature, pressure and composition. The formation of SMEDDS is spontaneous, and SNEDDS need high-energy methods for their fabrication, but both systems need some external energy to overcome kinetic energy barriers and support mass transport. In comparison, SNEDDS need lesser surfactant-to-oil ratio than SMEDDS. The preparation of SNEDDS involve specific mixing order in which surfactant must be mixed first with oil phase, whereas SMEDDS do not need any specific mixing order for their preparation. Ternary phase diagrams are required to have a suitable selection of both systems which should be coherent with different phases involved in preparation.

An important best-known example is Sandimmune Neoral® which was introduced in 1994 became the turning point for development of SMEDDS in oral lipid-based formulations of PWSD [30]. This formulation contains Cremophor RH40 (polyoxyl hydrogenated castor oil), corn oil glycerides, propylene glycol and ethanol, which emulsifies spontaneously into a microemulsion with a particle size smaller than 100 nm. This new formulation (Sandimmune Neoral®) resulted in a twofold increase in the bioavailability compared to the earlier product Sandimmune® [31]. Recent years, SMEDDS and SNEDDS have gained lots of interest as potential drug delivery vehicles largely due to their clarity, simplicity of preparation, thermodynamic stability and their abilities to be filtered and to incorporate a wide range of drugs of varying lipophilicity.

4.1.1. SMEDDS/SNEDDS within lipid formulation classification systems

By considering several factors in mind, Pouton [20, 32] introduced a lipid formulation classification system (LFCS) into four Types (I–IV) which differentiate lipid-based formulations from one to another that is being used as a framework to categorize nanoformulations. These four Types of formulations were classified on the basis of formulation compositions, their aqueous dispersibility and the potential effects of lipid digestion and possible drug precipitation from lipids. Among the LFCS, Type III systems are the most attractive formulations as they produce microemulsions/nanoemulsions (SMEDDS and SNEDDS) of lipid-surfactant mixtures with particle sizes in the range of 0–250 nm upon dispersion. The microemulsions can be used for many other drug delivery/application systems, such as topical, intra venous, trans-dermal, etc. There are several marketed products available which were developed as Type III formulations since the drugs may be absorbed from the microemulsions and or nanoemulsions without the digestion of lipids and/or surfactants present. Type III systems further divided into subtype IIIA and IIIB according to the hydrophilic content of the SMEDDS and SNEDDS. Type IV systems are efficient formulations as they also produce SMEDDS and/or SNEDDS and have high drug loading ability but may loss solvent capacity upon dilution with aqueous media.

4.2. Solidification of SMEDDS/SNEDDS

The excipients commonly used in designing SNEDDS are liquid at room temperature, and their compatibility with semi-solid and solid dosage forms allows encapsulating into soft/hard gelatin capsules for oral delivery. This could be a great challenge as the interaction between liquid formulation and capsule shell may result in either brittleness or softness of the shell [33]. In addition, the stability of liquid formulations could be another major issue (e.g., leaching and rancidity) since some drugs might suffer significant chemical instability in both aqueous and oily formulations. Apart from that, manufacturing liquid-filled soft gelatin capsules is a slow process and requires specialized equipment, having risk of formulation components migrating into capsule shell [23].

Therefore, to address this limitation, incorporation of liquid lipid formulations into a solid dosage form is convincing and desirable. Liquid lipid formulations could be transformed into acceptable free flowing fine powder by loading the formulation on a suitable solid carrier as solid SNEDDS [34, 35]. Only few studies have attempted to investigate the conversion of such formulations into free flowing powders by adsorption using various inorganic high surface area materials (i.e., neusilin, syloid, aeroperal and aerosol) that are amenable to encapsulation or tableting [36, 37]. On the other hand, the final powder preparation should have acceptable flow properties to achieve the best content uniformity and weight variation. The current interest in solidification technique by both the industry and academia is raised enormously due to the attractive properties including independence of gastric transit, flexibility in dose dividing, decrease in intra- and inter-subject variability, highest safety profile and physical/chemical stability improvement.

5. Equilibrium solubility of diluted nanoformulations

For lipid nanoformulations, drug solubility determines the maximum drug loading capacity (single unit dose) and is increased when the drug is highly lipid soluble or when the formulation contains high proportions of surfactant or cosolvent. The solubilization capacity of the nanoformulations (SNEDDS) is likely to decrease when excipients are dispersed and digested in the GI tract. As a result, the drug concentrations in the GI fluids are elevated from the equilibrium solubility and could cause extreme precipitation.

To predict the likely fate of the drug on dispersion effectively, one should investigate its solubility in the formulations during aqueous dilution. The solubility of PWSDs within the diluted nanoformulations can be determined using a shake-flask method to observe how the drug solubility is changed as water is incorporated into the system. The samples are prepared by adding an excess amount of drug to the formulation, which is then shaken and thoroughly mixed with a vortex mixer. The samples are incubated in a dry heat incubator at 37°C for 7 days and centrifuged to separate excess solid drug from the dissolved drug. An aliquot of the supernatant is weighed and diluted in an appropriate solvent. The dissolved drug concentration can be analyzed by UV-vis spectrophotometer.

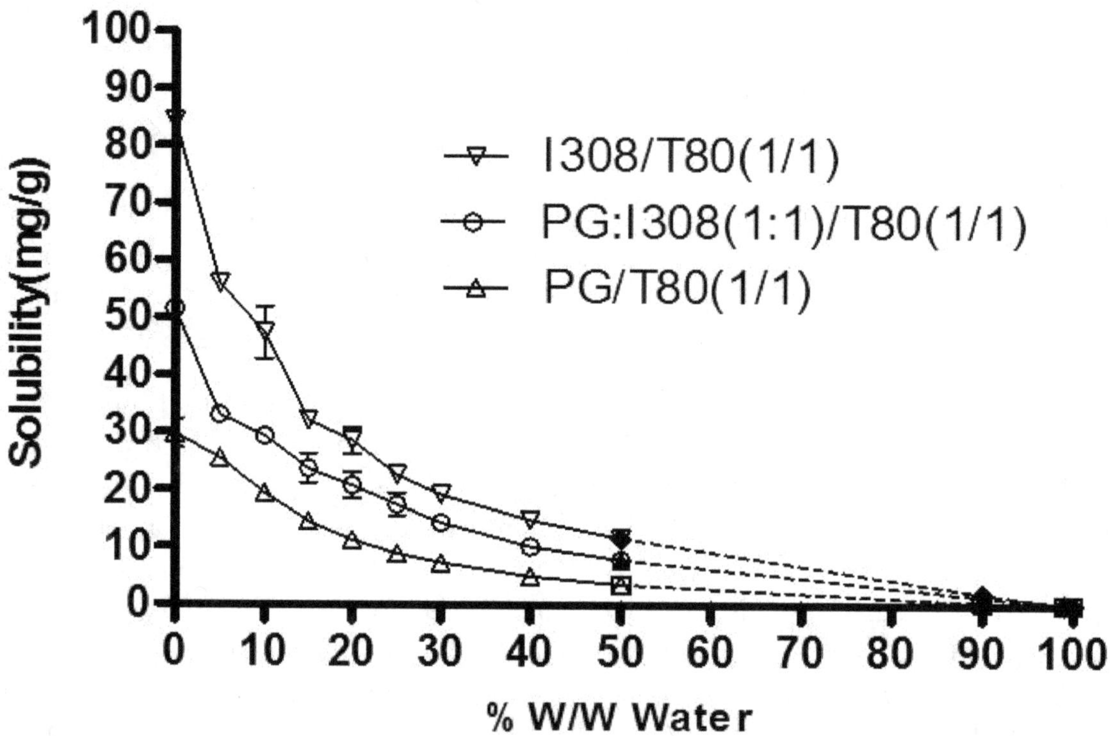

Figure 2. Effect of aqueous dilution on solubility of fenofibrate in nanoformulations representing LFCS Types IIIB and IV systems. Data are presented as mean ± SD (n = 3).

Figure 2 shows the fenofibrate solubility in nanoformulations (SMEDDS/SNEDDS) of LFCS Type IIIB and IV systems which was studied over 10–100 dilution with water. The results suggest how fenofibrate solubility decreased markedly, with several Type IIIB and IV nanoformulations, as the formulation was diluted with water [12]. After adding only 10% w/w water to the anhydrous formulation (drug dissolved at 80% of its equilibrium solubility), the one-third drug solubility had dropped down from the initial solubility of the formulation. The data predict that if fenofibrate was dissolved at its equilibrium solubility in the anhydrous formulations, its solubility would be exceeded in all cases when the formulation is diluted 1 in 10 or 1 in 100.

6. Drug release and the justification of dispersion test for nanoformulations

In vitro release studies assess the ability of lipid-based nanoformulations to disperse into various types of media and to evaluate whether the drug partitions from the vehicle into the aqueous medium. It can estimate how much drug will be in solution before absorption thus predicts the fate of the drug *in vivo*. A range of biorelevant dissolution test media and experimental methodologies has been developed by Dressman's group that have established application in drug release studies from lipid-based oral formulations [38, 39].

Technically, it is difficult to characterize drug release from emulsions *in vitro*, particularly under sink condition. Since solubility of the drug in sink phase may be poor, large volumes of aqueous content may be needed to maintain the sink conditions. It is hard to separate the oil droplets due to their smaller size from the dissolved or released drug in the sink solution levy. In a previous study, our group has conducted an *in vitro* dissolution of anti-histaminic drug, cinnarizine (CN, week base) from various SNEDDS systems and commercial product Stugeron® tablet [4]. Dissolution was carried out in simulated gastric fluid (SGF, pH 1.2) for first 2 h and subsequently shifted into simulated intestinal fluid (SIF, pH 6.8) for another 2 h.

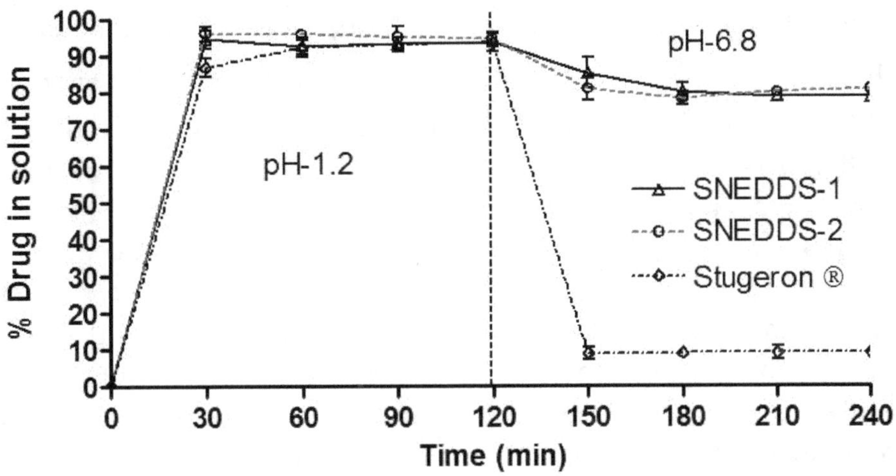

Figure 3. Dissolution profiles of cinnarizine SNEDDS 1 [MCT/MCDM/T85 (25/25/50)], SNEDDS 2 [MCT/MCM/T85 (25/25/50)] and Stugeron® tablets. Data are expressed as mean ± S.E, n = 3. **Abbreviations: MCT—medium-chain triglycerides (M810); MCDM—mixture of medium-chain di- and monoglycerides (I988); MCM—medium-chain monoglycerides (I308); T85—Tween 85.

In SGF, all the SNEDDS showed superior dissolution profiles with respect to Stugeron® tablet (**Figure 3**). At 15 min, Stugeron® tablet managed to release only 66.5% drug in solution where the optimal formulations were able to release 84–95% drug in solution. This indicates the ability of these formulations to provide more efficient and rapid release of CN with respect to the marketed tablet. Upon shifting from SGF to SIF, Stugeron® showed significant precipitation (87–92% precipitated), while the SNEDDS were able to hold high amount of CN (78–93%) in solution (**Figure 3**). This finding suggests the immense need for developing a SNEDDS that could enhance the drug dissolution profile and resist the sharp pH-dependent changes particularly for week bases.

A standard USP dissolution apparatus is suitable for the establishment of a dispersion test, but emphasis should be on precipitation rather than dissolution [4]. This is why, dynamic dispersion test is highly considered for the prediction of whether precipitation is likely to occur prior to digestion. In the dispersion study, samples are removed from the dispersion vessel at various intervals for at least 24 h and analyzed to determine the likelihood of precipitation during GI transit. Dispersion testing is vital for LFCS Types III and IV formulations (produce SNEDDS), which may loss solvent capacity on dispersion due to migration of water soluble components into the bulk aqueous phase. Care is needed in the design of lipid-based nanoformulations to ensure that the precipitation of the drug is minimized.

7. Mechanism of drug supersaturation: role of SMEDDS/SNEDDS

When the lipid nanoformulations approach to the high volume of gastric fluid, it is dispersed rapidly and reduces solubilization capacity of the drug due to the high content of surfactant/water soluble cosolvent, thus potentially generates supersaturation. Even though supersaturation in the stomach is not desirable as most of the drugs are absorbed in the small intestine, it poses threat for drug precipitation before the drug enters to small intestine. Therefore, SMEDDS/SNEDDS should be designed to minimize supersaturation in the stomach or at least to maintain a period sufficient to allow gastric emptying prior to drug precipitation.

Correlations between the investigations of the equilibrium solubility of the drug in the aqueous diluted formulation (10–99% diluted) and corresponding dynamic dispersion tests could help to predict whether precipitation is likely to take place, and whether it would affect bioavailability [12]. The imbalance between high initial solubilized drug concentrations and lower equilibrium drug solubilities during lipid dispersion and digestion *in vivo* does not immediately result in precipitation but stimulates drug supersaturation. This supersaturation is more likely to occur in the formulations that contain high proportions of water soluble surfactants or cosolvent. In some cases, during the process of lipid (or surfactant) digestion where hydrolysis occurs to form more polar post digestion products also stimulates changes to colloidal structure, thus lead to changes in drug solubility and may facilitate drug precipitation.

This is why, SNEDDS must contain drugs less than equilibrium solubility (approximately 50–90% of the equilibrium solubility) to avoid any precipitation. In recent studies, precipitation inhibitors have been introduced in supersaturated SNEDDS to overcome the risk of precipitations [40]. Supersaturated SNEDDS inhibit and minimize the nucleation process and subsequent drug precipitation in GIT by achieving and then sustaining the metastable supersaturated state. The commonly used water soluble precipitation inhibitors are PVP, HPMC, NaCMC and MC polymers [41].

7.1. The risk of drug precipitation from nanoformulations

Triglycerides alone (LFCS Type I) are poor solvents for most of the hydrophobic drugs but suitable for highly lipophilic compounds. If lipid-based formulations contain mixed glycerides, polar oils, surfactants and/or cosolvents (LFCS Type II and III), it is likely to improve the solvent capacity of the formulation. Therefore, formulators are always preferred to add water soluble surfactants and cosolvents against pure oils, ultimately sometimes resulting in the complete exclusion of oily excipients to produce oil-free formulations (LFCS Type IV). However, the formulator must keep well balance between oils and surfactants/cosolvents in the formulation to avoid risk of drug precipitation on aqueous dispersion. Several studies showed that small changes in formulation compositions are not expected to cause large changes in drug solubility, but there could be a dramatic drop in solvent capacity upon aqueous dilution [4, 12, 42]. Dilution of a cosolvent implies a substantial loss of solvent capacity, while the loss of solvent capacity may not be suffered with the use of surfactant. This could be possible due to the linearity between solubilized drug to the number of micelles present and therefore to the surfactant concentration. Drugs which are more soluble in surfactant or cosolvent than pure oil are at high precipitation risk because solvent capacity of surfactant and cosolvent decreases upon dilution but not pure oil. Hence, increasing the solubility of a drug by including a cosolvent is generally a poor strategy than using a nonionic surfactant [11, 43]. **Figure 4** shows the extreme precipitation of an anticancer drug, paclitaxel using LFCS Types III and IV formulations.

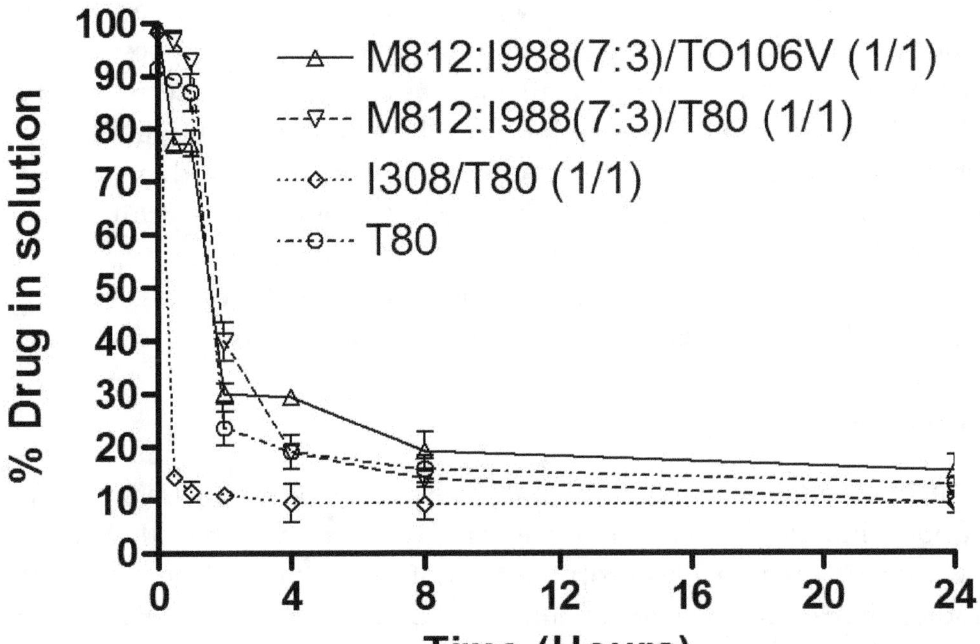

Figure 4. Percentage of the original dose of paclitaxel remaining in solution after 1:100 dilutions in the dispersion medium (paclitaxel was originally dissolved at 80% of the equilibrium solubility in the anhydrous mixture). One gram formulation was dispersed in 100 ml water, and then, the samples were withdrawn periodically over 24 h to examine the drug precipitations. Data are presented as mean ± SD (n = 3).

It is quite difficult to predict the fate of the PWSDs on dispersion of a typical LFCS Type IIIA lipid formulation. The hydrophilic surfactant used in Type IIIA systems is substantially separated from the oily components, forming a micellar solution in the continuous phase.

Hence, one might question: does this system lower the overall solvent capacity for the drug or not? However, this may depend on the log *P* of the drug, and to what extent the surfactant was contributing to its solubilization within the formulation. At present, there are no established techniques available to help formulators assessing the risk of precipitation. It is worth mentioning that in some cases, Type III formulations can take several days to reach equilibrium and the drug remains in a supersaturated state for up to 24 h time [12]. It could be argued that such formulations are not likely to cause precipitation in the gut before the drug is absorbed, and possibly the supersaturation acts as an absorption enhancer by increasing the thermodynamic stability of the drug [44].

8. Lipid digestion and drug absorption: mechanism

8.1. Lipid metabolism

Following ingestion of a lipid-based dosage form (capsule/tablet), the formulation is initially dispersed in the stomach where the digestion of exogenous dietary lipid is started by the action of gastric lipase on the lipid-water interface. Gastric lipase releases about 15% of free fatty acids from lipids [45]. Within the small intestine, pancreatic lipase together with its co-lipase completes the breakdown of dietary glycerides to diglyceride, monoglyceride and fatty acid. The presence of exogenous lipids in the small intestine also stimulates secretion of endogenous biliary lipids including bile salt, phospholipid and cholesterol from the gallbladder [45]. In the presence of elevated bile salts concentrations, lipid digestion products are subsequently incorporated into a series of colloidal structures including multilamellar/unilamellar vesicles, bile salt phospholipid mixed micelles and micelles [46]. Together these species significantly expand the solubilization capacity of the small intestine for both lipid digestion products and drugs, and this can be studied relatively easily as a preformulation exercise.

8.2. Drug absorption

Sufficient aqueous solubility along with good intestinal permeability is crucial for adequate drug absorption, ultimately leading to sufficient bioavailability. On the other hand, PWSDs are associated with poor and variable absorption and often affected by the various food intakes. Several studies have already documented lipid-based nanoformulations, particularly SNEDDS, as an absorption enhancer for PWSDs when administered orally [4, 47]. Possible mechanisms for improving drug absorption include: (i) an increase in the membrane fluidity facilitating transcellular absorption, (ii) larger surface area provided by the fine emulsion droplets, hydrolysis and formation of mixed micelles, (iii) paracellular transport by opening tight junction mainly for ionized drugs or hydrophilic macromolecules, (iv) inhibition of P-gp and/or CYP450 to increase intracellular concentration and residence time, and (v) stimulation of lipoprotein/chylomicron production. The natural process of digestion offers the possibility that very lipophilic drugs could be taken up into the lymphatic system by partitioning into chylomicrons in the mesentery. This is expected to be a mechanism of absorption for drugs with log *P* values >6.0 and has been demonstrated to be crucial in a past study for the absorption of the antimalarial compound halofantrine [48, 49].

The mixed micelles substantially transport digestion products across the unstirred water layer and reach the vicinity of the aqueous-microvillus interface to allow for lipid absorption through the mucosal cells. However, it is possible that digestion of a lipid formulation could reduce the solubility of the drug in the gut lumen, which would result in the precipitation of the drug and a decrease in the absorption rate. Therefore, more investigation on *in vitro* lipolysis is needed to clearly understand drug precipitation during digestion for better absorption.

9. *In vitro* digestion (lipolysis): significance

The fate of the lipid carrier in the GI tract is essentially important for the absorption of the incorporated drug and therefore has to be closely analyzed. It is evident that the solvent capacity of the formulation can be lost on digestion, leading to drug precipitation [26, 50]. However, the investigation of the lipolysis by *in vivo* experiments is complex, costly and time-consuming. Thus, the *in vitro* model simulating the enzymatic degradation of lipid-based formulations is highly significant as an alternative method of monitoring the digestion process in the simulated gastrointestinal media under fed and fasted conditions.

Lipolysis can be carried out as an *in vitro* test using a pH-stat titration unit to maintain pH and using the lipase/co-lipase content of porcine pancreatin to serve as model for human pancreatic juice. Bile salt lecithin-mixed micelles are used in the reaction mixture to provide a sink for solubilization of degradation products. Composition of mixture that used in the *in vitro* lipolysis studies is provided in **Table 2**.

Substance of the mixture for 10 ml aqueous media		
Lipid 250 mg		
Pancreatic lipase 1 ml (800 TBU/ml)		
Lipolysis buffer 9 ml		
Composition of the lipolysis buffer	**Concentration (fed state)**	**Concentration (fasted state)**
Bile salt (BS, mM)	20	5
Phospholipid (PL, mM)	5	1.25
Trizma maleate (mM)	0.5	0.5
Ca^+ (mM)	0.05	0.05
Na^+ (mM)	1.5	1.5

Table 2. Composition of mixture for *in vitro* lipolysis experiments. *Adapted with permission from Ref. [51].

Lipolysis is allowed to proceed for a fixed time (30–60 min), the reaction is then subjected to high-speed ultracentrifugation, and further drug analysis in the various phases allows predicting whether the drug will remain solubilized in the intestinal lumen after digestion of the formulation. However, if the drug is partially precipitated, then drug will be found in the pellet, which may be still in solution. The rate and extent of lipolysis can be quantified by the data generated from the pH-stat. This technique was recently applied in LFCS Types I–IV formulations to predict the effect of formulation on the fate of a number of drug compounds and assumed that surfactants are subjected to digestion, probably for SMEDDS and SNEDDS, where water soluble surfactants are used predominantly. Lipolysis experiments may play a vital role in the near future for establishing strong methods for *in vitro in vivo* correlations (*IVIVCs*).

10. *In vitro in vivo* correlation (*IVIVC*) for lipid nanoformulations

The *IVIVCs* play a major role in drug development, particularly on the optimization of suitable formulations which is time-consuming and a highly expensive process. Formulation optimization requires modifications in composition, equipment, manufacturing process and batch sizes. If such changes applied to the formulation, the *in vivo* bioequivalence studies in human are necessary to be conducted to confirm the similarity of the new formulation. This process will increase the load of carrying out a number of bioequivalence studies and therefore will increase the cost of process optimization and marketing of the new formulation.

To overcome these issues, it is necessary to develop *in vitro* tests that can imitate the bioavailability data. The *IVIVC* can be used in the development of new pharmaceuticals to decrease the number of human trials during the formulation development and to support biowaivers.

In the beginning of 1980s, the *IVIVC* theory was established based on many published research studies, which can be used as a prediction tool for correlating *in vitro* and *in vivo* data. The *IVIVC* is usually used in the development stages of pharmaceuticals to enhance the formulation and dosage optimization with fewer trials in human [51–56] or additional bioavailability studies. The FDA defines *IVIVC* as "a predictive mathematical model describing the relationship between an *in vitro* property of a dosage form (usually the rate or extent of drug dissolution or release) and a relevant *in vivo* response (e.g., plasma drug concentration or amount of drug absorbed)." For drugs that are administered orally, dissolution and intestinal permeation are considered as the rate-limiting steps for the absorption. Therefore, if an excellent correlation exists between *in vitro* dissolution test and a bioavailability parameter, then controlling the dissolution profile will permit the evaluation of bioavailability [57–59].

There are several tools which can be used to establish *IVIVC*. The *in vitro* drug release studies of the formulations can be performed using dissolution, dynamic dispersion and digestion tests, whereas the *in vivo* pharmacokinetic studies can be performed on various animal models. However, there are only a limited number of *IVIVC* studies so far have been conducted using lipid formulations. To obtain more robust *in vitro* and *in vivo* relationship, a large number of model compounds should be explored along with more human clinical data sets and complete characterizations of *in vitro* and *in vivo* solubilization of PWSDs formulated in lipid vehicles.

11. Conclusion

For many drugs with poor aqueous solubility, the technique of developing SMEDDS/SNEDDS provides a powerful and effective solution to improve their solubility in the aqueous contents of the GI tract that is the main obstacle for such drugs. The most critical step in designing the nanoformulations of lipid-based systems for PWSDs is the selection of the most suitable oil, surfactant and/or cosolvent for a particular drug with certain physicochemical properties. So, the formulators must keep a balance and make compatibility between the factors of different formulations such as self-emulsification efficiency, drug loading capacity, droplet size distribution, *in vitro* dispersion/release profile in acidic and basic media and *in vitro* digestion by using fed and fasted state. In summary, SMEDDS/SNEDDS provide a robust formulation approach to enhance GI solubilization and to promote drug absorption after oral administration. If there is a successful *IVIVC* made for lipid nanoformulations, confidence in the development of the pharmaceutical product and its quality are likely to improve, and the drug development time may be shortened.

Author details

Mohsin Kazi

Address all correspondence to: mkazi@ksu.edu.sa

Department of Pharmaceutics, College of Pharmacy, King Saud University, Riyadh, Kingdom of Saudi Arabia

References

[1] Lei, Y., et al., Solid self-nanoemulsifying cyclosporin A pellets prepared by fluid-bed coating: preparation, characterization and *in vitro* redispersibility. Int. J. Nanomed., 2011. 6: p. 795–805.

[2] Kommuru, T.R., et al., Self-emulsifying drug delivery systems (SEDDS) of coenzyme Q10: formulation development and bioavailability assessment. Int. J. Pharm., 2001. 212(2): p. 233–246.

[3] Mohsin, K., A.A. Shahba, and F.K. Alanazi, Lipid based self emulsifying formulations for poorly water soluble drugs-an excellent opportunity. Indian J. Pharm. Educ. Res., 2012. 46(2): p. 88–96.

[4] Shahba, A.A., K. Mohsin, and F.K. Alanazi, Novel self-nanoemulsifying drug delivery systems (SNEDDS) for oral delivery of cinnarizine: design, optimization, and *in-vitro* assessment. AAPS PharmSciTech, 2012. 13(3): p. 967–977.

[5] Mueller, E.A., et al., Improved dose linearity of cyclosporine pharmacokinetics from a microemulsion formulation. Pharm. Res., 1994. 11(2): p. 301–304.

[6] Date, A.A., et al., Self-nanoemulsifying drug delivery systems: formulation insights, applications and advances. Nanomedicine (Lond), 2010. 5(10): p. 1595–1616.

[7] Date, A.A. and M.S. Nagarsenker, Design and evaluation of self-nanoemulsifying drug delivery systems (SNEDDS) for cefpodoxime proxetil. Int. J. Pharm., 2007. 329(1–2): p. 166–172.

[8] Charman, S.A., et al., Self-emulsifying drug delivery systems: formulation and biopharmaceutic evaluation of an investigational lipophilic compound. Pharm. Res., 1992. 9(1): p. 87–93.

[9] Charman, W.N., et al., Effect of food and a monoglyceride emulsion formulation on danazol bioavailability. J. Clin. Pharmacol., 1993. 33(4): p. 381–386.

[10] Gursoy, R.N. and S. Benita, Self-emulsifying drug delivery systems (SEDDS) for improved oral delivery of lipophilic drugs. Biomed. Pharmacother., 2004. 58(3): p. 173–182.

[11] Pouton, C.W., Formulation of poorly water-soluble drugs for oral administration: physicochemical and physiological issues and the lipid formulation classification system. Eur. J. Pharm. Sci., 2006. 29(3–4): p. 278–287.

[12] Mohsin, K., M.A. Long, and C.W. Pouton, Design of lipid-based formulations for oral administration of poorly water-soluble drugs: precipitation of drug after dispersion of formulations in aqueous solution. J. Pharm. Sci., 2009. 98(10): p. 3582–3595.

[13] Duro, R., et al., Interfacial adsorption of polymers and surfactants: implications for the properties of disperse systems of pharmaceutical interest. Drug Dev. Ind. Pharm., 1999. 25(7): p. 817–829.

[14] Floyd, A.G., Top ten considerations in the development of parenteral emulsions. Pharm. Sci. Technol. Today, 1999. 4(2): p. 134–143.

[15] Pouton, C.W., Effects of the inclusion of a model drug on the performance of self emulsifying formulations. J. Pharm. Pharmacol., 1984. 36: p. 51.

[16] Pouton, C.W., Self emulsifying drug delivery systems: assessment of the efficiency of emulsification. Int. J. Pharm., 1985. 27: p. 335–348.

[17] Tarr, B.D. and S.H. Yalkowsky, Enhanced intestinal absorption of cyclosporine in rats through the reduction of emulsion droplet size. Pharm. Res., 1989. 6(1): p. 40–43.

[18] Humberstone, A.J. and W.N. Charman, Lipid based vehicles for the oral delivery of poorly water soluble drugs. Adv. Drug Deliv. Rev., 1997. 25(1): p. 103–128.

[19] Jannin, V., J. Musakhanian, and D. Marchaud, Approaches for the development of solid and semi-solid lipid-based formulations. Adv. Drug Deliv. Rev., 2008. 60(6): p. 734–746.

[20] Pouton, C. and C. Porter, Formulation of lipid-based delivery systems for oral administration: materials, methods and strategies. Adv. Drug Deliv. Rev., 2008. 60(6): p. 625–637.

[21] Mohsin, K., et al., Development of self-nanoemulsifying drug delivery systems for the enhancement of solubility and oral bioavailability of fenofibrate, a poorly water-soluble drug. Int. J. Nanomed., 2016. 11: p. 2829–2838.

[22] Cerpnjak, K., et al., Lipid-based systems as a promising approach for enhancing the bioavailability of poorly water-soluble drugs. Acta Pharm., 2013. 63(4): p. 427–445.

[23] Perry, C.M. and S. Noble, Saquinavir soft-gel capsule formulation. A review of its use in patients with HIV infection. Drugs, 1998. 55(3): p. 461–486.

[24] Hoffmann-La-Roche, *Fortovase (saquinavir) Soft Gelatin Capsules. Product Information.* (CAS registry number: 127779-20-8), 2003; http://www.medicines.org.au/files/ropforto.pdf

[25] Martin-Facklam, M., et al., Dose-dependent increase of saquinavir bioavailability by the pharmaceutic aid cremophor EL. Br. J. Clin. Pharmacol., 2002. 53(6): p. 576–581.

[26] Porter, C.J. and W.N. Charman, *In vitro* assessment of oral lipid based formulations. Adv. Drug Deliv. Rev., 2001. 50(Suppl 1): p. S127–S147.

[27] Talegaonkar, S., et al., Microemulsions: a novel approach to enhanced drug delivery. Recent Pat. Drug Deliv. Formul., 2008. 2(3): p. 238–257.

[28] Singh, B., et al., Self-emulsifying drug delivery systems (SEDDS): formulation development, characterization, and applications. Crit. Rev. Ther. Drug Carrier Syst., 2009. 26(5): p. 427–521.

[29] Cherniakov, I., A.J. Domb, and A. Hoffman, Self-nano-emulsifying drug delivery systems: an update of the biopharmaceutical aspects. Expert Opin. Drug Deliv., 2015. 12(7): p. 1121–1133.

[30] Klyashchitsky, B.A. and A.J. Owen, Drug delivery systems for cyclosporine: achievements and complications. J. Drug Target, 1998. 5(6): p. 443–458.

[31] Mueller, E.A., et al., Influence of a fat-rich meal on the pharmacokinetics of a new oral formulation of cyclosporine in a crossover comparison with the market formulation. Pharm. Res., 1994. 11(1): p. 151–155.

[32] Pouton, C.W., Lipid formulations for oral administration of drugs: non-emulsifying, self-emulsifying and 'self-microemulsifying' drug delivery systems. Eur. J. Pharm. Sci., 2000. 11(Suppl 2): p. S93–S98.

[33] Nazzal, S. and M. Khan, Controlled release of a self-emulsifying formulation from a tablet dosage form: stability assessment and optimization of some processing parameters. Int. J. Pharm., 2006. 315(1–2): p. 110–121.

[34] Tang, B., G. Cheng, J-C. Gu, and C-H. Xu, Development of solid self-emulsifying drug delivery systems: preparation techniques and dosage forms. Drug Discov. Today, 2008. 13: p. 606–612.

[35] Katteboina, S., P. Chandrasekhar, and S. Balaji, Approaches for the development of solid self-emulsifying drug delivery systems and dosage forms. Asian J. Pharm. Sci., 2009. 4: p. 240–253.

[36] Agarwal, V., A. Siddiqui, H. Ali, and S. Nazzal, Dissolution and powder flow characterization of solid self-emulsified drug delivery system (SEDDS). Int. J. Pharm., 2009. 366: p. 44–52.

[37] Shazly, G. and K. Mohsin, Dissolution improvement of solid self-emulsifying drug delivery systems of fenofibrate using an inorganic high surface adsorption material. Acta Pharm., 2015. 65(1): p. 29–42.

[38] Dressman, J.B. and Klein, S., eds. Development of dissolution tests on the basis of gastrointestinal physiology. Pharmaceutical Dissolution Testing, eds. Dressman, J., and Krämer, J., 2005, Taylor and Francis: NY, USA. pp. 193–227.

[39] Dressman, J.B., Alsenz, J., Schamp, K., and Beltz, K., eds. Characterizing release from lipid-based formulations. Oral Lipid-based Formulations: Enhancing the Bioavailability of Poorly Water-soluble Drugs, eds. Hauss, DJ., 2007, Informa Healthcare, Inc.: NY, USA. pp. 242–245.

[40] Thomas, N., K. Richter, T.B. Pedersen, R. Holm, A. Müllertz, and T. Rades, *In vitro* lipolysis data does not adequately predict the *in vivo* performance of lipid-based drug delivery systems containing fenofibrate. AAPS J., 2014. 16(3): p. 539–549.

[41] Gao, P., et al., Enhanced oral bioavailability of a poorly water soluble drug PNU-91325 by supersaturatable formulations. Drug Dev. Ind. Pharm., 2004. 30(2): p. 221–229.

[42] Mohsin, K. and F. Alanazi, The fate of paclitaxel during *in vitro* dispersion testing of different lipid-based formulations. J. Drug Deliv. Sci. Technol., 2012. 22(2): p. 197–204.

[43] Devraj, R., et al., *In vitro* assessment of drug-free and fenofibrate-containing lipid formulations using dispersion and digestion testing gives detailed insights into the likely fate of formulations in the intestine. Eur. J. Pharm. Sci., 2013. 49(4): p. 748–760.

[44] Gao, P., B.D. Rush, W.P. Pfund, T. Huang, J.M. Bauer, W. Morozowich, M.S. Kuo, and M.J. Hageman, Development of a supersaturable SEDDS (S-SEDDS) formulation of paclitaxel with improved oral bioavailability. J. Pharm. Sci., 2003. 92: p. 2386–2398.

[45] Porter, C.J., N.L. Trevaskis, and W.N. Charman, Lipids and lipid-based formulations: optimizing the oral delivery of lipophilic drugs. Nat. Rev. Drug Discov., 2007. 6(3): p. 231–248.

[46] Kossena, G.A., et al., Influence of the intermediate digestion phases of common formulation lipids on the absorption of a poorly water-soluble drug. J. Pharm. Sci., 2005. 94(3): p. 481–492.

[47] Stegemann, S., et al., Self-emulsifying drug delivery systems facing the bioavailability challenge in drug delivery. Pharm. Ind., 2009. 71(8): p. 1409–1416.

[48] Humberstone, A.J., C.J. Porter, and W.N. Charman, A physicochemical basis for the effect of food on the absolute oral bioavailability of halofantrine. J. Pharm. Sci., 1996. 85(5): p. 525–529.

[49] Boyd, M., et al., A stepwise surgical procedure to investigate the lymphatic transport of lipid-based oral drug formulations: cannulation of the mesenteric and thoracic lymph ducts within the rat. J. Pharmacol. Toxicol Methods, 2004. 49(2): p. 115–120.

[50] Pouton, C.W. and C.J. Porter, Formulation of lipid-based delivery systems for oral administration: materials, methods and strategies. Adv. Drug Deliv. Rev., 2008. 60(6): p. 625–637.

[51] Uppoor, V.R., Regulatory perspectives on *in vitro* (dissolution)/*in vivo* (bioavailability) correlations. J. Control. Release, 2001. 72(1–3): p. 127–132.

[52] Ghosh, P., M. Milewski, and K. Paudel, *In vitro/in vivo* correlations in transdermal product development. Ther. Deliv., 2015. 6(9): p. 1117–1124.

[53] Anand, O., et al., Dissolution testing for generic drugs: an FDA perspective. AAPS J., 2011. 13(3): p. 328–335.

[54] FDA, Guidance for Industry: Dissolution Testing of Immediate Release Solid Oral Dosage Forms, Food and Drug Administration, Rockville, 1997.

[55] Committee, I.C.o.H.S. Pharmaceutical Development Q8; Draft Consensus Guideline, Released for Consultation at Step 2 of the ICH Process; International Conference on Harmonisation of Technical Requirements for Registration of Pharmaceuticals for Human Use in International Conference on Harmonisation. 2004.

[56] European Agency for the Evaluation of Medicinal Products, H.M.E.U., Committee for Proprietary Medicinal Products, CPMP/QWP/155/96, *Note for Guidance on Development Pharmaceutics*, H.M.E.U. European Agency for the Evaluation of Medicinal Products, Committee for Proprietary Medicinal Products, CPMP/QWP/155/96, Editor 1998: London, UK.

[57] Hwang, S.S., W. Bayne, and F. Theeuwes, *In vivo* evaluation of controlled-release products. J. Pharm. Sci., 1993. 82(11): p. 1145–1150.

[58] Abd-Elbary, A., M.I. Tadros, and A.A. Alaa-Eldin, Development and *in vitro/in vivo* evaluation of etodolac controlled porosity osmotic pump tablets. AAPS PharmSciTech, 2011. 12(2): p. 485–495.

[59] Benet, L.Z., Pharmacokinetics of sustained-release etodolac. Rheumatol. Int., 1993. 13(Suppl 2): p. S3–S5.

4

Drug Delivery Systems in Bone Regeneration and Implant Dentistry

Sukumaran Anil, Asala F. Al-Sulaimani,
Ansar E. Beeran, Elna P. Chalisserry,
Harikrishna P.R. Varma and Mohammad D. Al Amri

1. Introduction

Bone regeneration is a complex, well-orchestrated physiological process involving a number of cell types and intracellular and extracellular molecular signaling pathways [1]. Bone grafts provide a structural framework for clot development, maturation and remodeling that supports bone formation in osseous defects. These materials must possess biocompatibility and osteoconductivity, as well as the properties that support osteogenesis. The ideal characteristics of a bone graft are that it must be nontoxic, non-antigenic, resistant to infection, easily adaptable, readily and sufficiently available to stimulate new attachment and able to trigger osteogenesis [2].

Osseous defects in the oral cavity have been successfully managed with a variety of biological and synthetic materials, including autografts, allografts, xenografts and alloplastic materials. Although autografts are unequivocally accepted as the gold standard, donor site morbidity and limitations on the quantity of bone that can be harvested demand that clinicians seek alternatives [3]. In light of the immunological and disease transfer risks from allogeneic bone, research has focused extensively on developing alloplastic bone substitutes that are predominantly based on ceramics, such as calcium phosphates (CaP), calcium sulfates, and bioactive glasses [4]. In general, these ceramic materials are renowned for their osteoconductive and bioactive properties [5]. The most commonly used ceramics are the CaP-based ceramics hydroxyapatite (HA) and beta tricalcium phosphate [6].

Considering engineered grafts, the most important factor is to prepare a three-dimensional structure consisting of biodegradable material, generally called a scaffold [7]. The nature and structure of the scaffold should support cell proliferation and differentiation, accelerating the process of tissue regeneration. Furthermore, the growth factor providing a scaffold to an injury site should enhance progenitors, causing inflammatory cells to migrate and activate the healing process [8, 9]. However, among the basic challenges for scaffold implantation is to control infection due to bacterial load, which can create immune problems and finally result in implant rejection. To overcome implant-related infection and bacterial load on the scaffold, antibiotic drug incorporation and its controlled release have been suggested as a promising strategy [10]. Bone is among the few tissues of the human body that has high endogenous healing capacity. Various concepts for local drug delivery to bone have been developed in recent decades to overcome such healing deficits.

Several methods are used for drug loading and release from scaffolds. However, the basic aim for drug release is to reduce infections and bacterial load to the site of implant, but if the drug is released too quickly, there could be a chance of infection because the entire drug has drained from the scaffold in the initial time itself. Similarly, if there is too much delay to drug release, infection can set in further, making it more difficult to manage the healing of wounds. Hence, better options for drug release would incorporate higher antibiotic release at the initial time and sustained release at an effective rate to inhibit the risk of infection from bacteria in the scaffold at an effective level [11]. Different techniques have been used for drug loading to the scaffold, and controlled release has been studied. One of the simplest strategies is the application of biodegradable polymer coatings loaded with specific drugs onto the scaffold structure. The other methods reported for coating the drug-loaded polymer have included solvent casting, thermally induced phase separation, evaporation, freeze drying and foam coating. Among these methods, an interesting approach for drug loading and release consists of combining drug-loaded microspheres with a macroporous scaffold `matrix' [12-15].

In a recent study, a biodegradable nanoporous bioceramic system was used as a highly bioresorbable matrix for drug delivery. This study emphasized the efficacy of hydroxyapatite-based material having interconnected nanoporosity as a vehicle for a therapeutic agent. An in vitro experiment was conducted with the goal of assessing this material and comparing it with commercially available gentamicin-loaded PMMA cement. It was found that the nanoporous bioceramic granules could act as antibiotic carriers, exhibiting a high initial burst effect followed by sustained low-level release for 3 weeks. It was very effective, confirming that the concentration of drug eluted was greater than that needed to maintain bactericidal levels [16].

In addition to the above-mentioned technique, magnetic nanoparticle-incorporated materials have also been used as a bone regeneration scaffold, and they are schematically represented in figure 3 [17]. To obtain homogenous dispersion of magnetic particle loading and surfactant, a porous structure generated by ceramic crystals, the in-situ method was followed. Further, it was made to a specific shape, and the specific drug was loaded via dip loading or other methods. The drug-loaded scaffold was placed at the defective site in the presence of a magnetic field (MF), which facilitated easy drug release from the scaffold, helping to protect it from bacterial colonization, and the MF stimulated the scaffold for cell proliferation. Recently released in vitro results support MF-induced bone regeneration [18-20].

Engineered biomaterials combined with growth factors, such as bone morphogenetic protein-2 (BMP-2), have been demonstrated to constitute an effective approach in bone tissue engineering because they can act both as a scaffold and as a drug delivery system to promote bone repair and regeneration. Despite the substantial progress made in developing porous materials as bone substitutes, the realization of synthetic structure able to harness fully bone's capability of regenerating and remodeling itself and to mimic the complicated physiochemical attributes of bone continues to present challenges.

In the following sections of this chapter, the materials and drug delivery techniques used to enhance bone regeneration and to control infection are discussed. The methods to enhance the surface of titanium implants to promote osseointegration are also detailed.

2. Bone regeneration materials

2.1. Calcium phosphate ceramics

The calcium phosphates have been widely studied due to their biocompatibility, tailorable bioabsorbability and bioactivity. Calcium phosphates have been used as novel delivery carriers for antibiotics, anti-inflammatory agents, analgesics, anticancer drugs, growth factors, proteins and genes [21, 22]. Furthermore, they can be synthesized using simple methods, and these drugs can easily be incorporated via different routes, such as wet chemical processes, solid state reactions, hydrothermal and micelle-mediated processes, etc. [23, 24]. Most of the polymeric systems show an acidic nature, and their degradation by-products can alter drug activity. The major advantages of CaPs, compared with other biodegradable polymeric systems, is that the degradation ions are Ca^{2+} and PO_4^{3-} ions, which already exist in the body in higher concentrations [25].

Nanotechnology-derived calcium phosphates have also successfully maintained a sustained and steady drug release over time. Calcium phosphate scaffolds not only provide initial structural integrity for bone cells but also direct their proliferation and differentiation and assist in the ultimate assembly of new tissue. Therefore, ceramic nanoscaffolds are usually 3-D and porous, although in some cases they consist of 2-D coatings or films. They mimic the in vivo environment of cells more completely than nanoparticles.

Therefore, most drug-eluted ceramic nanoscaffolds serve multiple functions, such as drug delivery, directing cell growth or tissue generation, and mechanical support. Indeed, the mechanical support provided by ceramic scaffolds far exceeds that provided by polymeric scaffolds. Studies have shown that drug-release kinetics could be further controlled by tailoring calcium phosphate nanoparticle grain size, surface area and calcium-to-phosphorus ratios [26]. Hollow silica nanospheres have been fabricated into well-controlled shapes and sizes using self-templating molecules [20]. For example, studies have shown that hollow silica nanospheres were capable of entrapping an eight-fold greater quantity of drug species than solid silica nanospheres. Time-delayed multiple-stage release profiles were also possible with these hollow silica nanospheres [27].

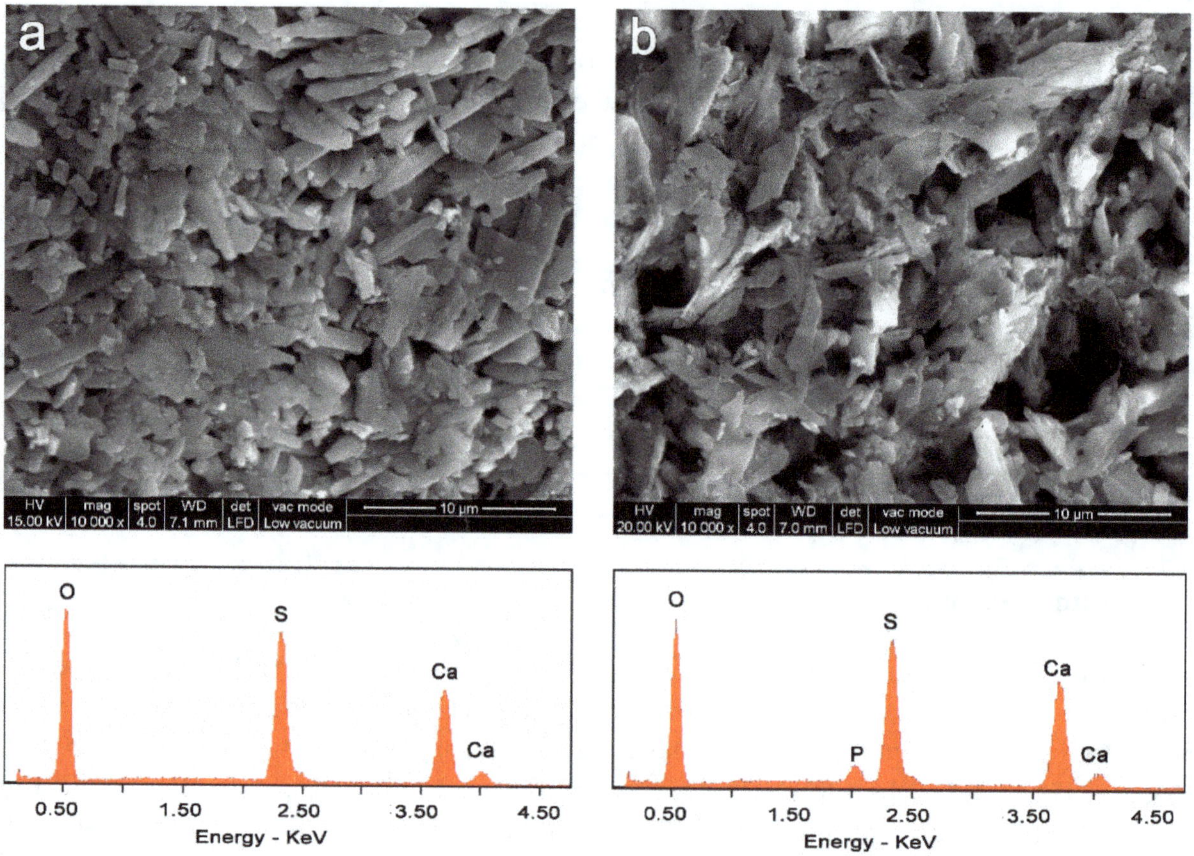

Figure 1. The micromorphology (SEM) of calcium sulfate-phosphate injectable cement. **a)** The set cement surface of unmodified low-dimensional medical grade calcium sulfate (crystal sizes less than 5 microns). **b)** The phosphate-containing material, which inhabits very small crystal formations grown into folding sheets. Energy dispersive (EDS) data, corresponding to the samples, are shown below each. The phosphorous content in the second sample is evident, whereas no separate phosphate phase appeared in XRD. The phosphate content resides as a substitution in the calcium sulfate crystals.

2.2. Porous spherical hydroxyapatite granules for drug delivery

Calcium phosphate-based bioceramics, such as hydroxyapatite (HA), are known for their excellent biocompatibility due to their similarity in composition to the apatite found in natural bone [28]. Various forms of HA bone grafts, such as dense and porous blocks, dense and porous granules, and powder forms, are available as bone substitutes [29]. The porous matrices enable cell migration and provide favorable conditions for nutrient transport, tissue infiltration, and vascularization [30, 31]. The spherically shaped particles are suitable for implantation as injectable bone cements, and the inter-granular space promotes cell migration and the growth of extracellular matrix [32, 33].

Porous HA is produced using methods such as ceramic slip foaming [34], positive replication of reticulated foam scaffolds [35], burnout of sacrificial porogens, such as polymer beads [3], and techniques that exploit naturally occurring porous calcium-based structures, such as the hydrothermal conversion of either coral or bone [36, 37]. Porous spherical HA granules can be used for drug delivery systems. The various pore and channel structures of spherical granules were obtained by adjusting the ratio of water to HA powder and the amount of sodium chloride (NaCl). Earlier studies focused on the use of anti-inflammatory or anti-bacterial drug release from HA, to control inflammation and infection at the site of implantation [38]. Currently, several drugs have been found to enhance bone formation, and the loading of HA with these drugs and agents could be a very effective method for enhancing bone formation at the site of implantation [39, 40]. Research is under way to control the drug release rate using the complex micro-channel structures of HA granules [41].

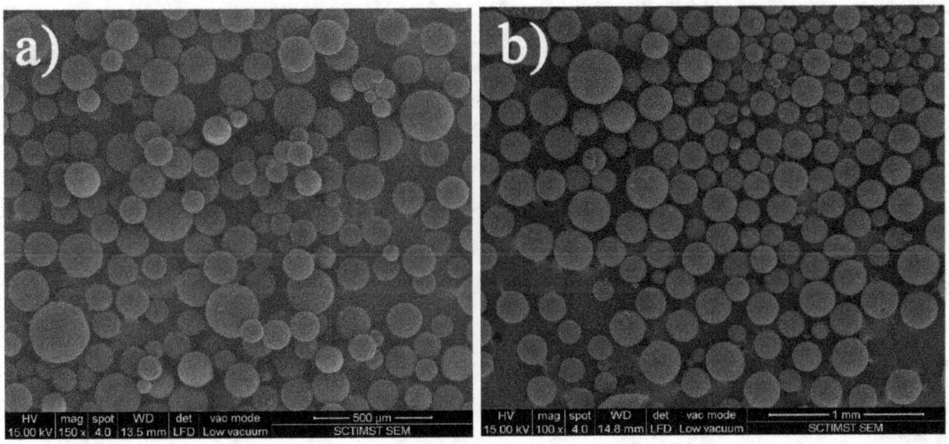

Figure 2. Scanning electron microscopic images of: a) polycaprolactone polymer microspheres; and b) magnetic hydroxyapatite-loaded polycaproctone polymer microspheres.

2.3. Demineralized bone matrix

Bone void fillers, such as demineralized bone matrix (DBM), offer a broad range of materials, structures and delivery systems to use in bone grafting procedures. Allogenic DBM possesses osteoinductive properties and could serve as an ideal drug delivery device for prophylactic treatment in a variety of different anatomical locations [42, 43]. The use of DBM would allow for the release of the entire quantity of antibiotic as the material is being remodeled.

2.4. Carriers and delivery systems for growth factors

Growth factors (GFs), such as bone morphogenetic protein, transforming growth factor-beta, fibroblast growth factor, platelet-derived growth factor, and insulin-like growth factor, are proteins secreted by cells that act on the appropriate target cell or cells to perform specific actions. A variety of so-called bone-graft substitutes, including demineralized bone matrix, calcium phosphate-containing preparations and Bioglass (BG), are also potential carriers for recombinant proteins [44]. Bioglass and calcium phosphate-based materials, such as hydroxyapatite, coralline hydroxyapatite, and tricalcium phosphate, have been shown to be biocompatible and to provide osteoconductive scaffolds that could potentially be combined with GFs to enhance bone repair [45].

Demineralized bone matrix preparations are particularly attractive as potential carriers for growth factors because they are osteoconductive and can have some osteoinductive potential as well. The disadvantages of these materials include poor handling characteristics and concerns about their overall bio-resorbability, as well as limited potential for remodeling and an unclear understanding of their effects on bone strength [46]. Recombinant bone morphogenetic protein (BMP) has been used to enhance the bone regeneration in graft and implant osseointegration in dentistry [47]. Recombinant human BMP-2 (rhBMP-2) has been shown to be effective in bone regeneration [48].

Among surface modification techniques, coating the implant surface with bone stimulating agents, such as GFs, is very promising. The most commonly used GFs include bone morphogenetic proteins (BMP-2), TGF-β1, platelet-derived growth factor, insulin-like growth factor and combinations [47, 49]. The actual mechanisms of GF combinations are not fully understood. From early reported studies, after implantation, both GFs (TGF-β and BMP) could directly increase the local pool of osteoprogenitor cells by stimulating their migration [50]. The circulation of pathways acts as a source of osteoprogenitor cells throughout ectopic BMP-induced bone regeneration. Similarly, the presence of both TGF-β1 and BMP-7 cooperatively interact to increase angiogenesis and vascular invasion after their co-administration increased vessel constitution [51]. The results demonstrated that the presence of GF associated with implant surfaces improved bone regeneration, vascular invasion and angiogenesis. Research is under way to optimize the carrier properties and the characteristics of the GF and its dose to maximize the regeneration potential.

2.5. Nanoscaffolds

The application of nanotechnology for drug delivery and the use of nanometer scale materials has helped to develop innovative approaches in this field. At this scale, materials display different physicochemical properties due to their small size, surface structure and high surface area. The nanoparticles based ceramic scaffolds have also demonstrated great potential for controlled drug delivery and is currently a fast growing research area. The ceramic nanoscaffolds have several advantages such as high porosity, high volume-to-area ratios, high surface area, high structural stability and long degradation times. These properties make them potent systems for controlled release of drugs. At the implantation sites drugs/chemical agents are applied for decreasing infection, reducing inflammation, and increasing bone growth on titanium surfaces. The nanotubular titania and calcium phosphate-based nanoscaffolds have showed good potential for drug and growth factor delivery.

2.6. Magnetic nanoparticles (FE-hydroxyapatite)

Superparamagnetic nanoparticles (MNPs) have been progressively explored for their potential in biomedical applications and in particular as contrast agents for diagnostic imaging, for magnetic drug delivery and, more recently, for tissue engineering applications [52-54]. MNPs have been used for biomedical applications, such as in hyperthermia [55], as a contrast agent for diagnostic imaging [56], for magnetic drug delivery [57, 58] [13], and for cell mechanosensitive receptor manipulation to induce cell differentiation [59].

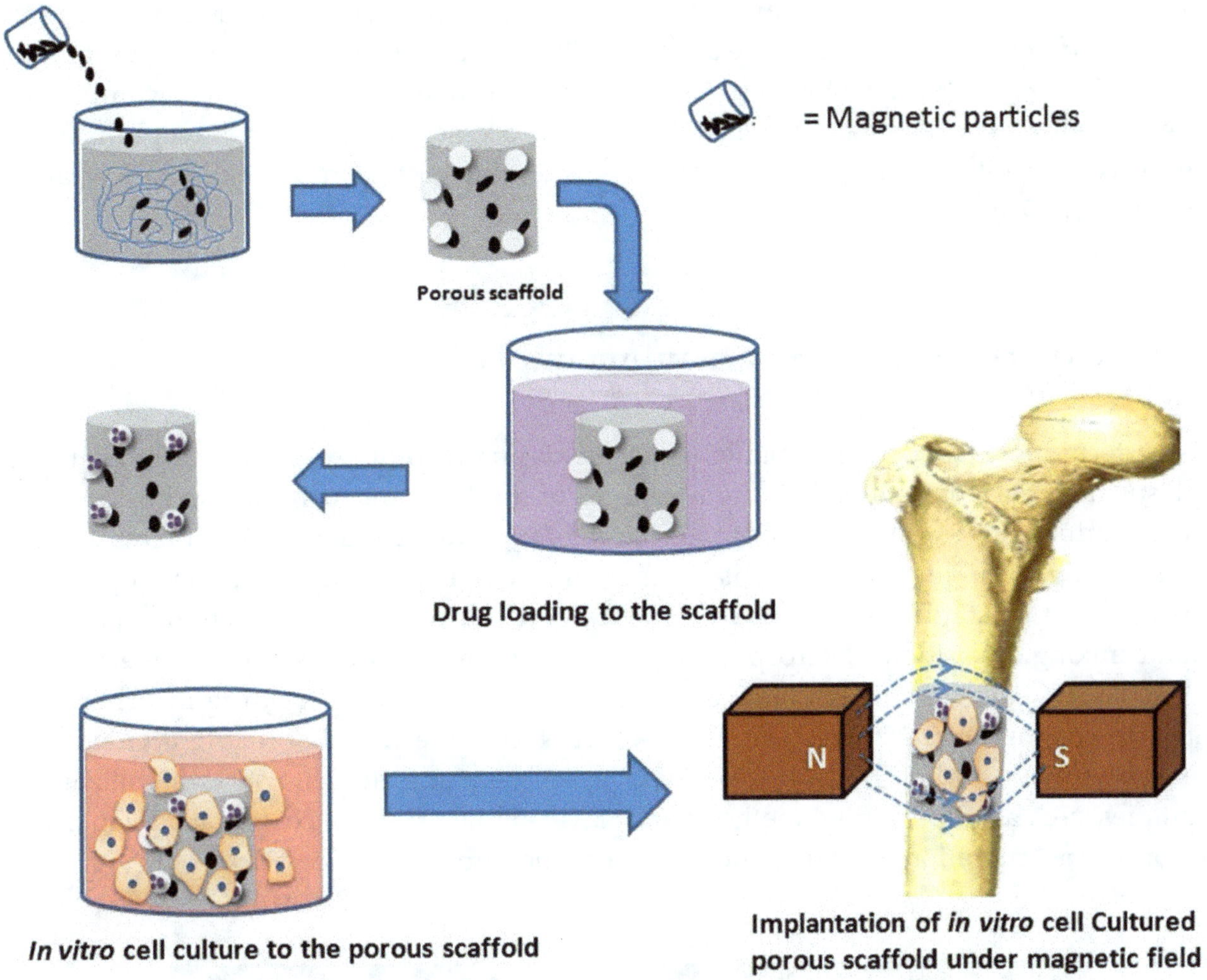

Figure 3. Schematic presentation of engineered magnetic scaffold preparation and implantation.

The most popular MNPs used in medicine and biotechnology are iron oxide-based phases, but their potential as a tissue engineering scaffold has not yet been fully assessed [60]. Although Fe is a vital element in the human body, its concentration within hard tissue is low, and its presence into the body scarcely affects bone remodeling [61]. In contrast, the biocompatibility and bioactivity of HA are already well established [62-64], and, in fact, more than 60% of the currently available bone graft substitutes involve calcium phosphate-based materials [65]. Hence, a Fe-HA phase endowed with superparamagnetic ability could be used as an active scaffold for bone and osteochondral regeneration or as a nontoxic, biodegradable, magnetic nanocarrier [17, 66, 67].

2.7. Chitosan hydroxy apatite

Chitosan is considered an appropriate functional material for biomedical applications because of its high biocompatibility, biodegradability, non-antigenicity and adsorption properties [68, 69]. The mechanical and biological properties of chitosan scaffolds could be improved by the incorporation of bioceramics, such as HA, β-tricalcium phosphate and calcium phosphate biomaterials, such as gelatin alginate, or inorganic material, such as wollastonite [70, 71]. Chitosan scaffolds are osteoconductive and can enhance bone formation both in vitro and in vivo [72]. Currently, the development of chitosan-nanohydroxyapatite (nHA) composites through in situ hybridization by ionic diffusion processes, freezing and lyophilization, stepwise co-precipitation, and mineralization via double diffusion are being undertaken successfully [73-75].

3. Surface functionalization of titanium implants

The long-term success of dental implants also depends on the complex **biointegration** of these alloplastic materials, determined by the responses of the different surrounding host tissues. The osteoinductivity of calcium phosphate coatings has attracted significant interest, using various coating techniques, including plasma spraying, magnetron sputtering, electrophoretic deposition, hot isostatic pressing, sol-gel deposition, pulsed laser deposition, ion beam dynamic mixing deposition, electrospray deposition, biomimetic deposition, and electrolytic deposition [76]. Non-ceramic implant coating is also used, allowing for drug incorporation during the coating process. The currently available techniques can be broadly divided into three categories, including hydrogel coatings, layer-by-layer coatings, and immobilization. Techniques such as 'dip-coating' methods and 'layer-by-layer' (LbL) coating techniques are used for the incorporation of BMP-2 and TGF-β1 to the implant surface [77].

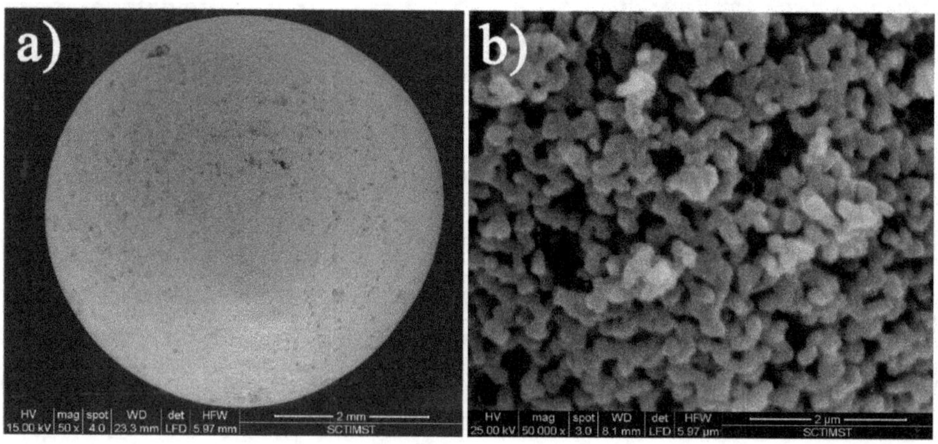

Figure 4. a) Scanning electron microscopic pictures of HAP microspheres; b) high-resolution SEM picture showing interconnected nanopores.

3.1. Nanotubular titanium surface

Nanotubular titania structures can be readily fabricated via direct anodization of titanium implants into an electrochemical cell that uses the titanium as an anode and platinum as a cathode in the presence of fluorine-based electrolytes [78, 79]. Penicillin-based antibiotics could be loaded to the nanotubular titania as a drug delivery platform by co-precipitating the drug and calcium phosphate crystals onto the nanostructures [80, 81].

Anodic oxidation has many advantages for surface modification, such as its ability to fabricate porous TiO_2 films through dielectric breakdown, the changeability of the crystalline structure and the chemical composition of the oxide film depending on the fabrication conditions, and it has been suggested to provide storage room for the delivery of GFs, such as rhBMP-2, to enhance osseointegration [82, 83]. In vitro studies have suggested that a dose response could be produced with appropriate period of delivery of the GF to the cells [84].

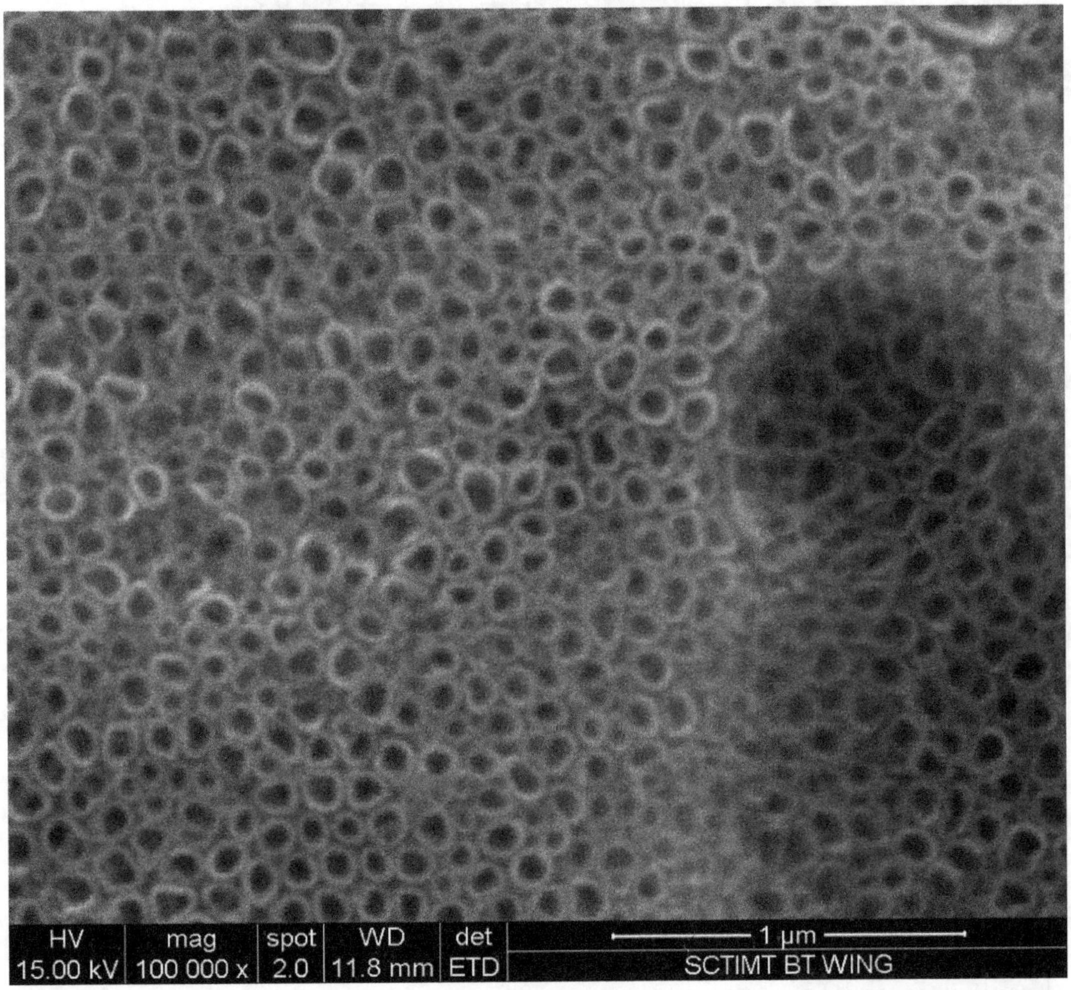

Figure 5. Scanning electron microscopic image of an anodized titanium implant surface showing uniform nano-tubules of titanium oxide throughout the surface.

3.2. Hydroxyapatite

Coating of titanium implant surfaces with HA has shown better integration with bone. HA can be coated to the surface by plasma spraying, sputtering, pulse laser deposition and electrostatic multilayer assemblies, fabricated using the layer-by-layer technique [85]. HA coatings enhance new bone formation on implant surfaces with a line-to-line fit, in areas with

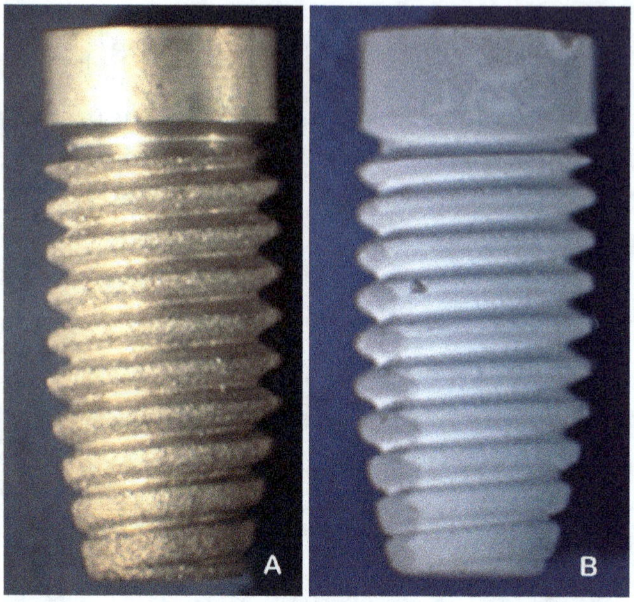

Figure 6. a) An anodized titanium implant; b) An anodized titanium implant coated with hydroxyapatite.

gaps of 1-2 mm between the coated implant and the surrounding bone. The coating also helps to prevent the formation of fibrous tissue that would normally result due to the micro-movements of an uncoated titanium implant [86].

HA coatings have been used as a method for the delivery of GFs, bioactive molecules, and DNA [85, 87, 88]. HA coatings augmented with bone morphogenetic protein-7 (BMP-7), placed on segmental femoral diaphyseal replacement prostheses, improved bone ingrowth in a canine extra-cortical bone-bridging model. Titanium alloy plasma-sprayed porous HA coatings, infiltrated with collagen, recombinant human bone morphogenetic protein (rhBMP-2) and RGD peptide, improved mesenchymal stem cell (MSC) adhesion, proliferation and differentiation in vitro and increased bone formation in ectopic muscle and intra-osseous locations in vivo [85].

Another group used hydroxyapatite nanoparticles complexed with chitosan into nanoscale non-degradable electrostatic multilayers, which were capped with a degradable poly(b-amino ester)-based film incorporating physiological amounts of rhBMP-2 [89]. Plasmid DNA, bound to calcium phosphate coatings deposited on poly-lactide-co-glycolide (PLG), was shown to be released in vitro according to the properties of the mineral and solution environment [87]. These methods of delivery of bioactive molecules extended the function of HA as a coating to enhance new bone formation around implants.

3.3. Antibiotics: Surface tethering of antibiotics

The initial adhesion and colonization of bacteria to an implant surface are considered to play key roles in the pathogenesis of infections related to biomaterials [90]. Two recent strategies are: (1) coating implants with antibiotics; and (2) covalently attaching antimicrobial molecules onto the implant surface. The objective of these bioactive surfaces is to disrupt the colonization

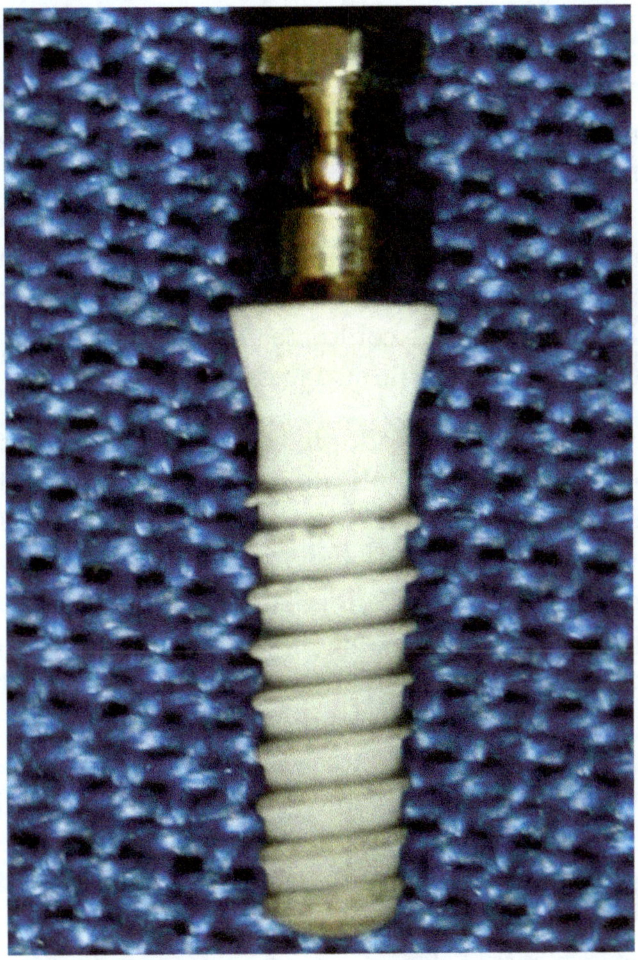

Figure 7. Hydroxyapatite-coated titanium implant.

of the microbes or to prevent bacterial adhesion to the implant and subsequent development of biofilm [91]. Hydrophilic surfaces have been shown to be less prone to become infected with microorganisms than hydrophobic surfaces [92]. The topical application of antibiotics on the implant surface might be more efficient because bacteria are killed locally directly upon binding, before the formation of biofilm. Local delivery of antibiotics has long been applied in bone cements used to repair orthopedic and dental implants [93].

Antibiotics such as gentamicin are incorporated into the cement, which slowly releases the drugs after setting *in situ*. Local delivery can prevent adhesion and growth of significant numbers of bacteria. HA coatings are frequently applied to dental implants to stimulate osseointegration and to accelerate bone formation. Antibiotics can be co-precipitated on titanium surfaces to obtain drug-releasing surface coatings. Studies have shown that antibiotics with optimal calcium-chelating properties had long lasting antimicrobial properties [94, 95]. Alt et al [96] demonstrated that both gentamicin-hydroxyapatite and gentamicin-RGD (arginine-glycineaspartate)-HA coatings could release antibiotics for up to twenty-four hours without inhibiting new bone formation. Erythromycin-impregnated strontium-doped calcium polyphosphate (SCPP) was found to inhibit bacterial growth completely for up to 14 days [97]

Nanoporous implants are suitable for the incorporation of antibiotics to obtain controlled release of drugs [98]. Nanostructured surfaces play a major role in advanced biomedical implant design because these surfaces have been studied for their enhanced bioactive properties, as well as their antagonistic behavior toward bacterial colonization. To maintain sustained drug elution properties and better bone bonding ability, significant efforts have been undertaken to develop bioactive hollow nanostructures on implant surfaces [99]. In this context, one of the implant titania nanotubular surfaces created via anodization showed enhanced bioactivity, conjugated with the capacity to store diverse compounds and control their elution. The anodization technique could create porous structures with controlled sizes of three-dimensional networks on metallic surfaces [100].

Anodization followed by HA coating was adopted as a surface modification technique to make drug-loadable Ti implants for dental applications. Self-organized titania nano-tubes were grown on titanium substrate as drug-carrying vehicles by coating HA ceramic using laser deposition. Nanostructured surfaces were achieved on titanium via anodization in a glycerol-NH_4F electrolyte system, followed by annealing. The nano-tubules were then capped with HA deposited with pulsed laser ablation. HA-coated polished titanium, nano-structured titanium and hydroxyapatite coated nano-structured titanium were analyzed for their drug-carrying capacity using gentamicin sulfate. The ceramic-coated anodized substrates were found to be most efficient among the aforementioned three compounds in controlled delivery for longer than 160 h, with drug content of 0.5 $\mu g/cm^2$, compared to the anodized substrate, which delivered the whole drug within 140 h. It was thus evident that laser deposition facilitated the controlled release of drug, compared to the anodized and bare substrates. This study proposed the application of laser deposition of bioceramics, such as HA, over nano-structured titanium for drug-eluting metallic implants [101].

3.4. Tan-Ag coatings

Due to the risk of the development of antibiotic resistance associated with antibiotic-loaded coatings, non-antibiotic agents in the coating have been used as alternatives. Among the various dopants, silver nanoparticles are among the most popular agents used due to their inhibition of bacterial adhesion, broad anti-bacterial spectrum, long lasting anti-bacterial effects, and propensity for being less prone to the development of resistance. Ag and Cu are known to be efficient antibacterial agents because of their specific antimicrobial activity and the nontoxicity of active Ag and Cu ions to human cells [102, 103]. Sputter coating of Ag, along with HA, resulted in an antibacterial-bioactive coating, which inhibited bacterial attachment without cytotoxic effects [104]. TaN-Ag nano-composite coating of titanium dental implants also showed significant antibacterial properties without any cytotoxic effects. Hence, it could be concluded that coating of titanium implants with materials having antimicrobial properties might be useful in preventing infection [105].

3.5. Bisphosphonate

Bisphosphonates (BPs) constitute a group of drugs that inhibit osteoclast action and the resorption of bone, and they are used to treat metabolic diseases such as osteoporosis, Paget's disease, hypercalcemia of malignancy and multiple myeloma [106]. The nitrogen-containing BPs are more potent, and they accumulate in maximum concentrations in the matrix and osteoclasts [107]. BPs have a high affinity for bone minerals and bind strongly to HA, resulting in selective uptake to the target organ and high local concentrations in bone, particularly at sites of active bone remodeling. The BPs have similar chemical structures to pyrophosphate, but their chemical stability is greater. In pyrophosphates, the phosphate group is bonded through phosphoanhydride bond (P-O-P), whereas in BP, P is bonded through a germinal carbon atom (P-C-P); hence, these bonds are resistant to hydrolysis under acidic conditions [108]. The affinity of BP to Ca^{2+} ions helps to target specific bony sites, and BP can be coupled with a gamma-emitting radioisotope, such as technetium, for simultaneous bone scanning [109]. BPs inhibit osteoclast differentiation, reduce their activity, and induce their apoptosis [110]. The nitrogen-containing BPs bind to and inhibit farnesyl pyrophosphate synthase (FPPS), a key enzyme of the mevalonate pathway, thereby preventing the prenylation and activation of small GTPases, which are essential for the bone-resorption activity and survival of osteoclasts [111].

Systemic and local delivery of BPs improved the osseointegration of dental implants in osteoporotic animal models [112-116]. Improved osseointegration and the mechanical stability of titanium implants were reported in ovariectomized rats supplemented with alendronate [112]. Kurth et al [113] showed enhanced integration of HA-coated titanium implants via the administration of ibandronate to osteoporotic rats. Similar observations of enhanced osseointegration have been reported in other studies via the local release of BPs (pamidronate and zoledronic acid) from the surface coatings of implants [115, 116]. An experimental study in an ovariectomized rabbit model showed that systemic zoledronic acid (ZA) administration improved the osseointegration of titanium implants [117].

3.6. Simvastatin

Statins are prescribed to decrease cholesterol biosynthesis by the liver, thereby reducing serum cholesterol concentrations and lowering the risk of heart attack. A liposoluble statin, simvastatin, could induce the expression of bone morphogenetic protein (BMP) 2 mRNA and, as a result, promote bone formation on the calvaria of mice following daily subcutaneous injections [118, 119]. Another study showed that the topical application of statins to alveolar bone increased bone formation and concurrently suppressed osteoclast activity at the bone healing sites [120]. Yang et al [119] demonstrated that simvastatin-loaded porous titanium surface potently increased ALP activity and the extracellular accumulation of proteins, such as osteocalcin and type I collagen, in mouse preosteoblast MC3T3-E1 cells. Du et al [121] demonstrated that administration of simvastatin resulted in significant improvement in the osseointegration of titanium implants in osteoporotic rats. This finding could be attributed to the increased expression of bone morphogenic protein 2, which stimulates osteoblast differentiation [118]. Statins are known to enhance the expression of VEGF (vascular endothelial growth factor), a bone anabolic factor, in osteoblasts and to regulate osteoblast function by increasing the expression of bone sialoprotein (BSP), osteocalcin (OCN), and type I collagen (COL-I), as well as suppressing the gene expression of collagenases, such as matrix metalloproteinase (MMP)-1 and MMP-13 [122, 123]. Thus the competitive inhibition of simvastatin interferes with the malevonate pathway, leading to decreased protein prenylation, which is necessary for normal osteoclast function [118].

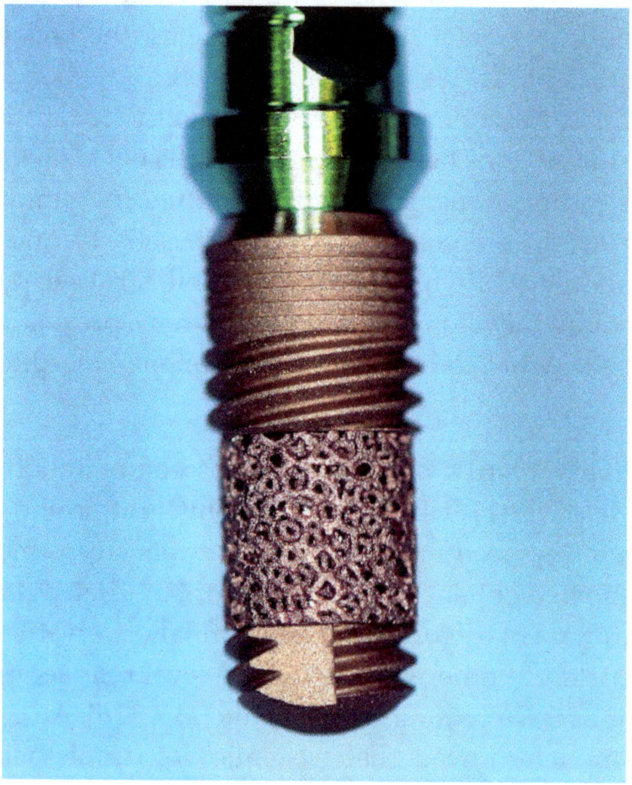

Figure 8. A trabecular implant that could be used to load drugs.

3.7. Calcitonin

Calcitonin (CT), produced by the C-cells of thyroid tissue, has been reported to stimulate hard tissue formation [124]. It acts on bone tissue via the suppression of osteolysis and the induction of Ca^{2+} release. It was reported that CT inhibited osteoclastic bone resorption by binding to specific cell surface receptors [125]. This hormone favors bone formation, inhibits osteoclastic activity and prevents osteopenia [126-128]. In vitro and in vivo studies have shown that this hormone stimulates the growth of bone tissue [40, 129, 130]. Calcitonin also showed increases in the amount and rate of bone formation, as observed in rat calvaria and extraction sockets in dogs [131].

3.8. Pantaprazole

A class of substituted benzimidazoles known as proton pump inhibitors (PPIs) have been shown to promote bone regeneration and peri-implant healing. Examples of these drugs include omeprazole and pantoprazole, which are employed clinically in the treatment of gastroesophageal reflux disorder (GERD). PPI-loaded calcium phosphate cements demonstrated not only inherent biocompatibility and osteoconductivity but also the ability to retard bone resorption through a drug delivery mechanism [132, 133]. Pantoprazole-loaded calcium phosphate cements inhibited osteoclastic resorption without interfering with the peri-implant bone resorption rate in a study performed rat femoral condyles [134]. Another advantage of the addition of omeprazole is that it inhibits osteoclastic acidification, which help to inhibit bone resorption and increases the lifespan of osteoclasts [135]. The drugs were dissolved in dimethyl sulfoxide to the desired concentration and were added to the liquid phase of the calcium phosphate.

4. Conclusions

Drug delivery systems (DDS) targeting specific organs and tissues and their bioavailability at specific sites have become critical issue in modern medicine. Local drug delivery systems in bone could be used to promote regeneration, prevent infection, or treat post-surgical pain. The quest for new bone scaffold materials to overcome the shortcomings of existing materials, such as ceramics and polymers, is undertaken to overcome the limited mechanical properties required for temporary bone substitutes. Mixing of polymers, natural or synthetic, and inorganic components, such as HA, TCP and BG, might help to develop better composite scaffolds that combine the advantages of both biodegradable polymers and bioactive ceramics [136].

If DDS are used in combination with implants, the coating strategies should allow for the choice of a drug or combination of drugs and their doses, localization and release due to intra-operative considerations. HA coatings on titanium implants themselves provide an osteoconductive and an osteoinductive approach for the enhancement of bone formation. These biological properties could be augmented further by adding growth factors and other molecules to produce a truly osteoinductive platform.

Proteins or glycosaminoglycans, such as collagen and chondroitin sulfate, provide a biomimetic coating on the surface of an implant, which can improve osseointegration [137]. Biomolecules such as GFs are also widely used for implant coatings, to modulate cellular functions, such as decreasing inflammation, enhancing stem cell differentiation, inducing blood vessel formation, or acting as chemoattractants for circulating osteoprogenitors [138, 139]. Although the implant materials available for the reconstruction of craniofacial bone defects have shown favorable results in most craniofacial and dental applications, the presence of complications related to infection and poor osseointegration still represent challenges in the biomedical field.

The current trend in the field of bone repair indicates that the tissue engineering field is moving toward the development of biomaterials with improved surfaces that will stimulate bone formation and avoid infections through the incorporation of surface modification techniques and antibacterial coatings and agents, as well as the incorporation of GFs, stem cells and other pharmacological drugs.

Author details

Sukumaran Anil[1*], Asala F. Al-Sulaimani[2], Ansar E. Beeran[3], Elna P. Chalisserry[4], Harikrishna P.R. Varma[3] and Mohammad D. Al Amri[5]

*Address all correspondence to: drsanil@gmail.com

1 Department of Periodontics and Community Dentistry, College of Dentistry, King Saud University, Riyadh, Saudi Arabia

2 King Saud University, Riyadh, Saudi Arabia

3 Biomedical Technology Wing, Sree Chitra Tirunal Institute for Medical Sciences & Technology, Poojappura, India

4 College of Dentistry, King Saud University, Riyadh, Saudi Arabia

5 Department of Prosthetic Dental Sciences, College of Dentistry, King Saud University, Riyadh, Saudi Arabia

References

[1] Kempene DH, Creemers LB, Alblas J, Lu L, Verbout AJ, Yaszemski MJ, Dhert WJ. Growth factor interactions in bone regeneration. Tissue engineering Part B, Reviews 2010; 16(6):551-566.

[2] Romagnoli C, D'Asta F, Brandi ML. Drug delivery using composite scaffolds in the context of bone tissue engineering. Clinical Cases in Mineral and Bone Metabolism 2013; 10(3):155.

[3] Moy PK, Lundgren S, Holmes RE. Maxillary sinus augmentation: histomorphometric analysis of graft materials for maxillary sinus floor augmentation. Journal of oral and maxillofacial surgery : official journal of the American Association of Oral and Maxillofacial Surgeons 1993; 51(8):857-862.

[4] Zamet JS, Darbar UR, Griffiths GS, Bulman JS, Bragger U, Burgin W, Newman HN. Particulate bioglass as a grafting material in the treatment of periodontal intrabony defects. Journal of clinical periodontology 1997; 24(6):410-418.

[5] Ignatius AA, Ohnmacht M, Claes LE, Kreidler J, Palm F. A composite polymer/tricalcium phosphate membrane for guided bone regeneration in maxillofacial surgery. Journal of biomedical materials research 2001; 58(5):564-569.

[6] Knabe C, Driessens FC, Planell JA, Gildenhaar R, Berger G, Reif D, Fitzner R, Radlanski RJ, Gross U. Evaluation of calcium phosphates and experimental calcium phosphate bone cements using osteogenic cultures. Journal of biomedical materials research 2000; 52(3):498-508.

[7] Langer R, Vacanti JP. Tissue engineering. Science 1993; 260(5110):920-926.

[8] Furth ME, Atala A, Van Dyke ME. Smart biomaterials design for tissue engineering and regenerative medicine. Biomaterials 2007; 28(34):5068-5073.

[9] Lee SH, Shin H. Matrices and scaffolds for delivery of bioactive molecules in bone and cartilage tissue engineering. Advanced drug delivery reviews 2007; 59(4-5): 339-359.

[10] Sussman C, Bates-Jensen BM: Wound care: a collaborative practice manual: Lippincott Williams & Wilkins; 2007.

[11] Adams CS, Antoci V, Jr., Harrison G, Patal P, Freeman TA, Shapiro IM, Parvizi J, Hickok NJ, Radin S, Ducheyne P. Controlled release of vancomycin from thin sol-gel films on implant surfaces successfully controls osteomyelitis. Journal of orthopaedic research : official publication of the Orthopaedic Research Society 2009; 27(6):701-709.

[12] Maquet V, Jerome R: Design of macroporous biodegradable polymer scaffolds for cell transplantation. In Materials Science Forum: 1997. Trans Tech Publ; 1997:15-42.

[13] Thomson RC, Yaszemski MJ, Powers JM, Mikos AG. Hydroxyapatite fiber reinforced poly(alpha-hydroxy ester) foams for bone regeneration. Biomaterials 1998; 19(21): 1935-1943.

[14] Zhang Y, Zhang M. Calcium phosphate/chitosan composite scaffolds for controlled in vitro antibiotic drug release. Journal of biomedical materials research 2002; 62(3): 378-386.

[15] Cabanas MV, Pena J, Roman J, Vallet-Regi M. Tailoring vancomycin release from beta-TCP/agarose scaffolds. European journal of pharmaceutical sciences : official journal of the European Federation for Pharmaceutical Sciences 2009; 37(3-4):249-256.

[16] Simon D, Manuel S, Varma H. Novel nanoporous bioceramic spheres for drug delivery application: a preliminary in vitro investigation. Oral surgery, oral medicine, oral pathology and oral radiology 2013; 115(3):e7-14.

[17] Panseri S, Cunha C, D'Alessandro T, Sandri M, Giavaresi G, Marcacci M, Hung CT, Tampieri A. Intrinsically superparamagnetic Fe-hydroxyapatite nanoparticles positively influence osteoblast-like cell behaviour. Journal of nanobiotechnology 2012; 10:32.

[18] Panseri S, Cunha C, D'Alessandro T, Sandri M, Russo A, Giavaresi G, Marcacci M, Hung CT, Tampieri A. Magnetic hydroxyapatite bone substitutes to enhance tissue regeneration: evaluation in vitro using osteoblast-like cells and in vivo in a bone defect. PloS one 2012; 7(6):e38710.

[19] Singh RK, Patel KD, Lee JH, Lee EJ, Kim JH, Kim TH, Kim HW. Potential of magnetic nanofiber scaffolds with mechanical and biological properties applicable for bone regeneration. PloS one 2014; 9(4):e91584.

[20] Yang L, Sheldon BW, Webster TJ. Nanophase Ceramics for Improved Drug Delivery: Current Opportunities and Challenges. American Ceramic Society Bulletin 2010; 89(2):24-31.

[21] Ginebra M, Traykova T, Planell J. Calcium phosphate cements as bone drug delivery systems: a review. Journal of Controlled Release 2006; 113(2):102-110.

[22] Kim K, Fisher JP. Nanoparticle technology in bone tissue engineering. J Drug Target 2007; 15(4):241-252.

[23] Barth BM, Sharma R, Altinoglu EI, Morgan TT, Shanmugavelandy SS, Kaiser JM, McGovern C, Matters GL, Smith JP, Kester M et al. Bioconjugation of calcium phosphosilicate composite nanoparticles for selective targeting of human breast and pancreatic cancers in vivo. ACS nano 2010; 4(3):1279-1287.

[24] Cheng X, Kuhn L. Chemotherapy drug delivery from calcium phosphate nanoparticles. International journal of nanomedicine 2007; 2(4):667-674.

[25] Wang S, McDonnell EH, Sedor FA, Toffaletti JG. pH effects on measurements of ionized calcium and ionized magnesium in blood. Archives of pathology & laboratory medicine 2002; 126(8):947-950.

[26] Melville AJ, Rodriguez-Lorenzo LM, Forsythe JS. Effects of calcination temperature on the drug delivery behaviour of Ibuprofen from hydroxyapatite powders. Journal of materials science Materials in medicine 2008; 19(3):1187-1195.

[27] Chen JF, Ding HM, Wang JX, Shao L. Preparation and characterization of porous hollow silica nanoparticles for drug delivery application. Biomaterials 2004; 25(4): 723-727.

[28] Suchanek W, Yoshimura M. Processing and properties of hydroxyapatite-based biomaterials for use as hard tissue replacement implants. Journal of Materials Research 2011; 13(01):94-117.

[29] Paul W, Sharma CP. Development of porous spherical hydroxyapatite granules: application towards protein delivery. Journal of materials science Materials in medicine 1999; 10(7):383-388.

[30] Jones AC, Milthorpe B, Averdunk H, Limaye A, Senden TJ, Sakellariou A, Sheppard AP, Sok RM, Knackstedt MA, Brandwood A et al. Analysis of 3D bone ingrowth into polymer scaffolds via micro-computed tomography imaging. Biomaterials 2004; 25(20):4947-4954.

[31] Karageorgiou V, Kaplan D. Porosity of 3D biomaterial scaffolds and osteogenesis. Biomaterials 2005; 26(27):5474-5491.

[32] Ribeiro CC, Barrias CC, Barbosa MA. Preparation and characterisation of calcium-phosphate porous microspheres with a uniform size for biomedical applications. Journal of materials science Materials in medicine 2006; 17(5):455-463.

[33] Zyman Z, Glushko V, Filippenko V, Radchenko V, Mezentsev V. Nonstoichiometric hydroxyapatite granules for orthopaedic applications. Journal of materials science Materials in medicine 2004; 15(5):551-558.

[34] Akao M, Aoki H, Kato K. Mechanical properties of sintered hydroxyapatite for prosthetic applications. Journal of Materials Science 1981; 16(3):809-812.

[35] Slosarczyk A. Highly Porous Hydroxyapatite Material. Powder Metall Int 1989; 21(4): 24-25.

[36] Roy DM, Linnehan SK. Hydroxyapatite formed from coral skeletal carbonate by hydrothermal exchange. Nature 1974; 247(5438):220-222.

[37] Dard M, Bauer A, Liebendorger A, Wahlig H, Dingeldein E. Preparation physiochemical and biological evaluation of a hydroxyapatite ceramic from bovine spongiosa. Act Odonto Stom 1994; 185:61-69.

[38] Schlapp M, Friess W. Collagen/PLGA microparticle composites for local controlled delivery of gentamicin. J Pharm Sci 2003; 92(11):2145-2151.

[39] Kim JH, Park YB, Li Z, Shim JS, Moon HS, Jung HS, Chung MK. Effect of alendronate on healing of extraction sockets and healing around implants. Oral diseases 2011; 17(7):705-711.

[40] Doğan H, Ozcelik B, Senel S. The effect of calcitonin on osseous healing in guinea pig mandible. Journal of endodontics 2001; 27(3):160-163.

[41] Hong MH, Son JS, Kim KM, Han M, Oh DS, Lee YK. Drug-loaded porous spherical hydroxyapatite granules for bone regeneration. Journal of materials science Materials in medicine 2011; 22(2):349-355.

[42] Sassard WR, Eidman DK, Gray PM, Block JE, Russo R, Russell JL, Taboada EM. Augmenting local bone with Grafton demineralized bone matrix for posterolateral lumbar spine fusion: avoiding second site autologous bone harvest. Orthopedics 2000; 23(10):1059-1064; discussion 1064-1055.

[43] Lewis CS, Supronowicz PR, Zhukauskas RM, Gill E, Cobb RR. Local antibiotic delivery with demineralized bone matrix. Cell Tissue Bank 2012; 13(1):119-127.

[44] Schmitt JM, Hwang K, Winn SR, Hollinger JO. Bone morphogenetic proteins: an update on basic biology and clinical relevance. Journal of orthopaedic research : official publication of the Orthopaedic Research Society 1999; 17(2):269-278.

[45] Lieberman JR, Daluiski A, Einhorn TA. The role of growth factors in the repair of bone. Biology and clinical applications. The Journal of bone and joint surgery American volume 2002; 84-A(6):1032-1044.

[46] Cornell CN. Osteoconductive Materials and Their Role as Substitutes for Autogenous Bone Grafts. Orthopedic Clinics of North America 1999; 30(4):591-598.

[47] Tatakis DN, Koh A, Jin L, Wozney JM, Rohrer MD, Wikesjo UM. Peri-implant bone regeneration using recombinant human bone morphogenetic protein-2 in a canine model: a dose-response study. Journal of periodontal research 2002; 37(2):93-100.

[48] Wikesjö UM, Sorensen RG, Wozney JM. Augmentation of Alveolar Bone and Dental Implant Osseointegration: Clinical Implications of Studies with rhBMP-2 A Comprehensive Review. The Journal of Bone & Joint Surgery 2001; 83(1_suppl_2):S136-S145.

[49] Bessho K, Carnes DL, Cavin R, Chen HY, Ong JL. BMP stimulation of bone response adjacent to titanium implants in vivo. Clinical oral implants research 1999; 10(3): 212-218.

[50] Janssens K, ten Dijke P, Janssens S, Van Hul W. Transforming growth factor-beta1 to the bone. Endocrine reviews 2005; 26(6):743-774.

[51] Duneas N, Crooks J, Ripamonti U. Transforming growth factor-beta 1: induction of bone morphogenetic protein genes expression during endochondral bone formation in the baboon, and synergistic interaction with osteogenic protein-1 (BMP-7). Growth factors 1998; 15(4):259-277.

[52] Jain TK, Reddy MK, Morales MA, Leslie-Pelecky DL, Labhasetwar V. Biodistribution, clearance, and biocompatibility of iron oxide magnetic nanoparticles in rats. Mol Pharm 2008; 5(2):316-327.

[53] Prijic S, Scancar J, Cemazar M, Bregar VB, Znidarsic A, Sersa G. Increased cellular uptake of biocompatible superparamagnetic iron oxide nanoparticles into malignant cells by an external magnetic field. The Journal of membrane biology 2010; 236(1): 167-179.

[54] Sun C, Du K, Fang C, Bhattarai N, Veiseh O, Kievit F, Stephen Z, Lee D, Ellenbogen RG, Ratner B. PEG-mediated synthesis of highly dispersive multifunctional superparamagnetic nanoparticles: their physicochemical properties and function in vivo. ACS nano 2010; 4(4):2402-2410.

[55] Amirfazli A. Nanomedicine: magnetic nanoparticles hit the target. Nat Nanotechnol 2007; 2(8):467-468.

[56] Glossop JR, Cartmell SH. Tensile strain and magnetic particle force application do not induce MAP3K8 and IL-1B differential gene expression in a similar manner to fluid shear stress in human mesenchymal stem cells. Journal of tissue engineering and regenerative medicine 2010; 4(7):577-579.

[57] Gupta AK, Gupta M. Synthesis and surface engineering of iron oxide nanoparticles for biomedical applications. Biomaterials 2005; 26(18):3995-4021.

[58] Arruebo M, Fernández-Pacheco R, Ibarra MR, Santamaría J. Magnetic nanoparticles for drug delivery. Nano Today 2007; 2(3):22-32.

[59] Kanczler JM, Sura HS, Magnay J, Green D, Oreffo RO, Dobson JP, El Haj AJ. Controlled differentiation of human bone marrow stromal cells using magnetic nanoparticle technology. Tissue engineering Part A 2010; 16(10):3241-3250.

[60] Singh N, Jenkins GJ, Asadi R, Doak SH. Potential toxicity of superparamagnetic iron oxide nanoparticles (SPION). Nano Rev 2010; 1.

[61] Morrissey R, Rodriguez-Lorenzo LM, Gross KA. Influence of ferrous iron incorporation on the structure of hydroxyapatite. Journal of materials science Materials in medicine 2005; 16(5):387-392.

[62] Landi E, Celotti G, Logroscino G, Tampieri A. Carbonated hydroxyapatite as bone substitute. Journal of the European Ceramic Society 2003; 23(15):2931-2937.

[63] Landi E, Tampieri A, Celotti G, Sprio S, Sandri M, Logroscino G. Sr-substituted hydroxyapatites for osteoporotic bone replacement. Acta biomaterialia 2007; 3(6): 961-969.

[64] Landi E, Tampieri A, Mattioli-Belmonte M, Celotti G, Sandri M, Gigante A, Fava P, Biagini G. Biomimetic Mg-and Mg, CO< sub> 3</sub>-substituted hydroxyapatites: synthesis characterization and in vitro behaviour. Journal of the European Ceramic Society 2006; 26(13):2593-2601.

[65] Laurencin C, Khan Y, El-Amin SF. Bone graft substitutes. Expert review of medical devices 2006; 3(1):49-57.

[66] Tampieri A, D'Alessandro T, Sandri M, Sprio S, Landi E, Bertinetti L, Panseri S, Pepponi G, Goettlicher J, Banobre-Lopez M et al. Intrinsic magnetism and hyperthermia in bioactive Fe-doped hydroxyapatite. Acta biomaterialia 2012; 8(2):843-851.

[67] Xu H-Y, Gu N. Magnetic responsive scaffolds and magnetic fields in bone repair and regeneration. Frontiers of Materials Science 2014; 8(1):20-31.

[68] Thein-Han WW, Misra RD. Biomimetic chitosan-nanohydroxyapatite composite scaffolds for bone tissue engineering. Acta biomaterialia 2009; 5(4):1182-1197.

[69] Muzzarelli R, Baldassarre V, Conti F, Ferrara P, Biagini G, Gazzanelli G, Vasi V. Biological activity of chitosan: ultrastructural study. Biomaterials 1988; 9(3):247-252.

[70] George M, Abraham TE. Polyionic hydrocolloids for the intestinal delivery of protein drugs: alginate and chitosan--a review. Journal of controlled release : official journal of the Controlled Release Society 2006; 114(1):1-14.

[71] Li Z, Ramay HR, Hauch KD, Xiao D, Zhang M. Chitosan-alginate hybrid scaffolds for bone tissue engineering. Biomaterials 2005; 26(18):3919-3928.

[72] Muzzarelli RA, Mattioli-Belmonte M, Tietz C, Biagini R, Ferioli G, Brunelli MA, Fini M, Giardino R, Ilari P, Biagini G. Stimulatory effect on bone formation exerted by a modified chitosan. Biomaterials 1994; 15(13):1075-1081.

[73] Hu Q. Preparation and characterization of biodegradable chitosan/hydroxyapatite nanocomposite rods via in situ hybridization: a potential material as internal fixation of bone fracture. Biomaterials 2004; 25(5):779-785.

[74] Manjubala I, Scheler S, Bossert J, Jandt KD. Mineralisation of chitosan scaffolds with nano-apatite formation by double diffusion technique. Acta biomaterialia 2006; 2(1): 75-84.

[75] Kong L, Gao Y, Cao W, Gong Y, Zhao N, Zhang X. Preparation and characterization of nano-hydroxyapatite/chitosan composite scaffolds. J Biomed Mater Res A 2005; 75(2):275-282.

[76] de Jonge LT, Leeuwenburgh SC, Wolke JG, Jansen JA. Organic-inorganic surface modifications for titanium implant surfaces. Pharmaceutical research 2008; 25(10): 2357-2369.

[77] Wildemann B, Bamdad P, Holmer C, Haas NP, Raschke M, Schmidmaier G. Local delivery of growth factors from coated titanium plates increases osteotomy healing in rats. Bone 2004; 34(5):862-868.

[78] Kim K-H, Kwon T-Y, Kim S-Y, Kang I-K, Kim S, Yang Y, Ong JL. Preparation and characterization of anodized titanium surfaces and their effect on osteoblast responses. Journal of Oral Implantology 2006; 32(1):8-13.

[79] Yao C, Webster TJ. Anodization: a promising nano-modification technique of titanium implants for orthopedic applications. J Nanosci Nanotechnol 2006; 6(9-10): 2682-2692.

[80] Yao C, Webster TJ. Prolonged antibiotic delivery from anodized nanotubular titanium using a co-precipitation drug loading method. Journal of Biomedical Materials Research Part B: Applied Biomaterials 2009; 91(2):587-595.

[81] Jia H, Kerr LL. Sustained ibuprofen release using composite poly (lactic-co-glycolic acid)/titanium dioxide nanotubes from Ti implant surface. Journal of pharmaceutical sciences 2013; 102(7):2341-2348.

[82] Kim HS, Yang Y, Koh JT, Lee KK, Lee DJ, Lee KM, Park SW. Fabrication and characterization of functionally graded nano-micro porous titanium surface by anodizing.ooJournal of biomedical materials research Part B, Applied biomaterials 2009; 88(2):427-435.

[83] Bae IH, Yun KD, Kim HS, Jeong BC, Lim HP, Park SW, Lee KM, Lim YC, Lee KK, Yang Y et al. Anodic oxidized nanotubular titanium implants enhance bone morphogenetic protein-2 delivery. Journal of biomedical materials research Part B, Applied biomaterials 2010; 93(2):484-491.

[84] Puleo DA, Huh WW, Duggirala SS, DeLuca PP. In vitro cellular responses to bioerodible particles loaded with recombinant human bone morphogenetic protein-2. Journal of biomedical materials research 1998; 41(1):104-110.

[85] He J, Huang T, Gan L, Zhou Z, Jiang B, Wu Y, Wu F, Gu Z. Collagen-infiltrated porous hydroxyapatite coating and its osteogenic properties: in vitro and in vivo study. J Biomed Mater Res A 2012; 100(7):1706-1715.

[86] Soballe K, Hansen ES, Brockstedt-Rasmussen H, Bunger C. Hydroxyapatite coating converts fibrous tissue to bone around loaded implants. The Journal of bone and joint surgery British volume 1993; 75(2):270-278.

[87] Choi S, Murphy WL. Sustained plasmid DNA release from dissolving mineral coatings. Acta biomaterialia 2010; 6(9):3426-3435.

[88] Saran N, Zhang R, Turcotte RE. Osteogenic protein-1 delivered by hydroxyapatite-coated implants improves bone ingrowth in extracortical bone bridging. Clinical orthopaedics and related research 2011; 469(5):1470-1478.

[89] Shah NJ, Hong J, Hyder MN, Hammond PT. Osteophilic multilayer coatings for accelerated bone tissue growth. Advanced materials 2012; 24(11):1445-1450.

[90] Ribeiro M, Monteiro FJ, Ferraz MP. Infection of orthopedic implants with emphasis on bacterial adhesion process and techniques used in studying bacterial-material interactions. Biomatter 2012; 2(4):176-194.

[91] Ketonis C, Parvizi J, Jones LC. Evolving strategies to prevent implant-associated infections. The Journal of the American Academy of Orthopaedic Surgeons 2012; 20(7): 478-480.

[92] Pavithra D, Doble M. Biofilm formation, bacterial adhesion and host response on polymeric implants—issues and prevention. Biomedical Materials 2008; 3(3):034003.

[93] Webb JC, Spencer RF. The role of polymethylmethacrylate bone cement in modern orthopaedic surgery. The Journal of bone and joint surgery British volume 2007; 89(7):851-857.

[94] Oosterbos CJ, Vogely H, Nijhof MW, Fleer A, Verbout AJ, Tonino AJ, Dhert WJ. Osseointegration of hydroxyapatite-coated and noncoated Ti6Al4V implants in the presence of local infection: a comparative histomorphometrical study in rabbits. Journal of biomedical materials research 2002; 60(3):339-347.

[95] Stigter M, Bezemer J, De Groot K, Layrolle P. Incorporation of different antibiotics into carbonated hydroxyapatite coatings on titanium implants, release and antibiotic efficacy. Journal of controlled release 2004; 99(1):127-137.

[96] Alt V, Bitschnau A, Bohner F, Heerich KE, Magesin E, Sewing A, Pavlidis T, Szalay G, Heiss C, Thormann U et al. Effects of gentamicin and gentamicin-RGD coatings on

bone ingrowth and biocompatibility of cementless joint prostheses: an experimental study in rabbits. Acta biomaterialia 2011; 7(3):1274-1280.

[97] Ren WP, Song W, Esquivel AO, Jackson NM, Nelson M, Flynn JC, Markel DC. Effect of erythromycin-doped calcium polyphosphate scaffold composite in a mouse pouch infection model. Journal of biomedical materials research Part B, Applied biomaterials 2014; 102(6):1140-1147.

[98] Zilberman M: Active Implants and Scaffolds for Tissue Regeneration. In Studies in Mechanobiology, Tissue Engineering and Biomaterials. Volume 8. Springer 2011:XII, 516

[99] Tovar N, Jimbo R, Witek L, Anchieta R, Yoo D, Manne L, Machado L, Gangolli R, Coelho PG. The physicochemical characterization and in vivo response of micro/nanoporous bioactive ceramic particulate bone graft materials. Materials science & engineering C, Materials for biological applications 2014; 43:472-480.

[100] Gultepe E, Nagesha D, Sridhar S, Amiji M. Nanoporous inorganic membranes or coatings for sustained drug delivery in implantable devices. Advanced drug delivery reviews 2010; 62(3):305-315.

[101] Rajesh P, Mohan N, Yokogawa Y, Varma H. Pulsed laser deposition of hydroxyapatite on nanostructured titanium towards drug eluting implants. Materials science & engineering C, Materials for biological applications 2013; 33(5):2899-2904.

[102] Zhang W, Chu PK. Enhancement of antibacterial properties and biocompatibility of polyethylene by silver and copper plasma immersion ion implantation. Surface and Coatings Technology 2008; 203(5-7):909-912.

[103] Huang H-L, Chang Y-Y, Lai M-C, Lin C-R, Lai C-H, Shieh T-M. Antibacterial TaN-Ag coatings on titanium dental implants. Surface and Coatings Technology 2010; 205(5):1636-1641.

[104] Chen W, Liu Y, Courtney HS, Bettenga M, Agrawal CM, Bumgardner JD, Ong JL. In vitro anti-bacterial and biological properties of magnetron co-sputtered silver-containing hydroxyapatite coating. Biomaterials 2006; 27(32):5512-5517.

[105] Chen Y, Zheng X, Xie Y, Ji H, Ding C, Li H, Dai K. Silver release from silver-containing hydroxyapatite coatings. Surface and Coatings Technology 2010; 205(7): 1892-1896.

[106] Cotte FE, Fardellone P, Mercier F, Gaudin AF, Roux C. Adherence to monthly and weekly oral bisphosphonates in women with osteoporosis. Osteoporosis international : a journal established as result of cooperation between the European Foundation for Osteoporosis and the National Osteoporosis Foundation of the USA 2010; 21(1): 145-155.

[107] Russell RG, Watts NB, Ebetino FH, Rogers MJ. Mechanisms of action of bisphosphonates: similarities and differences and their potential influence on clinical efficacy.

Osteoporosis international : a journal established as result of cooperation between the European Foundation for Osteoporosis and the National Osteoporosis Foundation of the USA 2008; 19(6):733-759.

[108] Russell RG. Bisphosphonates: mode of action and pharmacology. Pediatrics 2007; 119 Suppl 2:S150-162.

[109] Bisaz S, Jung A, Fleisch H. Uptake by bone of pyrophosphate, diphosphonates and their technetium derivatives. Clinical science and molecular medicine 1978; 54(3): 265-272.

[110] Drake MT, Clarke BL, Khosla S. Bisphosphonates: mechanism of action and role in clinical practice. Mayo Clinic proceedings Mayo Clinic 2008; 83(9):1032-1045.

[111] Schindeler A, Little DG. Bisphosphonate action: revelations and deceptions from in vitro studies. J Pharm Sci 2007; 96(8):1872-1878.

[112] Narai S, Nagahata S. Effects of alendronate on the removal torque of implants in rats with induced osteoporosis. Int J Oral Maxillofac Implants 2003; 18(2):218-223.

[113] Kurth AH, Eberhardt C, Muller S, Steinacker M, Schwarz M, Bauss F. The bisphosphonate ibandronate improves implant integration in osteopenic ovariectomized rats. Bone 2005; 37(2):204-210.

[114] Giro G, Sakakura CE, Goncalves D, Pereira RM, Marcantonio E, Jr., Orrico SR. Effect of 17beta-estradiol and alendronate on the removal torque of osseointegrated titanium implants in ovariectomized rats. J Periodontol 2007; 78(7):1316-1321.

[115] Yoshinari M, Oda Y, Inoue T, Matsuzaka K, Shimono M. Bone response to calcium phosphate-coated and bisphosphonate-immobilized titanium implants. Biomaterials 2002; 23(14):2879-2885.

[116] Peter B, Pioletti DP, Laib S, Bujoli B, Pilet P, Janvier P, Guicheux J, Zambelli PY, Bouler JM, Gauthier O. Calcium phosphate drug delivery system: influence of local zoledronate release on bone implant osteointegration. Bone 2005; 36(1):52-60.

[117] Yildiz A, Esen E, Kurkcu M, Damlar I, Daglioglu K, Akova T. Effect of zoledronic acid on osseointegration of titanium implants: an experimental study in an ovariectomized rabbit model. Journal of oral and maxillofacial surgery : official journal of the American Association of Oral and Maxillofacial Surgeons 2010; 68(3):515-523.

[118] Mundy G, Garrett R, Harris S, Chan J, Chen D, Rossini G, Boyce B, Zhao M, Gutierrez G. Stimulation of bone formation in vitro and in rodents by statins. Science 1999; 286(5446):1946-1949.

[119] Yang F, Zhao SF, Zhang F, He FM, Yang GL. Simvastatin-loaded porous implant surfaces stimulate preosteoblasts differentiation: an in vitro study. Oral surgery, oral medicine, oral pathology, oral radiology, and endodontics 2011; 111(5):551-556.

[120] Ayukawa Y, Yasukawa E, Moriyama Y, Ogino Y, Wada H, Atsuta I, Koyano K. Local application of statin promotes bone repair through the suppression of osteoclasts and

the enhancement of osteoblasts at bone-healing sites in rats. Oral surgery, oral medicine, oral pathology, oral radiology, and endodontics 2009; 107(3):336-342.

[121] Du Z, Chen J, Yan F, Xiao Y. Effects of Simvastatin on bone healing around titanium implants in osteoporotic rats. Clinical oral implants research 2009; 20(2):145-150.

[122] Maeda T, Kawane T, Horiuchi N. Statins augment vascular endothelial growth factor expression in osteoblastic cells via inhibition of protein prenylation. Endocrinology 2003; 144(2):681-692.

[123] Maeda T, Matsunuma A, Kurahashi I, Yanagawa T, Yoshida H, Horiuchi N. Induction of osteoblast differentiation indices by statins in MC3T3-E1 cells. Journal of cellular biochemistry 2004; 92(3):458-471.

[124] Ubios AM, Jares Furno G, Guglielmotti MB. Effect of calcitonin on alveolar wound healing. Journal of oral pathology & medicine : official publication of the International Association of Oral Pathologists and the American Academy of Oral Pathology 1991; 20(7):322-324.

[125] Rao LG, Heersche JN, Marchuk LL, Sturtridge W. Immunohistochemical demonstration of calcitonin binding to specific cell types in fixed rat bone tissue. Endocrinology 1981; 108(5):1972-1978.

[126] Dahlin C, Linde A, Gottlow J, Nyman S. Healing of bone defects by guided tissue regeneration. Plastic and reconstructive surgery 1988; 81(5):672-676.

[127] Ichikawa M, Nakamuta H, Hoshino T, Ogawa Y, Koida M. Anti-osteopenic effect of nasal salmon calcitonin in type 1 osteoporotic rats: comparison with subcutaneous dosing. Biological & pharmaceutical bulletin 1994; 17(7):911-913.

[128] Arisawa EA, Brandao AA, Almeida JD, da Rocha RF. Calcitonin in bone-guided regeneration of mandibles in ovariectomized rats: densitometric, histologic and histomorphometric analysis. International journal of oral and maxillofacial surgery 2008; 37(1):47-53.

[129] Reginster JY, Azria M, Gaspar S, Bleicher M, Franchimont N, Behhar M, Albert A, Franchimont P. Endogenous production of specific antibodies does not decrease hypocalcemic response to calcitonin in young rabbits. Calcified tissue international 1992; 50(6):518-520.

[130] Almeida JD, Arisawa EA, da Rocha RF, Carvalho YR. Effect of calcitonin on bone regeneration in male rats: a histomorphometric analysis. International journal of oral and maxillofacial surgery 2007; 36(5):435-440.

[131] Foster SC, Kronman JH. The effects of topical thyrocalcitonin on the extraction sites in the jaws of dogs. Oral surgery, oral medicine, and oral pathology 1974; 38(6): 866-873.

[132] Costa-Rodrigues J, Reis S, Teixeira S, Lopes S, Fernandes MH. Dose-dependent inhibitory effects of proton pump inhibitors on human osteoclastic and osteoblastic cell activity. The FEBS journal 2013; 280(20):5052-5064.

[133] Rzeszutek K, Sarraf F, Davies JE. Proton pump inhibitors control osteoclastic resorption of calcium phosphate implants and stimulate increased local reparative bone growth. The Journal of craniofacial surgery 2003; 14(3):301-307.

[134] Sheraly A, Lickorish D, Sarraf F, Davies J. Use of gastrointestinal proton pump inhibitors to regulate osteoclast-mediated resorption of calcium phosphate cements in vivo. Current drug delivery 2009; 6(2):192-198.

[135] Väänänen HK, Zhao H. Osteoclast function: biology and mechanisms. Principles of Bone Biology, 3rd ed Academic Press, San Diego, USA 2008:193-209.

[136] Porter JR, Ruckh TT, Popat KC. Bone tissue engineering: a review in bone biomimetics and drug delivery strategies. Biotechnology progress 2009; 25(6):1539-1560.

[137] Rammelt S, Illert T, Bierbaum S, Scharnweber D, Zwipp H, Schneiders W. Coating of titanium implants with collagen, RGD peptide and chondroitin sulfate. Biomaterials 2006; 27(32):5561-5571.

[138] Liu Y, de Groot K, Hunziker EB. BMP-2 liberated from biomimetic implant coatings induces and sustains direct ossification in an ectopic rat model. Bone 2005; 36(5): 745-757.

[139] Goodman SB, Yao Z, Keeney M, Yang F. The future of biologic coatings for orthopaedic implants. Biomaterials 2013; 34(13):3174-3183.

5

Biopolymer in Gene Delivery

Sakthivel Lakshmana Prabu and
Kandasamy Ruckmani

Abstract

Nowadays, biopolymers, a class of biomaterials, represent frontier area in the drug delivery systems. Drug release from nano- and microparticles is a complex process, which involves several steps. Uptake of nanoparticle in the intracellular is affected by numerous factors. Recently, gene delivery has been considered one of the promising approaches for the treatment of various diseases acquired genetically in human being. The use of biopolymers as nanoparticles in gene delivery can potentially avoid many of the safety concerns in the gene delivery system. In gene delivery, the genetic materials such as DNA plasmids, RNA and siRNA are either encapsulated inside or conjugated to the nanoparticles, which protects the genetic materials until the drug reaches its target site. Treatment of the diseases is based on the effective delivery of the genetic materials into specific cells that are responsible for disease development. Various properties such as particle size, surface charge, morphology of the surface and release rate of the loaded molecules are the important parameters in the gene delivery system. In this chapter, various biopolymers (cationic polymers) and inorganic non-viral-delivery vectors used in gene delivery used as therapeutic agents are discussed.

Keywords: gene delivery, polymers, biopolymers, delivery system, therapeutic effect

1. Introduction

Polymers are the materials that are either prepared/produced synthetically or isolated from natural sources. Polymers can respond based on their environmental conditions such as pH, temperature, ionic strength, electric field, magnetic field, chemical and biological stimuli to deliver the desired therapeutic agents. Recently, biopolymer is a biomaterial used in various delivery systems to interact with the biological system and release the therapeutic agent. These biopolymers are utilized in the various applications due to their biocompatibility, bio degradability and low immunogenicity. Among the various biopolymers, synthetic polymers have well-defined structure and fine-tunable degradation kinetic and mechanical properties compared to the natural polymers. Recently, biodegradable nanoparticles have a major role in the field of health sciences especially for treating various diseases through drugs, vaccines and genes [1–7]. Nanoparticle in gene-delivery system has been utilized for treating various diseases such as cancer and haemophilia. The major challenge in the gene delivery is delivering the genetic materials such as DNA, plasmids, RNA and siRNA into the target/special cells to replace the damaged genes or expression inhibition of undesired genes or expression and production of required proteins. In gene delivery, the genetic material is either encapsulated inside the nanoparticle or conjugated to the nanoparticle. The nature, source and their physico-chemical properties of the polymers play an important role in the formation of desired properties of nanoparticles and to achieve a better therapeutic effect [8–12].

2. Polymeric gene delivery vector

The important property in polymeric vector is that the polymer should be non-toxic (biocompatible), biodegradable (hence have less toxicity) and also help to release the DNA from the complex into the cytoplasm. In polymeric vector, the polymer must be condensate with the genetic material. Condensate between the cationic polymer and genetic materials can be done through electrostatic interactions. By modifying the surface of NP, NP-DNA complexes can be formed by electrostatic binding between the positive charges of the NPs and the negative charges of the DNA. Only when the medium is aqueous and hydrophilic, the polymeric vector will be mobile, because the vector needs hydrophobic and hydrophilic components and be stabilized in an aqueous solution by forming micelles [13].

2.1. Polymer properties in polymeric gene delivery

Polymers have permanent cationic charges on its surface and are not preferred due to its strong condensate property with DNA, which will not release DNA into the cell. Hence, ionizable cationic polymers with pK values between 5 and 7 are preferred in the polymeric vector delivery which is shown in **Figure 1**.

Other important factors to be considered for the polymer in the polymeric gene-delivery vector are its molecular weight, molecular structure and composition of the polymer. Increase in the polymer's molecular weight also increases its toxicity. Polymers of different molecular structures such as linear, branched, stars and dendrimers have an impact on the transfer genes into cells [14–18].

2.2. Preparation of polymeric gene vector

Polymeric vectors are prepared by mixing plasmid DNA with a cationic polymer. During condensation between plasmid DNA and polycation, plasmid DNA undergoes a conformational change from a hydrodynamic size of 200–300 nm to particles of less than 100 nm. Plasmid DNA has a highly organized chemical structure [19–22]. A condensation between plasmid DNA and polycation is shown in **Figure 2**.

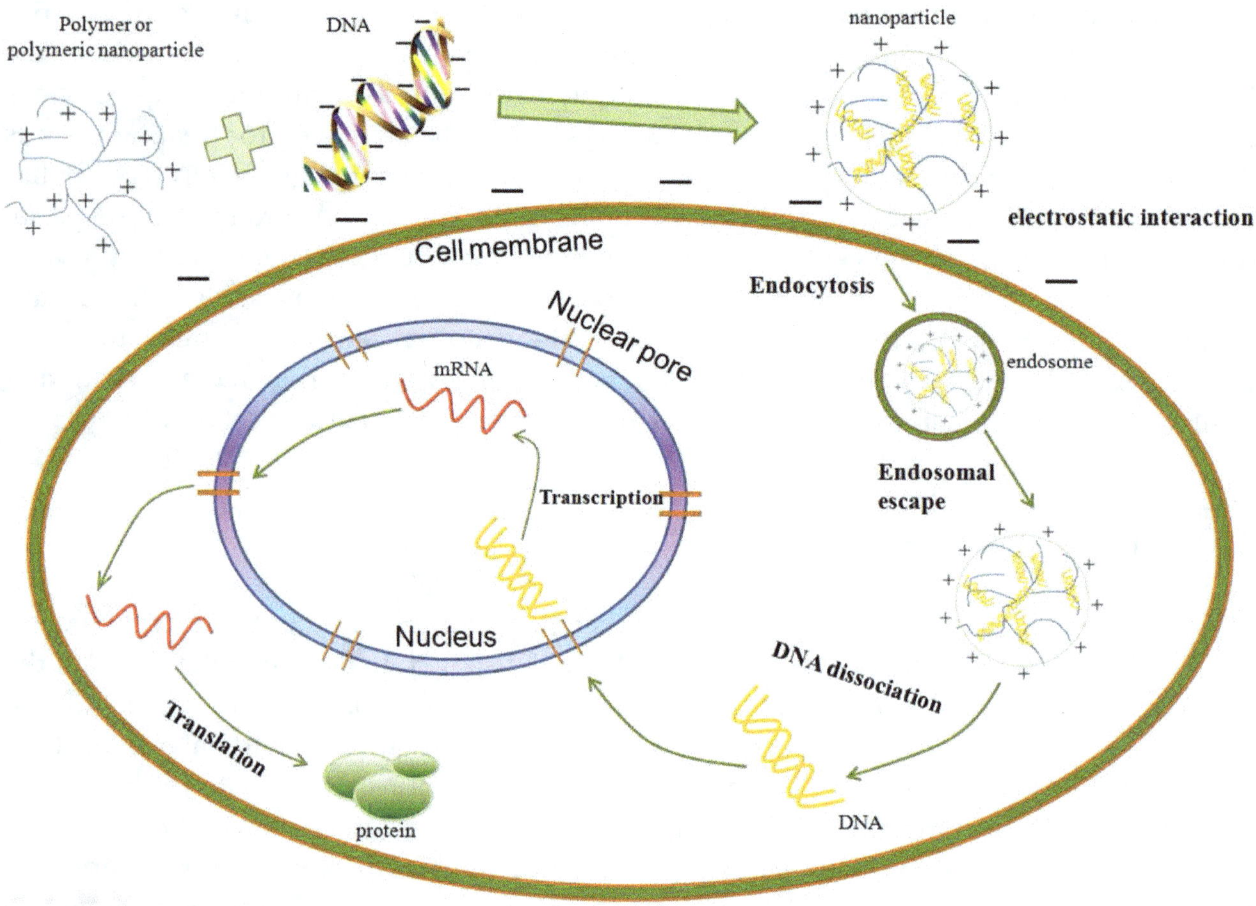

Figure 1. Gene delivery process of polymeric nanoparticle.

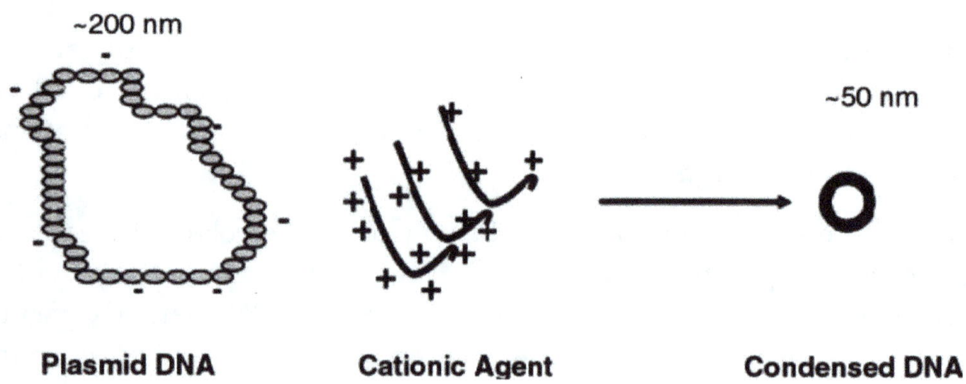

Figure 2. Condensation between plasmid DNA and polycation.

The order of mixing and vortex speed of mixing plays an important role in the size of the DNA nanoparticles. DNA can be condensate, either by evaporation under vacuum or by freeze drying. The freeze/thaw cycle can influence the particle size of DNA nanoparticles.

The charge ratio of DNA nanoparticles is the calculated ratio of amines on the polymer relative to the phosphates on DNA at a given stoichiometry of polymer to DNA. When a cationic polymer binds to plasmid DNA, sodium ions are displaced and the electronegative charge is partially satisfied. DNA condensates are normally prepared at near-neutral pH in low ionic strength buffer [23, 24].

3. Dendrimers

Dendrimer is a monodisperse macromolecule with perfectly branched regular structure and having at least one branched junction at each repeat unit 3. These dendrimers are used in gene delivery. The dendrimer/DNA complexes are encapsulated in a water-soluble polymer, and then deposited on or sandwiched in functional polymer films with a fast degradation by dehydration to mediate gene transfection.

Biodegradable dendrimers are commonly prepared by inclusion of ester groups in the polymer backbone, which will be chemically hydrolysed and/or enzymatically cleaved by esterases in physiological solutions. These dendrimers are large molecular weights which accumulate and retain in higher amounts in the tumour tissues. Dendrimer fragments are eliminated safely through urine.

Dendrimers are prepared through either a divergent method or a convergent method.

In the **divergent methods**, as given in **Figure 3**, dendrimer grows from a multifunctional core molecule to outwards. The first-generation dendrimers are derived from the core molecule that reacts with monomer molecules containing one reactive and two dormant groups. This periphery molecule is then activated to react with more monomers. This step is subsequently repetitive to produce layer-by-layer dendrimers for several generations.

In the` convergent approach, stepwise dendrimer is constructed, starting from the end groups and progressing inwards. The growing branched polymeric arms are called dendrons, which can attach to a multifunctional core molecule (**Figure 4**).

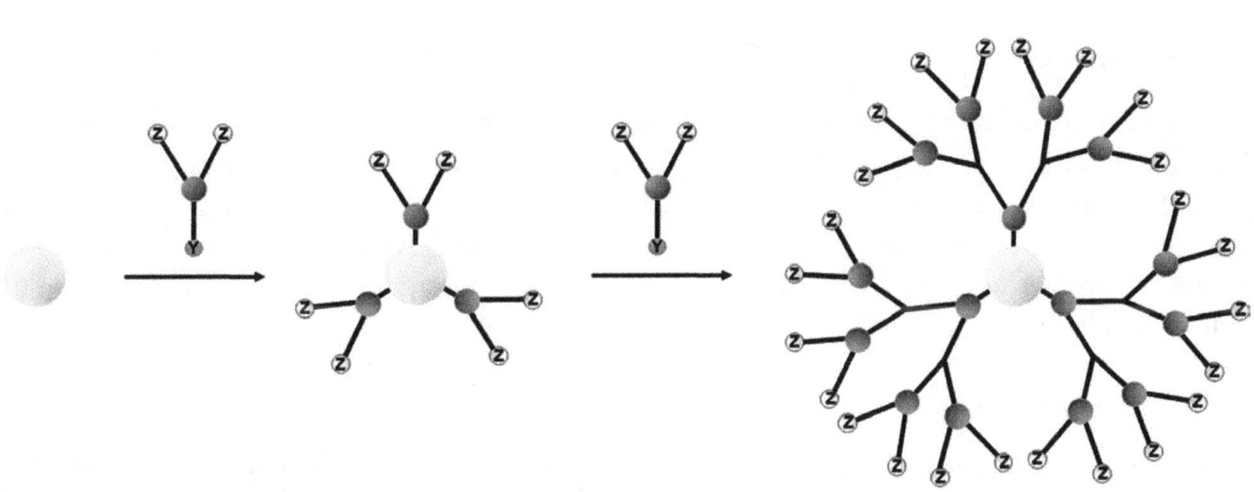

Figure 3. Formation of dendrimer by divergent methods.

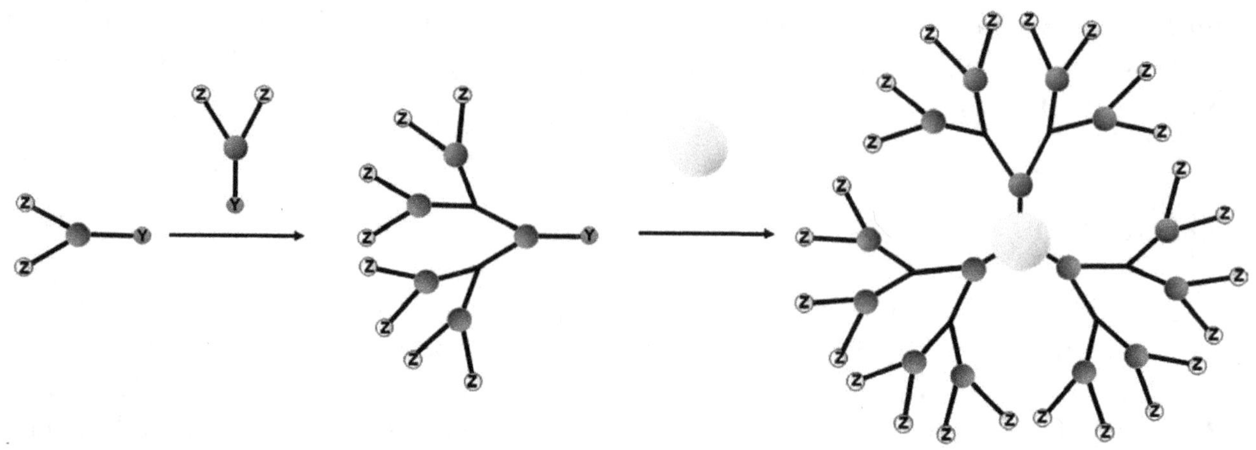

Figure 4. Formation of dendrimer by convergent method.

Whereas the structure Y in dendrimer is chemically active focal point and Z is the functional chemical group of another monomer.

3.1. Other types of dendrimers

3.1.1. Amino acid-based dendrimers

Amino acid-based dendrimers were developed to capitalize on the unique properties of the amino acid-building blocks, including chirality, hydrophilicity/hydrophobicity, biorecognition and optical properties. Optically active protein-mimetic dendrimers have been synthesized using various amino acids, such as tryptophan, phenylalanine, glutamic acid, aspartic acid, leucine, valine, glycine and alanine.

Amino acid-based dendrimers can be synthesized by

1. amino acid or peptide grafting and display on the surface of a conventional dendrimer
2. attachment of amino acids or peptides to an organic or a peptide core.

3.1.2. Glycodendrimers

Carbohydrate interactions with different receptors displayed at the cell surface control a number of normal (e.g., lymphocyte activation and cell-cell adhesion) and abnormal (e.g., cell-pathogen adhesion and cancer cell metastasis) biological processes. Glycodendrimers have been synthesized by coupling isothiocyanate-functionalized glycosyl and mannopyranoside ligands as well as an *N*-hydroxysuccinimide (NHS)-activated galactopyranosyl derivative to amine-terminated dendrimers.

3.1.3. Hydrophobic dendrimers

Dendrimers with hydrophobic interiors and a hydrophilic surface are called hydrophobic dendrimers. Hydrophobic dendrimer gives better encapsulation and efficient solubilization of hydrophobic drug molecules. Specifically, dendrimers with hydrophobic cores were proved to effectively retain hydrophobic drug molecules in the voids of their branching architecture, mimicking amphiphilic polymer micelles.

3.1.4. Asymmetric dendrimers

Asymmetric dendrimers are synthesized by coupling dendrons of different generations to a linear core, which yields a branched dendrimer with a nonuniform orthogonal architecture.

There are two different types of dendrimeric copolymers:

1. **Segment-block dendrimers**—segmented with segments of different constitution.
2. **Layer-block dendrimers**—concentric spheres of differing chemistry [25–42].

4. Cationic polymers

DNA, when combined with sufficient amounts of cationic polymers, will condense into discrete entities which are called as polyplexes [43]. The polyplexes are compact nanoparticles formed through electrostatic interactions between the positive charges of amines and the negative charges of DNA phosphates. The strength of DNA binding to the polymers is related to the N:P ratio.

The most common cationic polymers used as nonviral gene-delivery vectors include chitosan, PLL, polyethylenimine (PEI), poly(amido amine) (PAMAM) dendrimers and select polypeptides [24, 44, 45].

4.1. Chitosan

Chitosan is a polysaccharide copolymer composed of randomly distributed β-(1-4)-linked d-glucosamines and *N*-acetyl-d-glucosamines, obtained by partial alkaline deacetylation of chitin [46], with different molecular weights (50–200 kDa), degrees of deacetylation (40–98%) and viscosities [47]. Chitosan is a natural polymer, **Figure 5**, with linear polyamine, having reactive amino and hydroxyl groups, biodegradable to normal body constituent, safe and non-toxic, and binds to mammalian and microbial cells. The main commercial sources of chitosan are the crustacean shell wastes of crabs, shrimps and

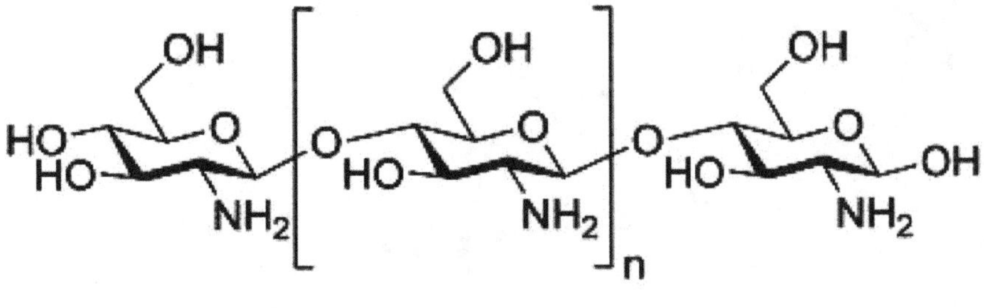

Figure 5. Structure of chitosan.

lobsters [48]. Chitosan is soluble in aqueous solutions of some acids and some selective N-alkylidination. Its solubility, biodegradability, reactivity and adsorptivity of many substrates depend on the amount of protonation of the $-NH_2$ function on the C-2 position of the D-glucosamine unit, whereby the polysaccharide is converted to a polyelectrolyte in acidic media. Chitosan is considered one of the most valuable polymers for biomedical and pharmaceutical applications due to its biodegradability, biocompatibility, antimicrobial, non-toxicity and anti-tumour properties.

Chitosan effectively condenses DNA and protects it from nuclease degradation. Various conjugates such as thiolation, glycolation and folate chitosan are available. Chitosan is biodegradable, biocompatible, low immunogenicity and non-toxic at low molecular weights (10–50 kDa). It has been suggested that the toxicity of chitosan is perhaps due to impurities in the chitosan polymers [49–60].

4.2. Poly-L-lysine

Poly-L-lysine (ε-poly-L-lysine), as given in **Figure 6**, is a small natural homopolymer of the essential amino acid L-lysine that is produced by bacterial fermentation. Poly-L-lysine is a positively charged amino acid polymer with approximately one HBr per lysine residue. The hydrobromide allows the poly-L-lysine to be in a crystalline form soluble in water. Adhesion

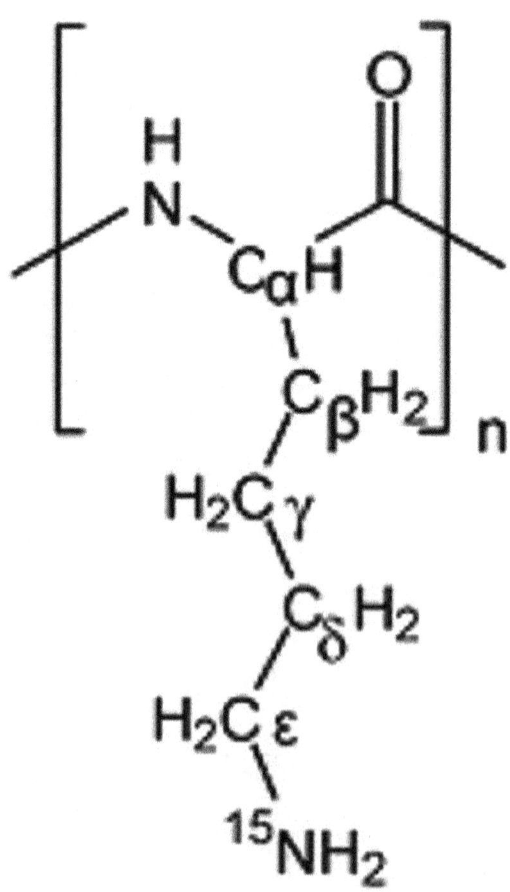

Figure 6. Structure of poly-L-lysine.

into the cell wall is based on the interaction between the negatively charged ions of the cell membrane and positive charge of poly-L-lysine. Simple electrostatic mixing of DNA and poly-L-lysine produces DNA particles with various structures. The mode of binding between the poly-L-lysine and DNA is cooperative and non-cooperative binding. Condensation between the DNA with the PLA depends upon the PLL chain length. Increase in the length of the PLL chain increases the condensation [61–68].

4.3. Polyethylenimine

Polyethylenimine (PEI), as given in **Figures 8** and **9**, is water-soluble, linear or branched polymers composed of the amine group and two carbon aliphatic CH_2CH_2 spacer. It is a weakly basic aliphatic polymer and polycationic one due to primary, secondary and tertiary amino groups. PEIs are available in different molecular masses and forms. Various forms of PEIs are shown in **Figure 7**–9. Linear polyethylenimines contain all secondary amines, whereas branched PEIs contain primary, secondary and tertiary amino groups. Due to their high cationic charge density at physiological pH, PEIs are able to form non-covalent complexes with DNA, siRNA and antisense oligodeoxynucleotide, and then brought into the cell via endocytosis. Once inside the cell, protonation of the amines results in an influx of counter-ions and a lowering of the osmotic potential, leading to bursts in the vesicle releasing the polymer-DNA complex (polyplex) into the cytoplasm. If the polyplex unpacks, then the DNA is free to diffuse to the nucleus; however, the long PEI chains have higher efficiency in gene transfection, and are more cytotoxic [69–93].

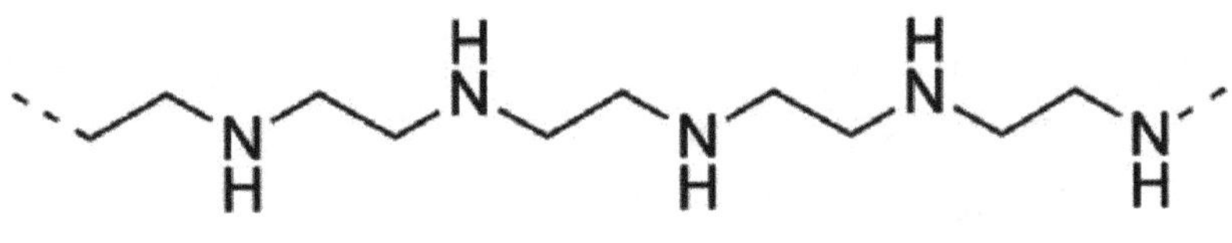

Figure 7. Structure of linear PEI.

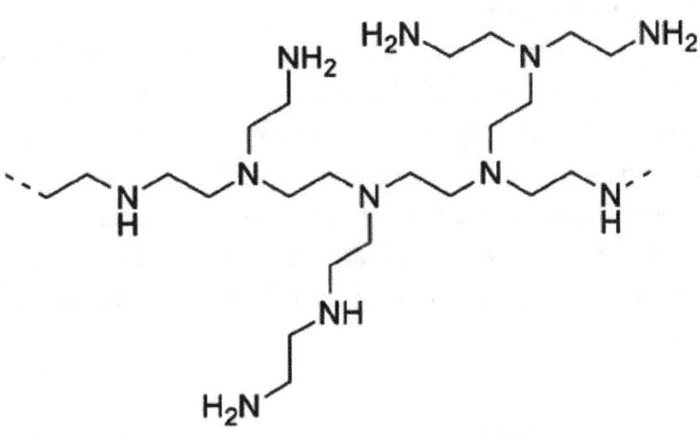

Figure 8. Structure of branched PEI.

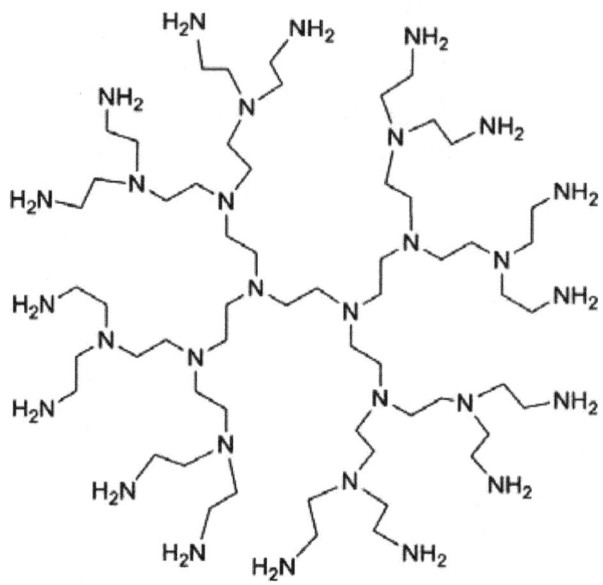

Figure 9. Structure of dendrimer PEI.

5. Cationic lipids

The four constituents are given as follows:

1. The cationic polar head group.
2. A hydrophobic chain that affects the physical properties of the lipid bilayer.
3. The space between two mentioned sections that improves chemical stability, biodegradability and gene transfection efficiency.
4. A backbone domain as a scaffold [19].

5.1. Monovalent cationic lipids

5.1.1. DOTMA

Chemically, it is N-[1-(2,3-dioleyloxy) propyl]-N,N,N-trimethylammonium chloride, as given in **Figure 10**, that consists of four different moieties: (1) a quaternary ammonium head group as the cationic head group, (2) a glycerol-based backbone, (3) two linkage bonds and (4) two hydrocarbon chains. Alternations can be made in the above moieties to reduce the toxicity and increase the gene transfection efficiencies. Replacement of a methyl group on the quaternary amine of DOTMA with a hydroxyl improves protein expression after gene transfection due to the replaced hydroxyl group in contact with the aqueous layer surrounding the liposome. Increase in the length of the aliphatic chain decreases the gene transfection and vice versa [94–98].

5.1.2. DOTAP

DOTAP, [1,2-bis(oleoyloxy)-3-(trimethylammonio) propane], as given in **Figure 11**, consists of a quaternary amine head group coupled to a glycerol backbone with two oleoyl chains.

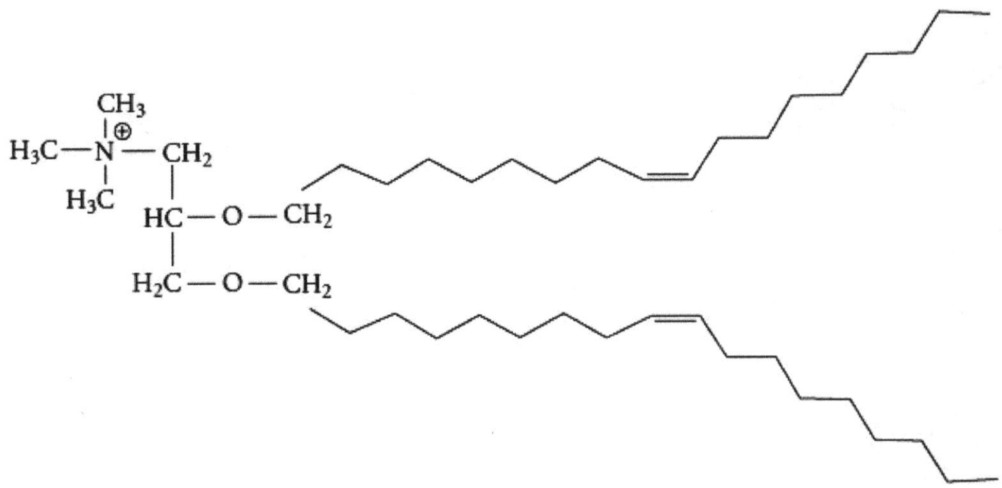

Figure 10. Structure of DOTMA.

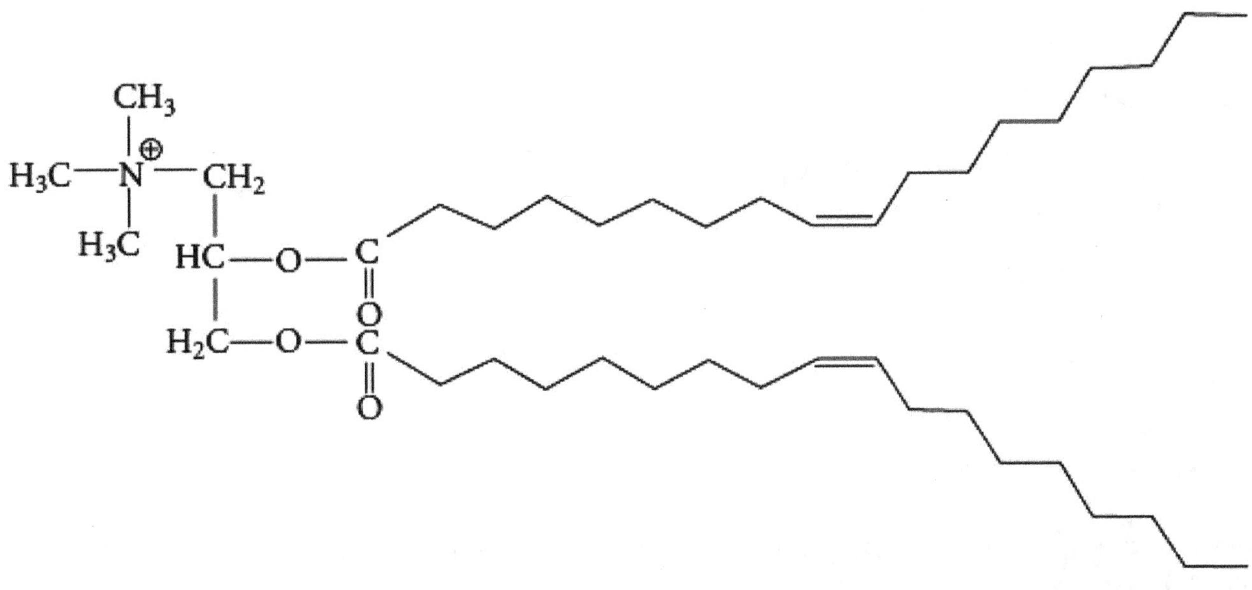

Figure 11. Structure of DOTAP.

The only differences between this molecule and DOTMA are that ester bonds link the chains to the backbone rather than ether bonds. The ester bonds present in the backbone are hydrolysable and lead to render the lipid biodegradable and reduce cytotoxicity. DOTAP cannot be used alone as a cationic liquid for gene delivery due to its dense positive charge, thereby preventing the ion exchange. Its gene-delivery efficiency can be changed by combining with other helper liquids [94, 99–103].

5.1.3. DC-Chol

3β[*N*-(*N′*,*N′*-dimethylaminoethane)-carbamoyl] cholesterol, as given in **Figure 12**, contains a cholesterol moiety attached by an ester bond to a hydrolysable dimethylethylenediamine. Due to the presence of cholesterol moiety, it is biocompatible and has good stability. The combination of DC-Chol and dioleoylphosphatidylethanolamine (DOPE) in the ratio 1:1

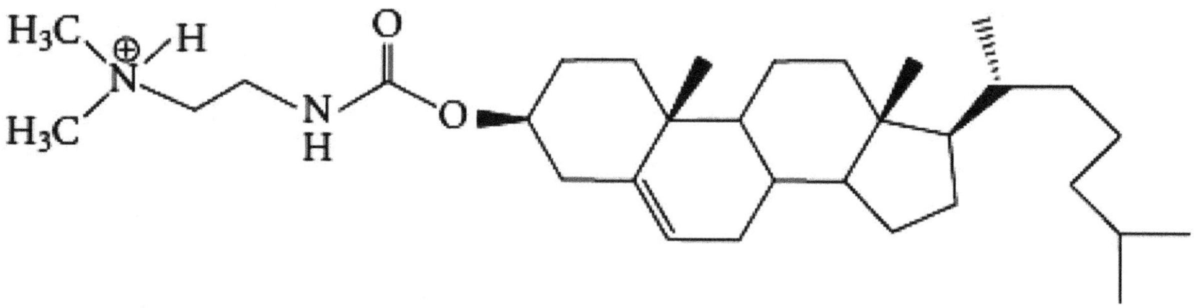

Figure 12. Structure of DC-Col.

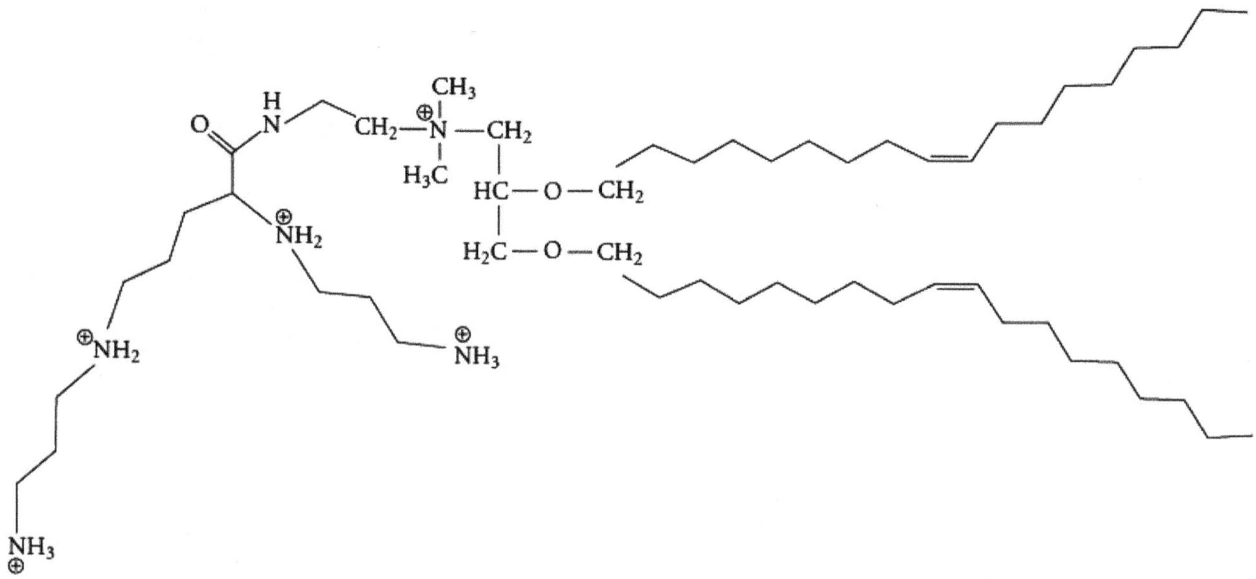

Figure 13. Structure of DOSPA.

reduces the lipoplex aggregation; it assists the DNA dissociation during gene delivery [94, 99, 100, 103, 104].

5.2. Multivalent cationic lipids

5.2.1. DOSPA

DOSPA is a derivative of DOTMA. Chemically, it is 2,3-dioleyloxy-N-[2(sperminecarboxamido) ethyl]-N,N-dimethyl-l-propanaminium trifluoroacetate, which is given in **Figure 13**. The difference between DOSPA and DOTMA is a spermine group, which is bound through a peptide bond to the hydrophobic chains. Spermine group allows more efficient packing of DNA due to its hydrogen bond interaction with the DNA [43, 94].

5.2.2. DOGS

DOGS, chemically it is di-octadecyl-amido-glycyl-spermine, structure of the DOGS is similar to DOSPA, as given in **Figure 14**. The molecular structures of both DOGS and DOSPA consist of a multivalent spermine head group and two 18-carbon alkyl chains. The saturated chains

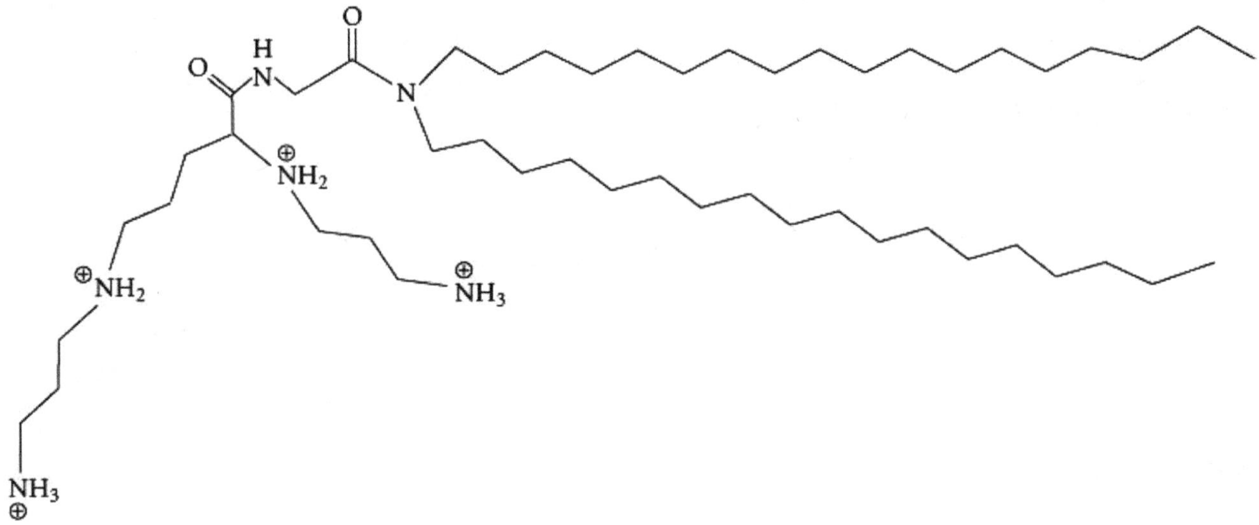

Figure 14. Structure of DOGS.

in DOGS are linked to the head group through a peptide bond. The packing ability of DNA by DOGS is due to its large head group molecule and the length of long unsaturated carbon chains. DOGS have efficient packing of DNA, due to its spermine head group. The presence of spermine head group in DOGS leads to efficient packing of DNA [94, 105–107].

6. Neutral lipids

The commonly used neutral lipids are dioleoylphosphatidylethanolamine (DOPE), as given in **Figure 15**, and dioleoylphosphatidylcholine (DOPC), as given in **Figure 16**. These neutral lipids are used in combination with the other cationic polymers. The gene transfection efficiencies of the cationic polymer are increased when it is used in combination with the helper neutral liquids. The increase in gene transfection efficiency is due to conformational shift to an inverted hexagonal packing structure like a honeycomb by DOPE at lower or acidic pH. The formation

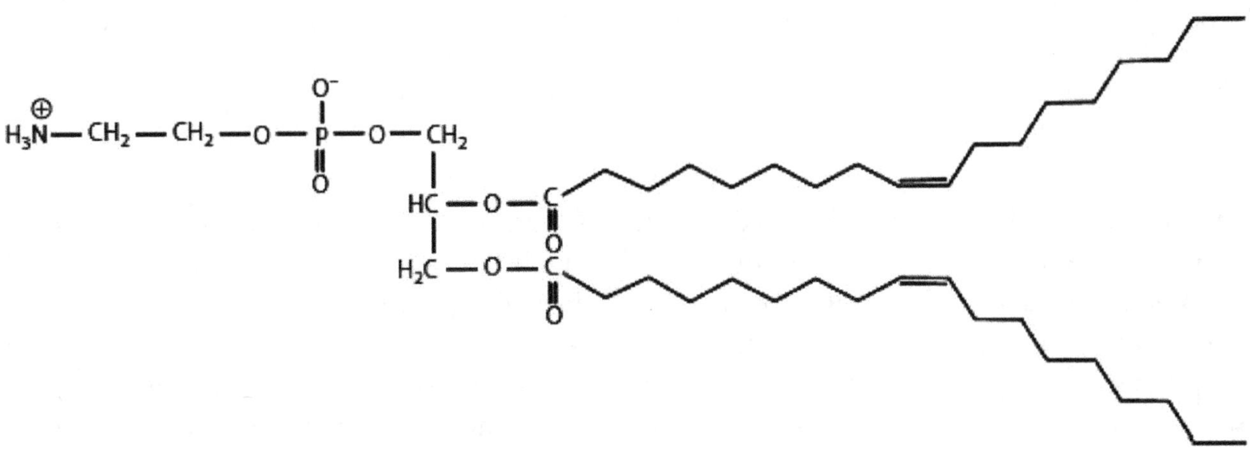

Figure 15. Structure of DOPE.

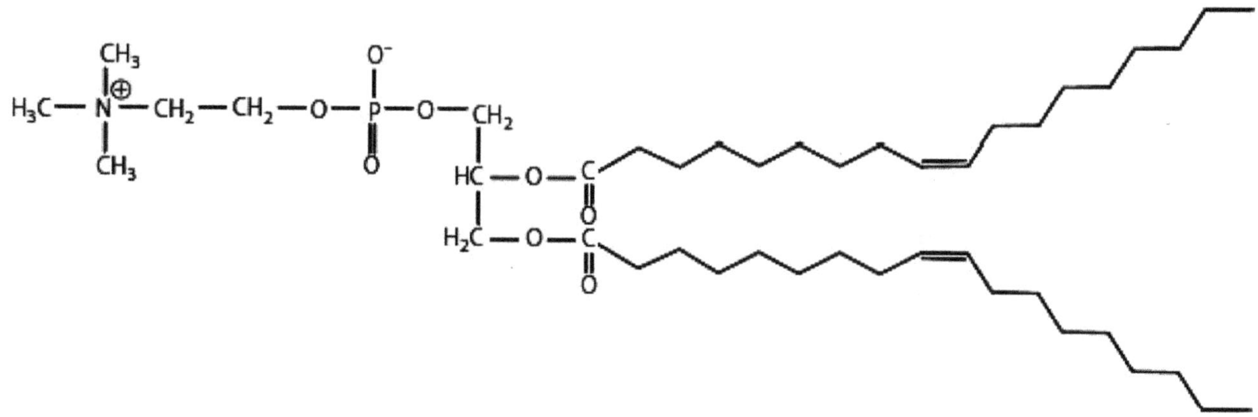

Figure 16. Structure of DOPC.

of inverted hexagonal-packing structure condenses the DNA inside by electrostatic interactions. During gene transfection, fusion and destabilization of the lipoplex occur which lead to the release of DNA from endosomal vesicles. Cationic polymers DOTAP, DC-Chol and other cholesterol derivatives have been incorporated with DOPE for gene transfection efficiency [94, 103, 108–114].

7. Poly(ethylene) glycol (PEG)

Chemically, poly(ethylene) glycol (PEG) ($C_{2n}H_{4n+2}O_{n+1}$) is a polyether or polymer of ethylene oxide.

The physical properties of PEG vary with respect to its chain length, whereas its chemical properties are almost the same. It is available in different molecular weights and different geometries such as branched PEG, star PEG and comb PEG. PEG is non-toxic and excreted through kidney. Degradation of the drug can be protected due to its surface modification property, and it has been extensively used as liposomal targeting by liposomal coating. The liposomes have longer circulation time in blood, reduced macrophage uptake, higher gene transfection efficiencies, larger available concentration and bioavailability [94, 115–120].

8. Conclusion

Nanotechnology is a science adapted in various research areas specifically in the drug-delivery system. At present, gene delivery system includes viral-based, non-viral-based and combined hybrid systems, which are widely used for the treatment of various diseases. To provide the desired concentration of the drug in the target site and therapeutic effect is critical of the drug-delivery system. Biopolymer is a biomaterial that has been utilized extensively for formulating genetic material into a nanoparticle either embedded or encapsulated within the polymeric matrix. Despite various biopolymers, choosing a suitable biopolymer, nanoparticle preparation procedure with desired properties can achieve the bio-distribution and effective delivery of the genetic material into the target site and regulate the damaged genes to produce the required proteins.

Author details

Sakthivel Lakshmana Prabu[1*] and Kandasamy Ruckmani[1,2]

*Address all correspondence to: slaxmanvel@gmail.com

1 Department of Pharmaceutical Technology, Bharathidasan Institute of Technology, Anna University, Tiruchirapalli, Tamil Nadu, India

2 Centre for Excellence in Nanobio Translational Research (CENTRE), National Facility on Drug Design (NFDD), Professor and Head, Department of Pharmaceutical Technology, Bharathidasan Institute of Technology, Anna University, Tiruchirapalli, Tamil Nadu, India

References

[1] Ward MA, Georgiou TK. Thermoresponsive polymers for biomedical applications. Polymers. 2011; 3: 1215–1242.

[2] Twaites BR, Alarcon CDH, Lavigne M, Saulnier A, Pennadam SS, Cunliffe D, et al., Thermoresponsive polymers as gene delivery vectors: Cell viability, DNA transport and transfection studies. J Control Release. 2005; 108: 472–473.

[3] Mahapatra A, Singh DK. Biodegradable nanoparticle are excellent vehicle for site directed in-vivo delivery of drugs and vaccines. J Nanobiotech. 2011; 9: 55.

[4] Mishra B, Vuppu S, Rath K. The role of microbial pullulan, a biopolymer in pharmaceutical approaches: A review. J Appl Pharm Sci. 2011; 1(6): 45–50.

[5] Eliyahu H, Barenholz Y, Domb AJ. Polymers for DNA delivery. Molecules. 2005; 10: 34–64.

[6] Pack DW, Hoffman AS, Pun S, Stayton PS. Design and development of polymers for gene delivery. Nature Rev Drug Discov. 2005; 4: 581–593.

[7] Dang JM, Leong KW. Natural polymers for gene delivery and tissue engineering. Adv Drug Del Rev. 2006; 58(4): 487–499.

[8] Nitta SK, Numata K. Biopolymer based nanoparticles for drug/gene delivery and tissue engineering. Int J Mol Sci. 2013; 14: 1629–1654.

[9] Harris TJ, Green JJ, Fung PW, Langer R, Anderson DG, Bhatia SN. Tissue specific gene delivery via nanoparticle coating. Biomaterials. 2010; 31(5): 998–1006.

[10] Labhasetwar V, Song C, Levy RJ. Nanoparticle drug delivery system for restenosis. Adv Drug Del Rev. 1997; 24(1): 63–85.

[11] Erdal C, Ali DS, Emre SC. Gene delivery systems: Recent progress in viral and non-viral therapy. In: Recent Advances in Novel Drug Carrier Systems, Ali DS (Ed.), 2012, InTech, Croatia, DOI: 10.5772/53392. http://www.intechopen.com/books/recent-advances-in-novel-drug-carrier-systems/gene-delivery-systems-recent-progress-in-viral-and-non-viral-therapy

[12] Liang GF, Zhu YL, Sun B, Hu FH, Tian T, Li SC, et al. PLGA-based gene delivering nanoparticle enhance suppression effect of miRNA in HePG2 cells. Nanoscale Res Lett. 2011; 6: 447.

[13] Jin S, Ye K. Mediated drug delivery and gene therapy. Biotechnol Prog. 2007; 23: 32–41.

[14] Georgiou TK, Vamvakaki M, Patrickios CS, Yamasaki EN, Phylactou LA. Nanoscopic cationic methacrylate star homopolymers: Synthesis by group transfer polymerization, characterization and evaluation as transfection reagents. Biomacromolecules. 2004; 5 (6):2221–2229.

[15] Godbey WT. Mikos AG. Recent progress in gene delivery using non-viral transfer complexes. J Cont Release. 2001; 72 (1–3):115–125.

[16] Xu FJ, Zhang ZX, Ping Y, Li J, Kang ET, Neoh KG. Star-shaped cationic polymers by atom transfer radical polymerization from beta-cyclodextrin cores for nonviral gene delivery. Biomacromolecules. 2009; 10 (2):285–293.

[17] Cloninger MJ. Biological applications of dendrimers. Curr Opin Chem Biol. 2002; 6 (6):742–748.

[18] Tang MX, Redemann CT, Szoka C. *In vitro* gene delivery by degraded polyamidoamine dendrimers. Bioconjug Chem. 1996; 7 (6):703–714.

[19] Dizaj SM, Jafari S, Khosroushahi AY. A sight on the current nanoparticle-based gene delivery vectors. Nanoscale Res Lett. 2014; 9: 252.

[20] Kabanov AV, Kabanov VA. DNA complexes with polycations for the delivery of genetic material into cells. Bioconjug Chem. 1995; 6: 7–20.

[21] Ledley FD. Pharmaceutical approach to somatic gene therapy. Pharm Res. 1996; 13: 1595–1614.

[22] Vijayanatham V, Thomas T, Thomas TJ. DNA nanoparticles and development of DNA delivery vehicles for gene therapy. Biochemistry. 2002; 41:14085–14094.

[23] Armstrong, TKC, Girouard LG, Anchordoquy TJ. Effects of PEGylation on preservation of cationic lipid/DNA complexes during freeze-thawing and lyophilization. J Pharm Sci. 2002; 91:2549–2558.

[24] Oyewumi MO, Rice KG. DNA nanoparticle gene delivery systems. In: Nanoparticle Technology for Drug Delivery. Gupta RB, Kompella UB (eds.). Marcel Dekker, New York, Vol. 159, 2006; pp. 361–379.

[25] Boas U, Heegaard PM. Dendrimers in drug research. Chem Soc Rev. 2004; 33: 43–63.

[26] Cheng Y, Wang J, Rao T, He X, Xu, T. Pharmaceutical applications of dendrimers: Promising nanocarriers for drug delivery. Front Biosci. 2008; 13: 1447–1471.

[27] Dufes C, Uchegbu IF, Schatzlein AG. Dendrimers in gene delivery. Adv Drug Deliv Rev. 2005; 57; 2177–2202.

[28] Gao Y, Gao G, He Y, Liu T, Qi R. Recent advances of dendrimers in delivery of genes and drugs. Mini Rev Med Chem. 2008; 8: 889–900.

[29] Gillies ER, Frechet JM. Dendrimers and dendritic polymers in drug delivery. Drug Discov Today. 2005; 10: 35–43.

[30] Svenson S, Tomalia DA. Dendrimers in biomedical applications--reflections on the field. Adv Drug Deliv Rev. 2005; 57: 2106–2129.

[31] Tomalia DA, Baker H, Dewald J, Hall M, Kallos G, Martin S, et al. Dendritic macromolecules: Synthesis of starburst dendrimers. Macromolecules. 1986, 19: 2466–2468.

[32] Klajnert B, Bryszewska M. Dendrimers: Properties and applications. Acta Biochem Polonica. 2001; 48: 199–208.

[33] Tomalia DA, Baker H, Dewald JR, Hall M, Kallos G, Martin S, Roeck J, Ryder, J., Smith P. A new class of polymers: Starburst-dendritic macromolecules. Polym J. 1985; 17: 117–132.

[34] Fischer M, Vogtle F. Dendrimers: From design to applications—A progress report. Angew Chem Int Ed. 1999; 38: 884–905.

[35] Zimmerman SC, Zeng F, Reichert DEC, Kolotuchin SV. Self-assembling dendrimers. Science. 1996; 271: 1095–1098.

[36] Frechet JMJ. Functional polymers and dendrimers: Reactivity, molecular architecture, and interfacial energy. Science. 1994; 263: 1710–1715.

[37] Tomalia DA, Dvornic PR. What promise for dendrimers? Nature. 1994; 372: 617–618.

[38] Twyman LJ, Beezer AE, Esfand R, Hardy MJ, Mitchell JC. The synthesis of water soluble dendrimers, and their application as possible drug delivery systems. Tetrahedron Lett. 1999; 40: 1743–1746.

[39] Waite CL, Sparks SM, Uhrich KE, Roth CM. Acetylation of pamam dendrimers for cellular delivery of sirna. BMC Biotechnol. 2009; 9: 38.

[40] Biswas S, Vladimir P. Torchilin. Dendrimers for siRNA delivery. Pharmaceuticals. 2013; 6: 161–183.

[41] Medina SH, El-Sayed MEH. Dendrimers as carriers for delivery of chemotherapeutic agents. Chem Rev. 2009; 109: 3141–3157.

[42] Tomalia DA, Frechet JMJ. Discovery of dendrimers and dendritic polymers: A brief historical perspective. J Polym Sci Part A: Polym Chem. 2002; 40(16): 2719–2728.

[43] Vuorimaa E, Urtti A, Seppänen R, Lemmetyinen H, Yliperttula M. Time-resolved fluorescence spectroscopy reveals functional differences of cationic polymer-DNA complexes. J Am Chem Soc. 2008; 130(35): 11695–11700.

[44] Guo P, Coban O, Snead NM, Trebley J, Hoeprich S, Guo S, et al. Engineering RNA for targeted siRNA delivery and medical application. Adv Drug Deliv Rev. 2010; 62: 650–666.

[45] Nimesh S, Gupta N, Chandra R. Cationic polymer based nanocarriers for delivery of therapeutic nucleic acids. J Biomed Nanotechnol. 2011; 7: 504–520.

[46] Synowiecki J, Al-Khateeb NA. Production, properties, and some new applications of chitin and its derivatives. Crit Rev Food Sci Nutr. 2003; 43(2): 145–171.

[47] Illum L. Chitosan and its use as a pharmaceutical excipient. Pharm Res. 1998; 15(9): 1326–1331.

[48] Hggard MK, Tubulekas I, Guan H, Edwards K, Nilsson M, Varum KM, et al., Chitosan as a nonviral gene delivery system. Structure property relationships and characteristics compared with polyethylenimine in vitro and after lung administration in vivo. Gene Ther. 2001; 8(14): 1108–1121.

[49] Lee M, Nah JW, Kwon Y, Koh JJ, Ko KS, Kim SW. Water-soluble and low molecular weight chitosan-based plasmid DNA delivery. Pharm Res. 2001; 18(4): 427–431.

[50] Lee D, Zhang W, Shirley SA, Kong X, Hellermann GR, Lockey RF, et al. Thiolated chitosan/DNA nanocomplexes exhibit enhanced and sustained gene delivery. Pharm Res. 2007; 24(1): 157–167.

[51] Mathur NK, Narang CK. Chitin and chitosan, versatile polysaccharides from marine animals. J Chem Educ. 1990; 67:938–42.

[52] Hudson SM, Jenkins DW. Chitin and chitosan. In: Encyclopedia of Polymer Science and Technology. Mark HF (ed.), New York, NY: Wiley; 2003. pp. 569–80.

[53] Krajewska B. Application of chitin- and chitosan-based materials for enzyme immobilizations: A review. Enzyme Microbiol Technol. 2004; 35: 126–139.

[54] Kanke M, Katayama H, Tsuzuki S, Kuramoto H. Application of chitin and chitosan to pharmaceutical preparations. Chem Pharm Bull. 1989; 37: 523–25.

[55] Kato Y, Onishi H, Machida Y. Application of chitin and chitosan derivatives in the pharmaceutical field. Curr Pharm Biotechnol. 2003; 4: 303–309.

[56] Anthonsen MW, Varum KM, Smidsrod O. Solution properties of chitosans: Conformation and chain stiffness of chitosans with different degrees of N-acetylation. Carbohyd Polym. 1993; 22: 193–201.

[57] Rinaudo M. Chitin and chitosan: Properties and applications. Prog Polym Sci. 2006; 31: 603–632.

[58] Alvarenga ES. Characterization and properties of chitosan. In: Biotechnology of Biopolymers. Elnashar M (ed.), InTech. 2011; pp. 91–108.

[59] Tungtong S, Okonogi S, Chowwanapoonpohn S, Phutdhawong W, Yotsawimonwat S. Solubility, viscosity and rheological properties of water-soluble chitosan derivatives. Maejo Int J Sci Technol. 2012; 6(2): 315–322.

[60] Pillai CKS, Paul W, Sharma CP. Chitin and chitosan polymers: Chemistry, solubility and fiber formation. Prog Polym Sci. 2009; 34: 641–678.

[61] Laemmli UK. Characterization of DNA condensates induced by poly(ethylene oxide) and polylysine. Proc Nat Acad Sci USA. 1975; 72(11): 4288–4292.

[62] Gonsho A, Irie K, Susaki H, Iwasawa H, Okuno S, Sugawara T. Tissue-targeting ability of saccharide-poly(L-lysine) conjugates. Biol Pharm Bull. 1994; 17(2): 275–282.

[63] Shima S, Sakai H. Polylysine produced by Streptomyces. Agric Biol Chem. 1977; 41: 1807–1809.

[64] Liu G, Molas M, Grossmann GA, Pasumarthy M, Perales JC, Cooper MJ, et al. Biological properties of poly-L-lysine-DNA complexes generated by cooperative binding of the polycation. J Biol Chem. 2001; 276(37): 34379–34387.

[65] Ferdous A, Watanabe H, Akaike T, Maruyama A. Comb-type copolymer: Stabilization of triplex DNA and possible application in antigene strategy. J Pharm Sci. 1998; 87(11): 1400–1405.

[66] Krikorian V, Kurian M, Galvin ME, Nowak AP, Deming TJ, Pochan DJ. Polypeptide-based nanocomposite: Structure and properties of poly(L-lysine)/Na_-montmorillonite. J Poly. Sci Part B: Poly Phys. 2002; 40: 2579–2586.

[67] Liu G, Molas M, Grossmann GA, Pasumarthy M, Perales JC, Cooper MJ, et al. Binding of the polycation complexes generated by cooperative biological properties of poly-l-lysine-DNA. J Biol Chem. 2001; 276: 34379–34387.

[68] Toncheva V, Wolfert MA, Dash PR, Oupicky D, Ulbrich K, Seymour LW, Schacht EH. Novel vectors for gene delivery formed by self-assembly of DNA with poly(L-lysine) grafted with hydrophilic polymers. Biochim Biophys Acta. 1998; 1380: 354–368.

[69] Boussif O, Zanta MA, Behr JP. Optimized galenics improve in vitro gene transfer with cationic molecules up to 1000-fold. Gene Ther. 1996; 3(12): 1074–1080.

[70] Godbey WT, Barry MA, Saggau P, Wu KK, Mikos AG. Poly(ethylenimine)-mediated transfection: A new paradigm for gene delivery. J Biomed Mater Res. 2000; 51(3): 321–328.

[71] Yao YH, Liu YB, Feng Y, Feng X, Xu DM, Yao SD. Synthesis and screening of polyethylenimine as a carrier for gene transfer into cultured human tumor cells. Ai Zheng. 2007; 26(7): 790–794.

[72] Sharma VK, Thomas M, Klibanov AM. Mechanistic studies on aggregation of polyethylenimine-DNA complexes and its prevention. Biotechnol Bioeng. 2005; 90(5): 614–620.

[73] Ogris M, Steinlein P, Kursa M, Mechtler K, Kircheis R, Wagner E. The size of DNA/transferrin-PEI complexes is an important factor for gene expression in cultured cells. Gene Ther. 1998; 5(10): 1425–1433.

[74] Lee H, Jeong JH, Park TG. A new gene delivery formulation of polyethylenimine/DNA complexes coated with PEG conjugated fusogenic peptide. J Con Rel. 2001; 76(1–2): 183–192.

[75] Aoki K, Furuhata S, Hatanaka K, Maeda M, Remy JS, Behr JP, et al. Polyethylenimine-mediated gene transfer into pancreatic tumor dissemination in the murine peritoneal cavity. Gene Ther. 2001; 8: 508–514.

[76] Boussif O, Lezoualc'h F, Zanta MA, Mergny MD, Scherman D, Demeneix B, et al. A versatile vector for gene and oligonucleotide transfer into cells in culture and in vivo: Polyethylenimine. Proc Natl Acad Sci USA. 1995; 92: 7297–7301.

[77] Lungwitz U, Breunig M, Blunk T, Gopferich A. Polyethylenimine-based non-viral gene delivery systems. Eur J Pharm Biopharm. 2005; 60: 247–266.

[78] Zintchenko A, Philipp A, Dehshahri A, Wagner E. Simple modifications of branched PEI lead to highly efficient sirna carriers with low toxicity. Bioconjug Chem. 2008; 19: 1448–1455.

[79] Lee M, Kim SW. Polyethylene glycol-conjugated copolymers for plasmid DNA delivery. Pharm Res. 2005; 22: 1–10.

[80] Nimesh S. Polyethylenimine as a promising vector for targeted sirna delivery. Curr Clin Pharmacol. 2012; 7: 121–130.

[81] Petersen H, Fechner PM, Martin AL, Kunath K, Stolnik S, Roberts CJ, Fischer D, Davies MC, Kissel T. Polyethylenimine-graft-poly(ethylene glycol) copolymers: Influence of copolymer block structure on DNA complexation and biological activities as gene delivery system. Bioconjug Chem. 2002; 13(4): 845–854.

[82] Godbey WT, Wu KK, Mikos AG: Poly (ethylenimine)-mediated gene delivery affects endothelial cell function and viability. Biomaterials. 2000; 22: 471–480.

[83] Godbey WT, Wu KK, Mikos AG. Size matters: Molecular weight affects the efficiency of poly(ethylenimine) as a gene delivery vehicle. J Biomed Mater Res. 1999; 45: 268–275.

[84] Fischer D, Bieber T, Li Y, Elsässer HP, Kissel T. A novel non-viral vector for DNA delivery based on low molecular weight, branched polyethylenimine: Effect of molecular weigh on transfection efficiency and cytotoxicity. Pharm Res. 1999; 16:1273–1279.

[85] Furgeson DY, Chan WS, Yockman JW, Kim SW. Modified linear polyethylenimine-cholesterol conjugates for DNA complexation. Bioconjugate Chem. 2003; 14: 840–847.

[86] Furgeson DY, Yockman JW, Janat MM, Kim SW: Tumor efficacy and biodistribution of linear polyethylenimine-cholesterol/DNA complexes. Mol Ther. 2004; 9: 837–845.

[87] Thomas M, Lu J, Ge Q, Zhang C, Chen J, Klibanov AM. Full deacylation of polyethylenimine dramatically boosts its gene delivery efficiency and specificity to mouse lung. Proc Natl Acad Sci USA. 2005; 102: 5679–5684.

[88] Jeon O, Yang HS, Lee TJ, Kim BS. Heparin-conjugated polyethylenimine for gene delivery. J Control Release. 2008; 132: 236–242.

[89] Xu Z, Shen G, Xia X, Zhao X, Zhang P, Wu H, et al. Comparisons of three polyethylenimine-derived nanoparticles as a gene therapy delivery system for renal cell carcinoma. J Transl Med. 2011; 9: 46.

[90] Felt O, Buri P, Guruy R. Chitosan: A unique polysaccharide for drug delivery. Drug Dev Ind Pharm. 1998; 24: 979.

[91] Tang MX, Szoka FC. The influence of polymer structure on the interactions of cationic polymers with DNA and morphology of the resulting complexes. Gene Ther. 1997; 4: 823–832.

[92] Fischer D, Bieber T, Li YX, Elsasser HP, Kissel T. A novel non-viral vector for DNA delivery based on low molecular weight, branched polyethylenimine: Effect of molecular weight on transfection efficiency and cytotoxicity. Pharm Res. 1999; 16: 1273–79.

[93] Von Harpe A, Petersen H, Li YX, Kissel T. Characterization of commercially available and synthesized polyethylenimines for gene delivery. J Control Release. 2000; 69: 309–322.

[94] Zhang X, Balazs DA, Godbey WT. Nanobiomaterials for nonviral gene delivery. In: Nanobiomaterials Hand Book, Balaji Sitharaman (ed.). CRC press, Taylor & Francis, 2011, pp.13–1 to 13–25.

[95] Ren T, Song YK, Zhang G, Liu D. Structural basis of DOTMA for its high intravenous transfection activity in mouse. Gene Therapy. 2000; 7: 764–768.

[96] Leventis R, Silvius JR. Interactions of mammalian cells with lipid dispersions containing novel metabolizable cationic amphiphiles. Biochim Biophys Acta. 1990; 1023: 124–32.

[97] Gao X, Huang L. A novel cationic liposome reagent for efficient transfection of mammalian cells. Biochem Biophys Res Commun. 1991; 179: 280–285.

[98] Malone RW, Felgner PL, Verma IM. Cationic liposome-mediated RNA transfection. Proc Natl Acad Sci USA. 1989; 86: 6077–6081.

[99] Zuidam NJ, Barenholz Y. Electrostatic and structural properties of complexes involving plasmid DNA and cationic lipids commonly used for gene delivery. Biochim Biophys Acta. 1998; 1368: 115–128.

[100] Zabner J, Fasbender AJ, Moninger T, Poellinger KA, Welsh MJ. Cellular and molecular barriers to gene transfer by a cationic lipid. J Biol Chem. 1995; 270: 18997–9007.

[101] Yang JP, Huang L. Time-dependent maturation of cationic liposome-DNA complex for serum resistance. Gene Ther.1998; 5: 380–387.

[102] Marchini C, Montani M, Amici M, Amenitsch H, Marianecci C, Pozzi D, et al. Structural stability and increase in size rationalize the efficiency of lipoplexes in serum. Langmuir. 2009; 25: 3013–3021.

[103] Gao X, Huang L. A novel cationic liposome reagent for efficient transfection of mammalian cells. Biochem Biophys Res Commun. 1991; 179(1): 280–285.

[104] Zuidam NJ, Barenholz Y. Electrostatic parameters of cationic liposomes commonly used for gene delivery as determined by 4-heptadecyl-7-hydroxycoumarin. Biochim Biophys Acta. 1997; 1329(2): 211–222.

[105] Behr JP, Demeneix B, Loeffler JP, Perez-Mutul J. Efficient gene transfer into mammalian primary endocrine cells with lipopolyamine-coated DNA. Proc Natl Acad Sci USA. 1989; 86(18): 6982–6986.

[106] Boukhnikachvili T, Aguerre-Chariol O, Airiau M, Lesieur S, Ollivon M, Vacus J. Structure of in-serum transfecting DNA-cationic lipid complexes. FEBS Lett. 1997; 409(2): 188–194.

[107] Remy JS, Sirlin C, Vierling P, Behr JP. Gene transfer with a series of lipophilic DNA-binding molecules. Bioconjug Chem. 1994; 5(6): 647–654.

[108] Farhood H, Gao X, Son K, Yang YY, Lazo JS, Huang L, et al. Cationic liposomes for direct gene transfer in therapy of cancer and other diseases. Ann N Y Acad Sci. 1994; 716: 23–34.

[109] Farhood H, Serbina N, Huang L. The role of dioleoyl phosphatidylethanolamine in cationic liposome mediated gene transfer. Biochim Biophys Acta. 1995; 1235(2): 289–295.

[110] Chesnoy S, Huang L. Structure and function of lipid-DNA complexes for gene delivery. Annu Rev Biophys Biomol Struct. 2000; 29: 27–47.

[111] Hui SW, Langner M, Zhao YL, Ross P, Hurley E, Cha K. The role of helper lipids in cationic liposome-mediated gene transfer. Biophys J. 1996; 71(2): 590–599.

[112] Kawakami S, Yamashita F, Nishikawa M, Takakura Y, Hashida M. Asialoglycoprotein receptor-mediated gene transfer using novel galactosylated cationic liposomes. Biochem Biophys Res Commun. 1998; 252(1): 78–83.

[113] Legendre JY, Szoka Jr FC. Delivery of plasmid DNA into mammalian cell lines using pH-sensitive liposomes: Comparison with cationic liposomes. Pharm Res. 1992; 9(10): 1235–1242.

[114] Zuhorn IS, Bakowsky U, Polushkin E, Visser WH, Stuart MC, Engberts JB, Hoekstra D. Nonbilayer phase of lipoplex-membrane mixture determines endosomal escape of genetic cargo and transfection efficiency. Mol Ther. 2005; 11(5): 801–810.

[115] Decastro M, Saijoh Y, Schoenwolf GC. Optimized cationic lipid-based gene delivery reagents for use in developing vertebrate embryos. Dev Dyn. 2006; 235(8): 2210–2219.

[116] Ishida O, Maruyama K, Tanahashi H, Iwatsuru M, Sasaki K, Eriguchi M, et al., Liposomes bearing polyethyleneglycol-coupled transferrin with intracellular targeting property to the solid tumors in vivo. Pharm Res. 2001; 18(7): 1042–1048.

[117] Huang RQ, Qu YH, Ke WL, Zhu JH, Pei YY, Jiang C. Efficient gene delivery targeted to the brain using a transferrin conjugated polyethyleneglycol-modified polyamidoamine dendrimer. FASEB J. 2007; 21(4): 1117–1125.

[118] Kim JK, Choi SH, Kim CO, Park JS, Ahn WS, Kim CK. Enhancement of polyethylene glycol (PEG)-modified cationic liposome-mediated gene deliveries: Effects on serum stability and transfection efficiency. J Pharm Pharmacol. 2003; 55(4): 453–460.

[119] Kim TI, Seo HJ, Choi JS, Jang HS, Baek JU, Kim K, et al. PAMAM-PEG-PAMAM: Novel triblock copolymer as a biocompatible and efficient gene delivery carrier. Biomacromolecules. 2004; 5(6): 2487–2492.

[120] Metselaar JM, Bruin P, de Boer LW, de Vringer T, Snel C, Oussoren C, et al. A novel family of L-amino acid-based biodegradable polymer-lipid conjugates for the development of long-circulating liposomes with effective drug-targeting capacity. Bioconjug Chem. 2003; 14(6): 1156–1164.

6

Numerical Simulation and Experimental Testing to Improve Olfactory Drug Delivery with Electric Field Guidance of Charged Particles

Jinxiang Xi and Xiuhua April Si

Abstract

Even though the direct nose-to-brain drug delivery has many clinical benefits, there are limited successes in delivering medication aerosols to the olfactory mucosa with standard inhalation devices. In this study, different delivery techniques were assessed in terms of their capacities to deliver drug aerosols to the olfactory epithelium. Specifically, the feasibility of electric field guidance of charged aerosols to the olfactory mucosa was evaluated in an image-based nose model both numerically and experimentally. Multi-sectional nasal cast replicas were fabricated using a 3-D printer to measure the olfactory deposition rates and visualize the deposition distributions. An intranasal deposition test platform was developed that comprised an electric field guidance system, a dry powder charging device, and a point-release nozzle. Numerical simulations were conducted using both ANSYS Fluent and COMSOL. We demonstrated that it is feasible to control charged particles inside the human nose use an external electric field. Both the point-release technique and electric field guidance of drug particles are essential in attaining optimal olfactory doses. Consistent deposition patterns were achieved between in vitro experiments and computational simulations. Future investigations are warrnated for further improvements of olfactory delivery through refining the particle generation, charging, and releasing, and navigation systems.

Keywords: intranasal drug delivery, olfactory region, particle point release, electric field guidance, charged particles, nose-to-brain drug delivery

1. Introduction

Drug delivery for treating neurological disorders such as brain tumors is often forestalled by the blood-brain-barrier (BBB), a network of endothelial cells with tight junctions in the brain's capillaries. The BBB, which can effectively protect the central nervous system (CNS) from pathogens, also prevents therapeutically agents from the diseased tissues in the CNS [1]. For years, the BBB has thwarted the utilizations of many new neurological medications for the treatment of CNS diseases such as brain tumors, depression, and Alzheimer's disease [2, 3].

Intranasal drug delivery to the olfactory epithelium is a noninvasive technique in which medications can bypass the BBB and enter the brain, eliciting a quick uptake and action onset of the therapeutic agents [3, 4]. However, there are many challenges that preclude effective drug delivery to the olfactory region. Very low doses can be delivered to the olfactory region (<1%) via the nasal route using standard nasal devices such as nasal pumps and sprays [5, 6]. It is primarily due to the complicated structure of the human nose, which is composed of convoluted, narrow, and passages. The olfactory mucosa is located at the uppermost part of the nose and is poorly ventilated due to its secluded location [7, 8]. As a result, standard nasal devices have limited success in olfactory drug delivery in that they rely on aerodynamic forces or particle inertia to drive medications to the target area [9]. After administration, particles travel passively with the nasal airflow. Thus, the behavior and fate of these aerosols are primarily dependent on their release positions and initial speeds. Due to the complex nasal structure, most of the medications will be trapped by the nasal valve and turbinate, with very few left that can make their final journey to the olfactory mucosa [10].

Nasal deposition of inhaled aerosols in humans has been extensively investigated both experimentally and numerically. Despite the high variability among subjects, these studies have persistently demonstrated that intranasal drug delivery can be influenced by multiple factors, including patient breathing, nasal devices, administration technique, and drug formulation. Furthermore, local or cellular-level deposition has been shown to be a more appropriate parameter than the total deposition in predicting adverse health effects or therapeutic outcomes. However, reports of local doses are still rare in comparison with extensive reports of total deposition fractions in the literature.

New techniques have been under active investigation to improve the olfactory delivery efficiency. Wang et al. [11] proposed to insert a catheter into the nose and administer drugs beneath the olfactory region. However, due to its invasive nature, this method has the risk to damage the wall tissues when guiding the catheter to the olfactory proximity, and patient compliance is expected to be low. Gizurarson [12] tested a nozzle with a narrow spray angle in hope that aerosols can penetrate into the posterior nose and the olfactory mucosa. A high pressure was necessary for this technique to overcome the nasal resistance so that particles can penetrate into the superior meatus. Hoekman and Ho [13] proposed to use a swirling flow in additional to the narrow spray plume so that particles can penetrate deeper into the upper posterior nose. Persistent higher doses in the olfactory region with swirling flows were measured in rats relative to nonswirling flows. However, extrapolating rat data to humans is difficult because of large interspecies discrepancies [14]. For instance, the olfactory region of a Sprague-Dawley rat covers 45% of the nasal surface, while only 5.2% of the human nasal surface is lined by the olfactory epitheliums in humans [15]. Realizing that a particle released into the nostril at a different location will follow a specific path, Si et al. [6] release drug particles from a selected site in the nostril (termed as point release). Improved dosage in the olfactory region was demonstrated using the point releasing than the traditional whole nostril releasing; however, the improvements are limited and still fall short of the doses to be clinically significant. Considering all the techniques aforementioned, it is noticed that once the particles are released into the nose the particle motions are dictated solely by the aerodynamic force. Due to the complex structure of the nasal structure, most particles will deposit in the nasal valve and turbinate region and only a low percentage of particles penetrate into the olfactory region.

Previous studies have suggested that charged particles under an appropriate electric field can improve nasal and pulmonary drug deliveries [16–18]. Improved dosing of charged particles has been demonstrated in the respiratory tract of both humans and animals [19–29]. Noticing that low olfactory deposition mainly result from the lack of control over particle dynamics in the nose, Xi et al. [25] numerically investigated the transport and deposition of charged particles under different electric strengths and showed that significantly enhanced olfactory dosage is practical by optimizing the electric field strength and particle releasing locations. Similarly, enhanced olfactory dosing can also be attained by using magnetic control of ferromagnetic particles. Preliminary computational simulations predicted a 45.0% deposition fraction for ferromagnetic particles, and the optimal particle diameter is around 15 μm [25].

One issue of intranasal drug delivery of nebulized droplets or small particles is the unwanted dosages into the lungs. One strategy to address this issue is the bi-directional delivery method, which administers medications into one nostril when the patient blows into the apparatus [30]. This method takes advantage of the nature that the soft palate lifts up during exhalation through the mouth, which closes the oropharynx and separates the nasal cavity from the rest of the respiratory tract. As a result, particle penetration into the lungs can be avoided. Moreover, the particles enter one nostril and exit from the other, which allows an increased time for drug deposition. This method did show an increase in medications depositing in the nasal cavity but failed to provide a practical way of dispensing an appreciable amount of medications to the olfactory region [31, 32]. It is hypothesized that by combining the electric guidance of charged particles with the bi-directional strategy, the olfactory dosage can be further enhanced.

The objective of this chapter is to improve the targeted delivery of neurological medications to the olfactory region using both computational modeling and *in vitro* experiments in an image-based nasal airway model. Different strategies were explored to control the intranasal particle motions in order to maximize the dose to the olfactory region and minimize the drug losses in other regions. These strategies include point release, vestibular intubation, deep intubation, and electric guidance of charged particles. Effect of breathing conditions, such as normal inhalation and bi-directional breathing, was also considered.

2. Design of experiments

2.1. Image-based reconstruction of nasal airway model

First, building anatomically accurate airway models is crucial for the assessment of the health outcomes of inhalation therapies. **Figure 1** illustrates the procedures of the translation from medical images into a high-quality computational mesh or *in vitro* casts of the nose-pharynx. To reconstruct the 3-D nasal airway model, MRI scans (512 × 512 pixel resolution) of a healthy 53-year-old male were used. The multislice MRI images were segmented using MIMICS (Materialise, Ann Arbor, MI) to convert the raw image data into a set of cross-sectional contours that define the solid geometry (**Figure 1a**). A surface geometry was reconstructed based on these contours in Gambit (Ansys, Inc.). This surface geometry as shown in **Figure 1b** was subsequently imported into ANSYS ICEM (Ansys, Inc.) for meshing. In general, unless for extremely high-quality image data, a solid model that is directly reconstructed from medical images cannot be used for computational meshing due to the artifacts and resolution limits inherent in current imaging techniques. Considering the high complexity of the nasal airway structure, an unstructured mesh was generated with fine boy-fitted cells in the near-wall region (**Figure 1c**). This nasal geometry has been reconstructed with minimal surface smoothing and was intended to accurately represent the nasal anatomy of human adults. More details of image-based model development can be viewed in a recent video article from our group [33]. This model was also manufactured into hollow casts for *in vitro* studies using 3-D prototyping techniques (**Figure 1d**).

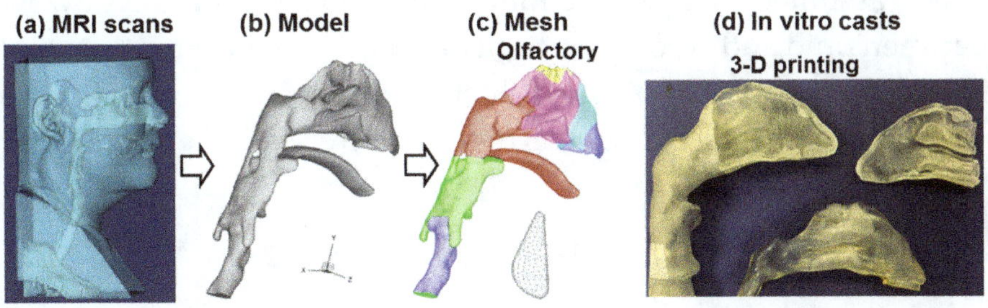

Figure 1. Procedures of translating medical images into computational mesh and *in vitro* casts. First, MRI scans were segmented to reconstruct the airway surface model. Second, high-quality computational mesh was generated with fine near-wall cells. Hollow *in vitro* cast replicas were also fabricated using 3-D printing technique and were used for experimental deposition studies. In order to study deposition distributions, the nasal cavity was divided into different regions: vestibule-valve region (VV), turbinate region (TR), nasopharynx (NP), and olfactory region (OL) that was at the very top of the nasal cavity (yellow color in middle panel).

2.2. Computational fluid-particle transport models

2.2.1. *Airflow and particle dynamics*

Depending on breathing activities, multiple flow regimes, such as laminar, transitional, or fully turbulent, can exist in the human respiratory tract. The two-order turbulence models have been shown to adequately capture the main flow features and particle transport if a fine body-fitted mesh is used near the wall [34]. In particular, the low Reynolds number (LRN) k-ω model has been widely adopted in computational studies of respiratory flows. It has been validated in many studies to be able to accurately predict the particle transport and deposition in the oral airway [35, 36], nasal cavity [8], and lungs [37, 38]. Moreover, the LRN k-ω model was demonstrated to accurately predict the flow regime transition when the turbulent viscosity approaches zero [39]. Governing equations for the turbulent kinetic energy (k) and dissipation rate (ω) can be found in Wilcox [39].

Transport of monodisperse aerosols was solved using the discrete Lagrangian tracking algorithm through the integration of the particle dynamic equation. Spherical shape was assumed for each particle. The particle diameters range from 0.2 to 5 μm, which have very low Stokes numbers ($St_k = \rho_p d_p^2 UC_c/18\mu D_h << 1$), with ρ_p being the density of the particles (1.0 g/cm^3), U being the fluid velocity, C_c being the Cunningham slip factor [40], and D_h being the nostril effective diameter. The governing equation of Lagrangian tracking is

$$\frac{dv_i}{dt} = \frac{f}{\tau_p C_c}(u_i - v_i) + g_i(1-\alpha) + f_{i,Brownian} + f_{i,lift} + f_{i,electric} \tag{1}$$

where u_i is the airflow velocity, v_i is the particle speed, f is the drag coefficient, and $\tau_p = \rho_p d_p^2/18\mu$ is the particle characteristic time to respond to flow variations. The drag coefficient f was based on the equation of Morsi and Alexander [41]. Gravity and Saffman lift force were also included for particles >1 μm [42]. Brownian motion effects were included for submicron particles [35]. It was assumed that particle motion had no effect on the flow field, i.e., a one-way coupling between fluid and aerosols in light of the dilute concentration of pharmaceutical aerosols. The impact of the anisotropic flow fluctuations near the wall was also included by applying an anisotropic turbulence model as described by Matida et al. [43]:

$$u'_n = f_v \xi \sqrt{2k/3} \quad \text{and} \quad f_v = 1 - exp(-0.002y^+) \tag{2}$$

In the above equation, f_v is a damping component normal to the airway wall and ξ is a random number generated by the Gaussian probability density function.

2.2.2. *Electric field and electric force*

For the direct current (DC) field, the electric potential, U_{DC}, is attained by solving the Poisson's equation,

$$-\nabla \cdot \varepsilon_0 \varepsilon_r \nabla U = 0 \tag{3}$$

where ε_0 and ε_r are the absolute (F/m) and (dimensionless) permittivity of the free space, respectively. The zero value on the right-hand side of the equation means no space charge. For the alternating current (AC) field, the AC potential is computed by solving the conservation of electric currents [44]:

$$-\nabla\cdot(\sigma + j\omega\varepsilon_0\varepsilon_r)\nabla V = 0 \tag{4}$$

In the above equation, σ is the electrical conductivity and ω is the alternating frequency (Hz). Considering that the equations for both DC and AC fields are linear, the total electric field can be obtained by superposing the DC and AC fields.

The electric force as a function of the electric field can be expressed as

$$f_{i,electrophoretic} = neE = ne\left(E_{DC} + E_{AC}\right) \tag{5}$$

where n is the nondimensional charge number and e is the elementary charge (e = 1.6 × 10^{-19} C). E_{DC} and E_{AC} are the intensity of the DC and AC electric fields, respectively, which are calculated as follows:

$$E_{DC} = -\nabla U;\ E_{AC} = -real[\nabla\tilde{V}e^{(j\omega t)}] \tag{6}$$

The symbol $\tilde{V}$ means that the AC potential is a complex variable.

2.2.3. *Numerical methods*

To solve the concomitant flow-electric-particle multiphysics involved in each of the cases considered, ANSYS Fluent (Canonsburg, PA) and COMSOL (Burlington, MA) were employed to simulate the airflow, electric field, and particle tracing. User-supplied functions (UDFs) in the language of Fortran ad C were developed for the calculation of mass flux to the wall, initial particle profile, Brownian force [45], near-wall velocity interpolation [36], and anisotropic turbulence effect [43]. Body-fitted computational mesh was generated to resolve the large gradients of flow velocities near the airway surface. Local mesh refinement was made considering the complex anatomy of the nasal cavity. A grid independence study was performed by evaluating various grid densities, such as 0.4, 0.8, 1.2, and 2.2 million computational cells. The variation in predicted deposition fraction was 1% or less when changing the grid density from 1.2 to 2.4 million. Therefore, the computational mesh of 1.2 million cells was implemented for all subsequent simulations.

2.3. Experimental setup and materials

2.3.1. *In vitro test platform*

The *in vitro* test platform for intranasal delivery of charged particles has four components: a particle charging apparatus (**Figure 2a**), a three-dimensional replica of a normal human nasal cavity, voltage supplies to induce electric fields, and a scale to quantify deposition. A powder coating system (Powder System Solutions, Nolensville, TN) was modified to charge the dry powders. Copper plates and DC power supplies (MPJA, Lake Park, FL) were implemented to produce external electric fields. A high-precision electronic scale (Sartorius) was utilized to quantify the deposited mass of aerosols. A microscope (AmScope B120C-E1) was used to estimate the diameter of the charged particles. Details of the sectional nasal cast preparation and experimental procedures are described below.

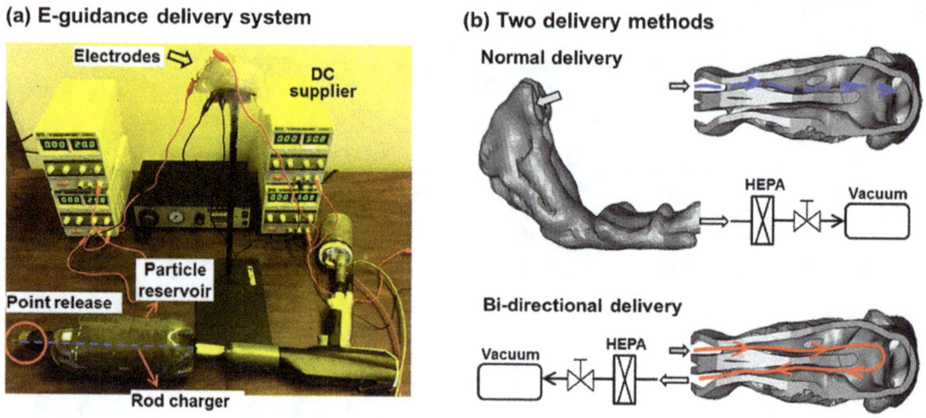

Figure 2. *In vitro* experiments to test the feasibility of electric-guided olfactory drug delivery: (a) experimental setup and (b) two delivery strategies: normal and bi-directional. In both delivery strategies, drug particles are administered into the right-side nostril. However, particles exit the airway through the trachea in the normal delivery and exit through the left nostril in the bi-directional delivery.

2.3.2. Multisectional nasal cast

A multisectional nasal replica was prepared that allows quantitative measurement of regional deposition as well as direct visualization of deposition distributions. After developing the nasal airway geometry model as listed in 2.1, Magics (Materialise, Ann Arbor, MI) was utilized to create the nasal cast wall with a constant layer of 4 mm. The nasal replica was divided into several parts: the nasal vestibule and valve, turbinate, and nasopharynx, as shown in **Figure 1b**. Step-shaped grooves were created at the ends of each replica section for proper sealing and easy assembly. To visualize deposition distributions within the nasal cavity, the nasal replica was cut open along the top ridge of the right nasal passage to disclose the septum and turbinate in the right nose. In order to characterize the olfactory doses, the section representing the olfactory mucosa was separated from the other region. An in-house 3-D printer with a resolution of 16 μm (0.0006 in) (Stratasys Objet30 Pro, Northville, MI) was utilized to fabricate the nasal casts using polypropylene (Veroclear, Northville, MI) that has a clear color and allows for a smooth surface.

2.3.3. Experimental procedures

Dry powders of 30 μm in size (matte black powder coat paint) were selected in this study for their easy availability and excellent charging properties. and easy ava. The modification made to the powder coating system integrated a charging reservoir (a 2-L bottle) to the nozzle of the charging gun (**Figure 2a**). An additional metal wire was added to extend the charging rod to the reservoir exit, with the wire's length being parallel with the direction of the flow of solid particles. A high voltage supply (Spectracoat coating system), which has an adjustable potential output of 0–100 kV, was connected to the rod. The solid particles were distributed out of a 4-mm-diameter nozzle and subsequently distributed into a multisectional nasal cast replica. Three copper-plated electrodes (A, B, C) were attached to the top of the nose replica, and one copper-plated electrode (D) was attached to the bottom of the replica. Charged dry powders were distributed from the powder coat gun for 20 seconds per trial. For the normal delivery, particles were administered into one nostril and exited through the nasopharynx (**Figure 2b**, upper panel). In contrast, for the bi-directional delivery, the bottom of the pharynx was blocked to simulate the uplifted soft palate, while particles were administered into one nostril and exited through the other (**Figure 2b**, lower panel). A vacuum pump (Robinair 3 CFM, Warren, MI) was connected to the exit of the nasal replica in each test case to simulate the respiration. An in-line flow meter (Omega, FL-510, Stamford, CT) was used to monitor the volumetric flow rate.

2.3.4. Statistical analysis

The variable of interest in this study was the ratio of the olfactory dosage to the vestibule-turbinate dosage (i.e., olfactory-nasal dosage ratio). Results were represented as the main ± standard deviation (SD), with SD being calculated from five trials for each scenario. Statistical analysis software Minitab (State College, PA) was applied to analyze the deposition data. Tukey's method and analysis of variance (ANOVA) were implemented to assess the data variances. The difference was considered statistically significant if the *p*-value was <0.05.

3. Results

3.1. Numerical (ANSYS Fluent) assessment of olfactory delivery with nasal intubations

Figure 3a shows the motion of 1 μm particles inside the nasal airway predicted using ANSYS Fluent. It is observed that particles that are released from the tip of the nostril move along the upper nasal cavity, while particles from the base of the nostril move along the nasal floor. At an inhalation rate of 20 L/min (normal breathing condition), it takes around 0.02–0.03 seconds for the particles to be delivered to the olfactory region after administration (**Figure 3a**). Faster movements of particles are noted in the middle passages and slow-moving aerosols are observed in the near-wall region. The numerical model in this study had been validated by comparing to *in vitro* deposition data measured in a comparable nasal replica. Good agreement was obtained between the numerically predicted and *in vitro* measurements in comparable nasal casts by Cheng et al. [46, 47] (**Figure 3b**). It is emphasized that the computational nasal airway model in this study and the *in vitro* nasal casts in Cheng et al. [46] were reconstructed from the same set of MRI images.

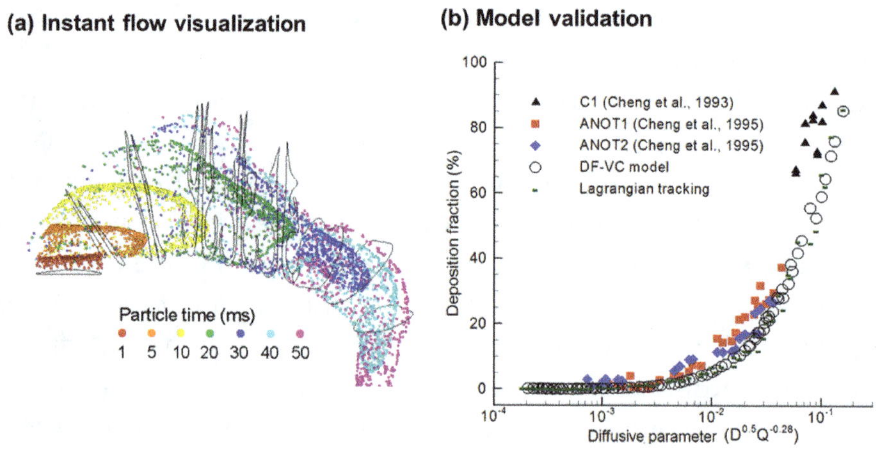

Figure 3. Nasal particle motion and model validation. (a) Snapshots of particle motion at varying instants. (b) Good agreement in nasal deposition between the numerical predictions and experimental measurements of Cheng et al. [46, 47].

In this study, we first tested the feasibility of optimizing particle release positions (smart delivery concept) for intranasal olfactory drug delivery. Two protocols were tested, with the first termed as "vestibular intubation" where particles are released from a selective point in the vestibule (**Figure 4a**), while the second protocol being the "deep intubation" with the nebulizer nozzle inserted directly below the olfactory mucosa (**Figure 4a**). In principle, particles released into the upper vestibule moves along the upper nasal passage and therefore are more likely to deposit in the olfactory region. The computational simulations also confirm that it can deliver higher doses to the olfactory region for both particle sizes considered (150 nm and 1 μm). Furthermore, the deposition pattern appears to be focused close to the olfactory region. Considering the deep intubation protocol, the nozzle was inserted right below the olfactory mucosa so that filtration by the nasal valve and turbinate can be avoided. Therefore, elevated doses were predicted in the olfactory proximity with nonsignificant doses in the middle and inferior turbinate regions.

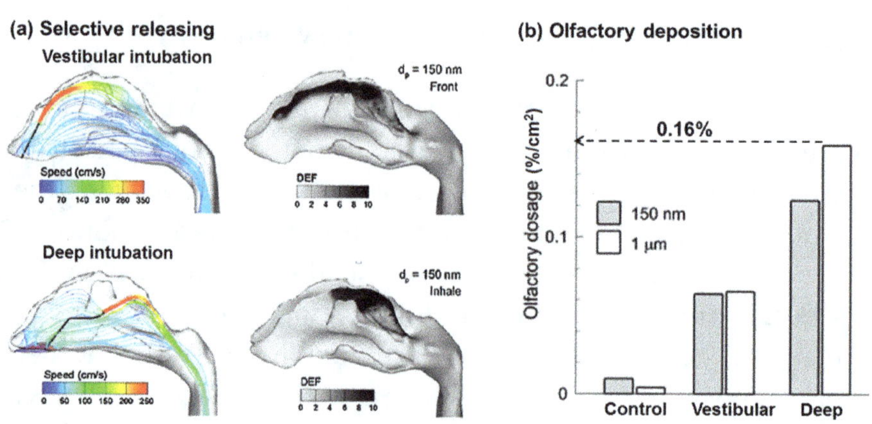

Figure 4. Two delivery protocols with selective particle releasing: vestibular intubation and deep intubation. (a) Streamlines and surface deposition. (b) Olfactory deposition rate with the vestibular and deep intubations in comparison to the conventional delivery method, which releases drugs to the entire nostril (control case).

The olfactory doses between the vestibular and deep intubation protocols, as well as the conventional delivery method, were compared on the basis of deposition fraction per area (%/cm^2) (**Figure 4b**). The surface area of the olfactory mucosa in this study (**Figure 1c**) is 6.8 cm^2. Overall speaking, both intubation protocols significantly enhanced the olfactory targeting while the deep intubation outperformed the vestibular intubation. However, it is noted that even using the deep intubation method, very low fractions of administered dose (0.16%/cm^2 or 1.09% in the olfactory region) were delivered to target, while nearly 99% was lost in other regions, causing tremendous waste and potentially significant unwanted side effects. Therefore, further efforts are needed to explore strategies that can precisely target drug particles to the olfactory region while minimizing drug loss to other tissues.

3.2. Sar-Gel visualization of nasal deposition distributions

Sar-Gel visualization of the local deposition inside the nasal replica is displayed in **Figure 5** for two common nasal spray products (Astelin and Nasonex). The angle of the spray plume was approximately 35° ± 0.8° for Astelin and 20° ± 0.5° for Nasonex. The majority of spray droplets were trapped by the narrow flow-limiting nasal valve. It is noted that the drug distribution is largely dictated by the physical properties of spray droplets. The high filtration by the slit-shaped nasal valve can be attributed to the high inertia of spray droplets that have large sizes (70–90 μm) and exit from the spray pumps with relatively high speeds. Dripping was absent in Astelin that had a wide spray plume angle, while dripping was observed in Nasonex that had a narrow plume and was prone to cause local droplet accumulation (**Figure 5a** vs. **5b**). Deposition of Astelin appeared to be more dispersed than Nasonex.

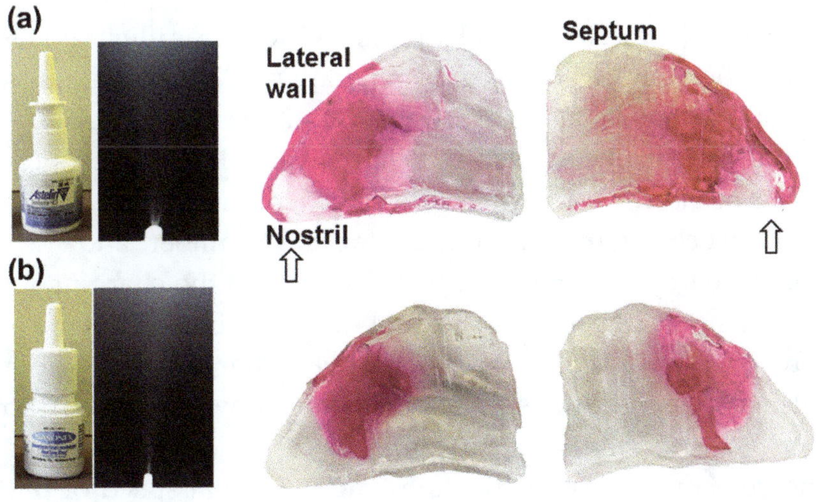

Figure 5. Deposition pattern in the nose with two nasal spray products: (a) Astelin and (b) Nasonex. The majority of spray droplets deposit in the nasal vestibule and valve region and cannot reach the olfactory region.

A commercially available jet nebulizer (Philips Respironics InnoSpire) was utilized to evaluate particle deposition in the nose. Nebulized aerosols were released into the nostril at an orientation 15° from the vertical direction. As shown in **Figure 6**, most administered droplets deposited in the anterior nose (vestibule and valve regions). Aerosol deposition in the middle and inferior turbinate was also observed, but at a lower level than the anterior nose. Almost no aerosol deposited in the superior meatus and olfactory region (dashed blue ellipse). The above deposition distribution is similar as that reported in Laube [48] who observed predominant doses in the anterior nose. Both **Figures 5** and **6** corroborate the observation that conventional nasal devices cannot deliver adequate doses to the olfactory mucosa, and thus advanced drug delivery systems are warranted in order to achieve clinical significant olfactory delivery.

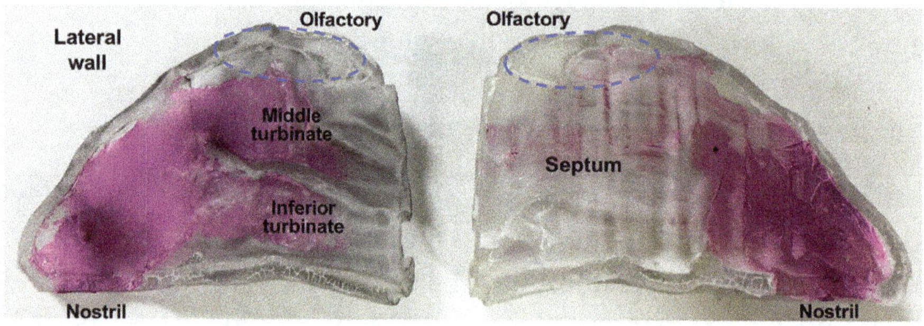

Figure 6. Sar-Gel visualization of the nasal deposition pattern using a standard nebulizer. Even though some nebulized aerosols escape the nasal valve filtration, most of them deposit in the turbinate region and only a very small fraction reaches the olfactory region.

3.3. Multiphysics (COMOL) simulations of olfactory dosing delivery of charged particles

3.3.1. Electric-guided olfactory delivery diagram

The principle of olfactory drug delivery under electric guidance is illustrated in **Figure 7**. There are four essential functions in this device: (1) generation, (2) charging, (3) focusing, and (4) navigation of the pharmaceutical aerosols (**Figure 7a**). A head brace can be added to fix the device relative to the patient's head. Commercially available nebulizers (droplets) and dry powder inhalers can be used to generate aerosolized particles [49]. Particle charging was achieved by letting particles going through a charging chamber, and the acquired charge number can be controlled by varying the voltage supply to the charging chamber [50]. The focusing chamber is composed of several slits [51], with the first slit having a positive voltage and the last one having zero voltage. When the positively charged dry powders travel through these slits, a repulsive force from the slit pushes the dry powders inward to form a focused beam; simultaneously, the forward component of the repulsion accelerates the aerosol beam to a certain exiting velocity. The benefit of knowing the initial speed of particles is that the deposition pattern can be estimated beforehand so that the optimal delivery protocol can be selected. Another benefit is that drug delivery will be more independent of the breathing condition if the initial particle velocities are much higher than the respiratory airflow velocities. This feature is very desirable for inhalation therapy for seniors or people with breathing problems or low compliance capability. After particles were administered into the nose, they will experience an external electric force and divert from their original course. For optimal drug delivery to the olfactory region, particles should move along the middle passage of the nose to minimize wall losses (**Figure 7b**). In this chapter, we will evaluate whether it is feasible to enhance the olfactory doing through electric guidance of charged particles with charge levels and electric potentials that are safe to humans.

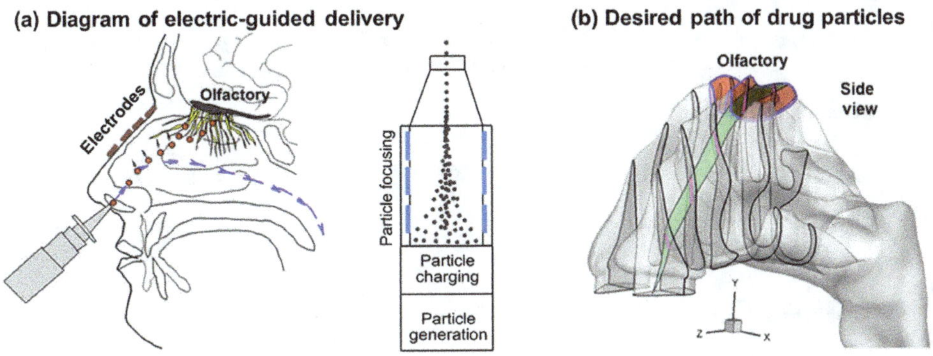

Figure 7. Diagram of electric-guided olfactory drug delivery. (a) Charged particles will be attracted toward the olfactory region by an applied electric field. (b) For optimal olfactory drug delivery, particles should travel along the middle plane of the nasal passage.

3.3.2. Idealized 2-D nose model

The proposed delivery protocol was first evaluated in an idealized 2-D nose configuration. The inhaled airflow field in the nose is shown in **Figure 8a**. There are three streams due to the obstruction of the inferior and middle turbinate. The upper flow stream is further divided by the superior turbinate. Only a small fraction of inhaled airflow was ventilated into the uppermost olfactory region. Due to poor olfactory ventilations, inhaled particles are unlikely to be conveyed to the olfactory region by convection or inertia. It is also observed in **Figure 8a** that stream traces initiating from the posterior naris move toward the nasal floor, while those from the anterior naris move toward the upper passage (superior meatus). It is hypothesized that pharmaceutical agents released into the at the naris tip have a larger chance to deposit into the olfactory mucosa.

To generate a desirable external electric field, four electrodes were put on top of the nose. The electrode voltages were specified to be −3, −8, −12, and 0 V, respectively (**Figure 8a**). The small electric potential (3 V) above the nasal vestibule was intended to impart particles an upward attraction. The electric potential above the middle nose was increased to −8 V to attract particles further toward the olfactory mucosa. The electric potential close to the olfactory region was around −12 V in order to catch the charged aerosols. **Figure 8b** shows the numerically predicted electric field (E-field), which changes from nearly 0 V at the nostrils to about −12 V at the olfactory region.

From **Figure 8c**, electric guidance of charged particles significantly increased the olfactory dosing, which was two orders of magnitude higher in comparison with that when an electric field was absent. **Figure 8d** displays particle transport in the nose 1 second after administration. The majority of particles (~95%) deposit in the olfactory mucosa. As a comparison, only 0.77% deposit in the olfactory region without an electric field.

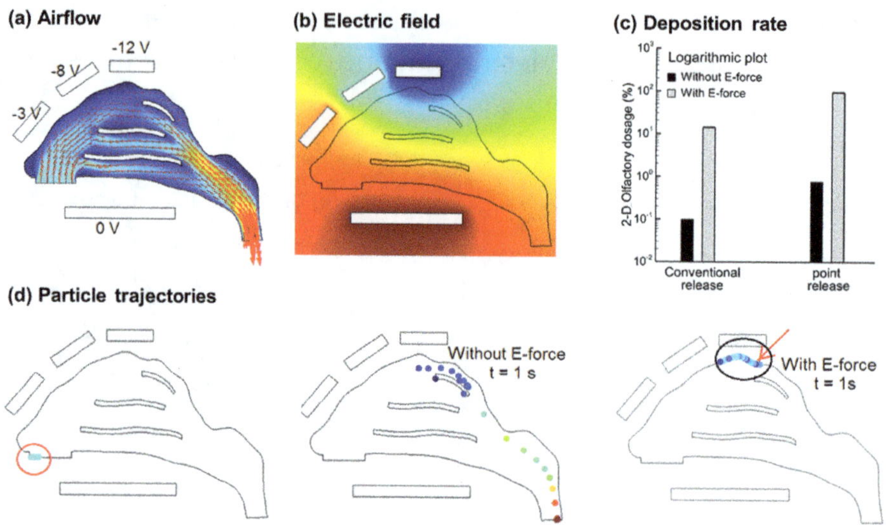

Figure 8. Computational modeling of electric-guided delivery in a 2-D nose model. (a) Airflow field, (b) electric field, (c) comparison of the olfactory deposition rates with and without electric guidance for conventional and point-release delivery techniques, and (d) particle trajectories with and without electric force for the point-release technique. Electric-guided delivery of charged particles can enhance the olfactory doses by two orders of magnitude relative to the case without an electric field.

3.3.3. Realistic 3-D nose model

A comparison of deposition patterns in the image-based 3-D nose model with and without electric guidance is shown in **Figure 9a**. The charge number of the particles is 5000, and the particle size is 0.5 μm. With an appropriate electric field, 3.7% of inhaled particles reached the olfactory mucosa (**Figure 9a**). However, only 0.06% of administered aerosols delivered to the olfactory mucosa without electric guidance.

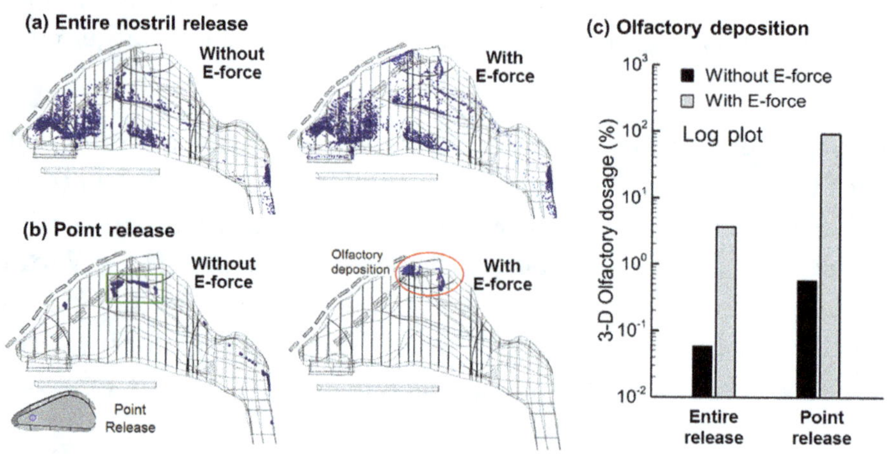

Figure 9. Computational modeling of electric-guided delivery in an anatomically accurate 3-D nose model. Particle deposition patterns were compared with and without electric forces for (a) the entire nostril release method (conventional delivery) and (b) the point-release method. (c) Significantly improved olfactory doses were achieved with electric guidance for both the conventional and point-release techniques. Electric-guided delivery increased the olfactory doses by approximately two orders of magnitude than without an electric field.

To further improve drug delivery to the olfactory mucosa, particles are released into a small point in the anterior nostril to minimize the filtration by the nasal valve and turbinate. With appropriate electric field strength, a majority (92%) of administered particles were dispensed to the olfactory region (red ellipse) that would have otherwise landed in the upper posterior nose in the absence of an electric field (**Figure 9b**, right vs. left). A careful study of the deposition distribution in the upper nose (green square, **Figure 9b**) shows that more aerosols are deposited on the turbinate wall (outer side) than on the septum (inner side). To minimize deposition in the turbinate, a lateral force is required to keep the aerosols from depositing onto the turbinate.

3.4. *In vitro* experiments of electric-guided olfactory delivery

3.4.1. *Normal inhalation delivery*

Particle deposition of charge particles was assessed in the realistic nose replicas. In order to generate a desirable electric field, two positive electrodes (25 and 100 V) were placed above the nose, and one electrode was placed below the nose as the ground. **Figure 10** compares deposition patterns of particles without and with electrostatic charges. For neutral particles, most inhaled particles deposited in the anterior nose while a small amount of particles reached the olfactory mucosa, which resembles the droplet deposition pattern visualized by Sar-Gel images (**Figure 5**). By contrast, significantly improved olfactory dosing was measured for charged particles under an external electric field (blue-dashed ellipse, **Figure 10b**). Meanwhile, filtration by the nasal vestibule and valve region was perceivably lower.

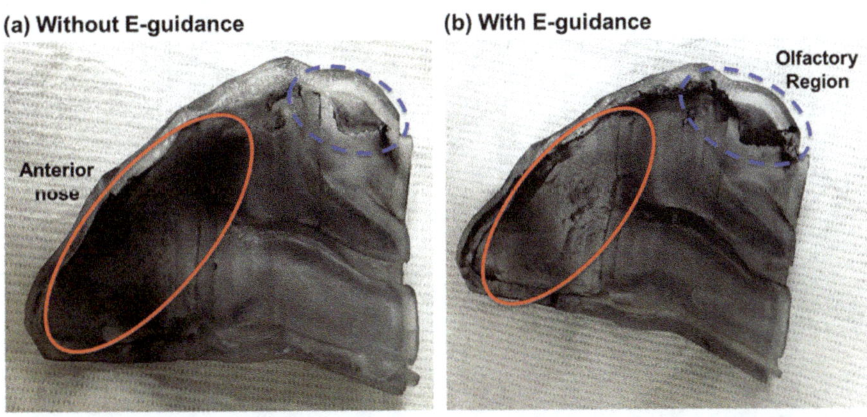

Figure 10. Particle deposition patterns in the 3-D nasal cast (a) without electric guidance versus (b) with electric guidance. Electric guidance of charged particles led to decreased deposition in the nasal valve region and noticeably enhanced deposition in the olfactory region.

3.4.2. *Bi-directional delivery*

The distribution of particle deposition using the bi-directional method is shown in **Figure 11**. High particle accumulations were observed in the upper nose of the right nasal passage, indicating there is an effective electric field guidance of charged particles to the olfactory region. It was also noted that particle deposition in the two passages was apparently different (right panel, **Figure 11**). In the right passage, particle deposition was more uniformly distributed, and a large portion of particles appeared to be pulled toward the electrodes. By contrast, the majority of particles in the left passage deposited in the inferior nose while much fewer particles reached the upper nose, presumably due to the gravitational effect.

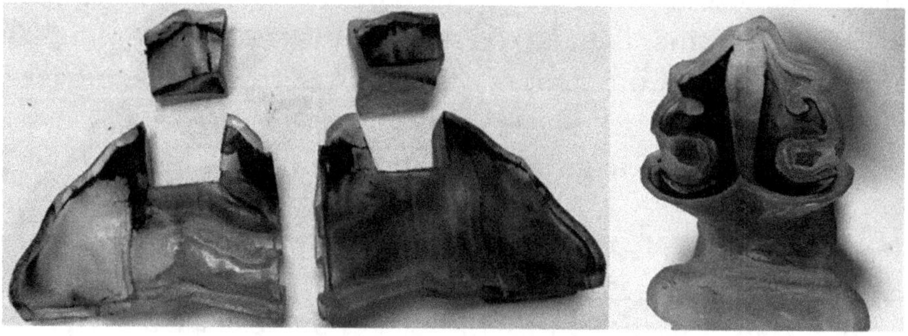

Figure 11. Deposition pattern in the right nasal passage and nasopharynx with the bi-directional delivery method. Appreciable deposition of particles was observed in the olfactory region. Because particles travel through the right and left passages in sequence, more particles were observed in the right passage than in the left passage.

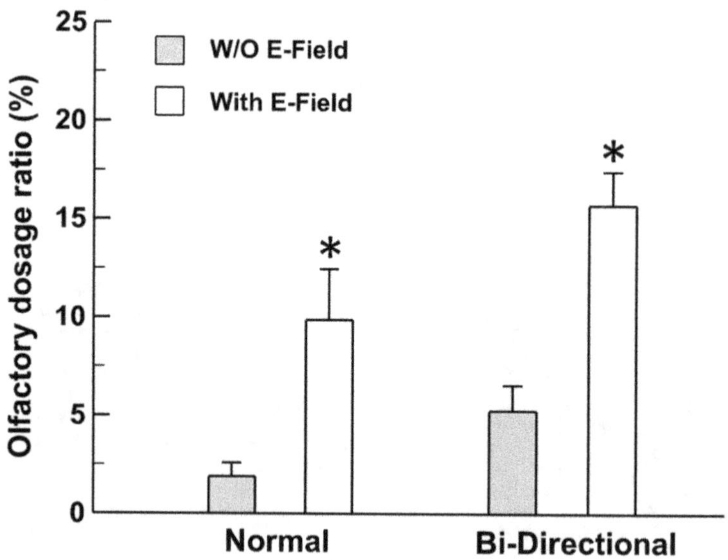

Figure 12. Comparison of the olfactory-to-nasal dosage ratio with and without electric guidance for the normal and bi-directional delivery strategies. *p-value < 0.05.

Figure 12 shows the comparison of the olfactory-to-nasal dosage ratio between the cases with and without the electric field guidance. The particle releasing time is 20 seconds, and the results are presented as the mean ± SD from five trials. With electric field guidance, significantly improved olfactory depositions were obtained for both delivery strategies, i.e., by a factor of 5 for the normal delivery and by a factor of 3 for the bi-directional delivery. The effect of the delivery method was also examined in the absence of an electric field; the olfactory dose using the bi-directional method was 2.8 times that under the normal method. However, with electric field guidance, the bi-directional olfactory dose was only 1.6 times the normal dose.

4. Discussion and conclusion

In this chapter, we presented a series of efforts in our lab aiming to improve the olfactory targeting of neurological medications. Both numerical and experimental tests were conducted to this aim by exploring various delivery strategies. Results of this study show that it is feasible to achieve clinically relevant olfactory doses using electric guidance of charged particles. All three protocols were demonstrated to give improved olfactory doses even though the improvement differs among the three. Compared to standard nasal devices, the point-release methods (vestibular and deep intubations) delivered approximately two order of magnitude higher doses to the olfactory region for both 150 nm and 1 μm particles. But even using the optimal delivery protocol (deep intubation), the olfactory dosage (1%) is still not adequate (~1%) to be clinically practical for the purpose of direct nose-to-brain drug delivery. In contrast, active control of drug particles using an externally applied electric field has been demonstrated to deliver much higher doses to target than the case without an electric field. An olfactory deposition fraction of 16% was measured with electric guidance under bi-directional breathing conditions.

The ability to dispense medications to the olfactory epithelium has tremendous superiority over convention inhalation devices in treating neurological diseases. A significantly enhanced olfactory dosing remits or eases the prevailing problem of too low olfactory doses. Second, reduced particle deposition in regions other than the olfactory region can minimize adverse side effects in those regions. Third, charged particles under the control of an external electric force will be are less dependent on respirations, making it suitable for seniors or subjects with comprised breathing capacities [52, 53]. The feature of robust delivery with electric guidance is especially appealing when the administration of medications requires long durations.

The electric delivery device is envisioned to have two major parts: a head-mounted nasal mask and a particle charging system. The nasal mask holds the electrodes and fixes the electrode relative to the patient head (**Figure 13a**). One example of the particle charging system is

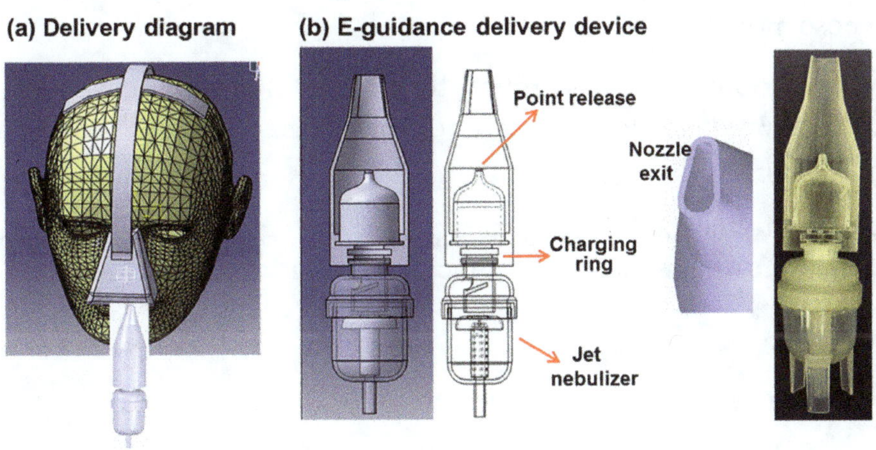

Figure 13. Electric-guidance olfactory delivery diagram and conceptual device designs. (a) A delivery system consists of two parts: a nose-mounted apparatus to generate desired electric field and a device to generate, charge, and point-release particles. (b) The conceptual delivery device uses a jet nebulizer and has an upright position.

illustrated in **Figure 13b** that contains a nebulizer, a charging ring, and a point-release nozzle. A prototype of this conceptual design was built using an Object30 Pro 3D printer (**Figure 13b**). An ideal design will generate small sized aerosols (<4 μm) at a slow speed and with high levels of electrostatic charges. Our preliminary test of this device, however, failed to produce such aerosols. Further testing and refinement are warranted to optimize the performance of this device.

Limitations of *in vitro* tests in this study include large particle size (30 μm), high exiting velocities of charge dry powders, large point-release area, and limited number of nasal models. Dry powders of 30 μm were selected because of the limited availability of dry powders satisfying both geometric and electrostatic requirements herein. Smaller aerosol particles are more sensitive to the guidance of electric forces and thus will lead to better doses in the olfactory region. A slow-moving particle will have longer residence time to respond to electric controls and is more likely to reach the target. In this study, the point-release catheter has a diameter of 4 mm and needs to be decreased to produce more site-specific doses. The nasal airway model was reconstructed from MRI images of one subject only and could not account intersubject variability. Future *in vitro* experiments and numerical simulations with more realistic scenarios are necessary to optimize the performance of electric-guidance delivery systems.

In conclusion, drug delivery of charged particles to the olfactory mucosa was assessed using both experiments and computations. Specific findings are as follows:

1. Complex nasal structure and no active control of particle motion in the nose are the two reasons lead to low doses in the olfactory region.
2. Conventional nasal devices, such as nasal drops, sprays, and nebulizers, fail to dispense clinically significant doses to the olfactory region.
3. The concomitant use of particle point release and electric field guidance can significantly enhance olfactory doses. With appropriate electric field and particle properties, a dose enhancement of two orders of magnitudes was predicted in both idealized 2-D and MRI-based 3-D nose models.
4. *In vitro* tests demonstrated a significantly higher olfactory dose using electric field guidance. There was a 5.2-fold increase for the normal delivery strategy and a 3.0-fold increase for the bi-directional strategy.
5. Future studies to refine the aerosol generation, charging, releasing, and guidance systems are warranted to further enhance the olfactory delivery.

Acknowledgements

Jun Lu at Central Michigan University, Linlin Zhao at Rutgers University, and Biwei Cao at Georgetown University are gratefully acknowledged for helpful discussions and for reviewing the manuscript.

Author details

Jinxiang Xi[1*] and Xiuhua April Si[2]

*Address all correspondence to: xi1j@cmich.edu

1 School of Engineering and Technology, Central Michigan University, Mount Pleasant, MI, USA

2 Department of Mechanical Engineering, California Baptist University, Riverside, CA, USA

References

[1] Bagger M, Bechgaard E. A microdialysis model to examine nasal drug delivery and olfactory absorption in rats using lidocaine hydrochloride as a model drug. Int. J. Pharm. 2004; 269: 311–322. doi: 10.1016/j.ijphann.2003.09.017

[2] Misra A, Kher G. Drug delivery systems from nose to brain. Curr. Pharm. Biotechnol. 2012; 13: 2355–2379. doi: 10.2174/138920112803341752

[3] Mistry A, Stolnik S, Illum L. Nanoparticles for direct nose-to-brain delivery of drugs. Int. J. Pharm. 2009; 379: 146–157. doi: 10.1016/j.ijpharm.2009.06.019

[4] Alam S, Khan ZI, Mustafa G, Kumar M, Islam F, Bhatnagar A, et al. Development and evaluation of thymoquinone-encapsulated chitosan nanoparticles for nose-to-brain targeting: a pharmacoscintigraphic study. Int. J. Nanomed. 2012; 7: 5705–5718. doi: 10.2147/ijn.s35329

[5] Shi H, Kleinstreuer C, Zhang Z. Laminar airflow and nanoparticle or vapor deposition in a human nasal cavity model. J. Biomech. Eng. 2006; 128: 697–706. doi: 10.1115/1.2244574

[6] Si X, Xi J, Kim J, Zhou Y, Zhong H. Modeling of release position and ventilation effects on olfactory aerosol drug delivery. Respir. Physiol. Neurobiol. 2013; 186: 22–32. doi: 10.1016/j.resp.2012.12.005

[7] Si X, Xi J, Kim J. Effect of laryngopharyngeal anatomy on expiratory airflow and submicrometer particle deposition in human extrathoracic airways. Open J. Fluid D. 2013; 3: 286–301. doi: 10.4236/ojfd.2013.34036

[8] Xi J, Longest PW. Numerical predictions of submicrometer aerosol deposition in the nasal cavity using a novel drift flux approach. Int. J. Heat Mass Transf. 2008; 51: 5562–5577. doi: 10.1016/j.ijheatmasstransfer.2008.04.037

[9] Illum L. Nasal drug delivery: new developments and strategies. Drug Discov. Today. 2002; 7: 1184–1189. doi: 10.1016/s1359-6446(02)02529-1

[10] El Taoum KK, Xi J, Kim JW, Berlinski A. In vitro evaluation of aerosols delivered via the nasal route. Respir. Care. 2015; 60: 1015–1025. doi: 10.4187/respcare.03606

[11] Wang J, Bentz J, Anderson R. Nasal device for delivery to the olfactory region. US 20070119451 A1. 2007.

[12] Gizurarson S. Method for administration of active substances to the olfactory region. Patents CA 2298596. 2003.

[13] Hoekman JD, Ho RJY. Effects of localized hydrophilic mannitol and hydrophobic nelfinavir administration targeted to olfactory epithelium on brain distribution. AAPS Pharmscitech. 2011; 12: 534–543. doi: 10.1208/s12249-011-9614-1

[14] Corley RA, Kabilan S, Kuprat AP, Carson JP, Minard KR, Jacob RE, et al. Comparative computational modeling of airflows and vapor dosimetry in the respiratory tracts of rat, monkey, and human. Toxicol. Sci. 2012; 128: 500–516. doi: 10.1093/toxsci/kfs168

[15] Xi J, Kim J, Si XA, Corley RA, Zhou Y. Modeling of inertial depositions in scaled models of rat and human nasal airways: towards in vitro regional dosimetry in small animals. J. Aerosol Sci. 2015; 99: 78–93. doi: 10.1016/j.jaerosci.2016.01.013

[16] Wilson IB. The deposition of charged particles in tubes, with reference to the retention of therapeutic aerosols in the human lung. J. Colloid Sci. 1947; 2: 271–276. doi: 10.1016/0095-8522(47)90028-7

[17] Bailey AG, Hashish AH, Williams TJ. Drug delivery by inhalation of charged particles. J. Electrostat. 1998; 44: 3–10. doi: 10.1016/S0304-3886(98)00017-5

[18] Wong J, Chan HK, Kwok PC. Electrostatics in pharmaceutical aerosols for inhalation. Ther. Deliv. 2013; 4: 981–1002. doi: 10.4155/tde.13.70

[19] Yu CP. Theories of electrostatic lung deposition of inhaled aerosols. Ann. Occup. Hyg. 1985; 29: 219–227. doi: 10.1093/annhyg/29.2.219

[20] Ferin J, Mercer TT, Leach LJ. The effect of aerosol charge on the deposition and clearance of TiO2 particles in rats. Environ. Res. 1983; 31: 148–151. doi: 10.1016/0013-9351 (83)90071-3

[21] Ali M, Reddy RN, Mazumder MK. Electrostatic charge effect on respirable aerosol particle deposition in a cadaver based throat cast replica. J. Electrostat. 2008; 66: 401–406. doi: 10.1016/j.elstat.2008.02.005

[22] Scheuch G, Gebhart J, Roth C. Uptake of electrical charges in the human respiratory tract during exposure to air loaded with negative ions. J. Aerosol Sci. 1990; 21: S439–S442. doi: 10.1016/0021-8502(90)90275-3

[23] Azhdarzadeh M, Olfert JS, Vehring R, Finlay WH. Effect of electrostatic charge on oral-extrathoracic deposition for uniformly charged monodisperse aerosols. J. Aerosol Sci. 2014; 68: 38–45. doi: 10.1016/j.jaerosci.2013.11.002

[24] Xi J, Si X, Longest W. Electrostatic charge effects on pharmaceutical aerosol deposition in human nasal-laryngeal airways. Pharmaceutics. 2014; 6: 26–35. doi: 10.3390/pharmaceutics6010026

[25] Xi J, Si XA, Gaide R. Electrophoretic particle guidance significantly enhances olfactory drug delivery: a easibility study. PLoS ONE. 2014; 9: e86593. doi: 10.1371/journal.pone.0086593

[26] Melandri C, Tarroni G, Prodi V, De Zaiacomo T, Formignani M, Lombardi CC. Deposition of charged particles in the human airways. J. Aerosol Sci. 1983; 14: 657–669. doi: 10.1016/0021-8502(83)90070-8

[27] Hashish AH, Bailey AG, Williams TJ. Selective deposition of pulsed charged aerosols in the human lung. J. Aerosol Med. 1994; 7: 167–171. doi: 10.1089/jam.1994.7.167

[28] Ali M. Engineered aerosol medicine and drug delivery methods for optimal respiratory therapy. Respir. Care. 2014; 59: 1608–1610. doi: 10.4187/respcare.03634

[29] Balachandran W, Machowski W, Gaura E, Hudson C. Control of drug aerosol in human airways using electrostatic forces. J. Electrostat. 1997; 40: 579–584. doi: 10.1016/S0304-3886(97)00106-X

[30] Djupesland PG, Skretting A, Winderen M, Holand T. Bi-directional nasal delivery of aerosols can prevent lung deposition. J. Aerosol Med. Pulm. Drug Deliv. 2004; 17: 249–259. doi: 10.1089/0894268042176355

[31] Luthringer R, Djupesland PG, Sheldrake CD, Flint A, Boeijinga P, Danjou P, et al. Rapid absorption of sumatriptan powder and effects on glyceryl trinitrate model of headache following intranasal delivery using a novel bi-directional device. J. Pharm. Pharmacol. 2009; 61: 1219–1228. doi: 10.1211/jpp/61.09.0012

[32] Djupesland PG, Docekal P, Czech Migraine Investigators G. Intranasal sumatriptan powder delivered by a novel breath-actuated bi-directional device for the acute treatment of migraine: a randomised, placebo-controlled study. Cephalalgia. 2010; 30: 933–942. doi: 10.1177/0333102409359314

[33] Si X, Xi J. Modeling and simulations of olfactory drug delivery with passive and active controls of nasally inhaled pharmaceutical aerosols. J. Vis. Exp. 2016. 111:e53902. doi: 10.3791/53902

[34] Xi J, Longest PW, Martonen TB. Effects of the laryngeal jet on nano- and microparticle transport and deposition in an approximate model of the upper tracheobronchial airways. J. Appl. Physilo. 2008; 104: 1761–1777. doi: 10.1152/japplphysiol.01233.2007

[35] Xi J, Longest PW. Effects of oral airway geometry characteristics on the diffusional deposition of inhaled nanoparticles. J. Biomech. Eng. Trans. ASME. 2008; 130: 011008. doi: 10.011008.1115/1.2838039

[36] Xi J, Longest PW. Transport and deposition of micro-aerosols in realistic and simplified models of the oral airway. Ann. Biomed. Eng. 2007; 35: 560–581. doi: 10.1007/s10439-006-9245-y

[37] Xi J, Longest PW. Evaluation of a drift flux model for simulating submicrometer aerosol dynamics in human upper tracheobronchial airways. Ann. Biomed. Eng. 2008; 36: 1714–1734. doi: 10.1007/s10439-008-9552-6

[38] Longest PW, Vinchurkar S. Validating CFD predictions of respiratory aerosol deposition: effects of upstream transition and turbulence. J. Biomech. 2007; 40: 305–316. doi: 10.1016/j.jbiomech.2006.01.006

[39] Wilcox DC. Turbulence Modeling for CFD. 3rd ed. California: DCW Industries, Inc. 2006.

[40] Hinds WC. Aerosol Technology: Properties, Behavior, and Measurement of Airborne Particles. New York: John Wiley and Sons. 1999.

[41] Morsi SA, Alexander AJ. An investigation of particle trajectories in two-phase flow systems. J. Fluid Mech. 1972; 55: 193–208. doi: 10.1017/S0022112072001806

[42] Xi J, Longest PW. Characterization of submicrometer aerosol deposition in extrathoracic airways during nasal exhalation. Aerosol Sci. Technol. 2009; 43: 808–827. doi: 10.1007/s10439-008-9552-6

[43] Matida EA, Finlay WH, Grgic LB. Improved numerical simulation of aerosol deposition in an idealized mouth-throat. J. Aerosol Sci. 2004; 35: 1–19. doi: 10.1016/S0021-8502(03)00381-1

[44] Ribeiro P, Si X Section 2: Electric and Magnetic Circuit. In: Beaty HW, Fink DG, editors. Standard Handbook for Electrical Engineering. 16 ed: McGraw Hill, New York. 2012. pp. 2.1-2.58.

[45] Longest PW, Xi J. Effectiveness of direct Lagrangian tracking models for simulating nanoparticle deposition in the upper airways. Aerosol Sci. Technol. 2007; 41: 380–397. doi: 10.1080/02786820701203223

[46] Cheng YS, Su YF, Yeh HC, Swift DL. Deposition of thoron progeny in human head airways. Aerosol Sci. Technol. 1993; 18: 359–375. doi: 10.1080/02786829308959610

[47] Cheng KH, Cheng YS, Yeh HC, Swift DL. Deposition of ultrafine aerosols in the head airways during natural breathing and during simulated breath-holding using replicate human upper airway casts. Aerosol Sci. Technol. 1995; 23: 465–474. doi: 10.1080/02786829508965329

[48] Laube BL. Devices for aerosol delivery to treat sinusitis. J. Aerosol Med. 2007; 20: S5–S18. doi: 10.1089/jam.2007.0569

[49] Geller DE. Comparing clinical features of the nebulizer, metered-dose inhaler, and dry powder inhaler. Respir. Care. 2005; 50: 1313–1322.

[50] Covert D, Wiedensohler A, Russell L. Particle charging and transmission efficiencies of aerosol charge neutralizers. Aerosol Sci. Technol. 1997; 27: 206–214. doi: 10.1080/02786829708965467

[51] Zeng Y, von Klitzing R. Scaling of layer spacing of charged particles under slit-pore confinement: an effect of concentration or of effective particle diameter? J. Phys. Condens. Matter. 2012; 24: 464125. doi: 10.1088/0953-8984/24/46/464125

[52] Dhand R. Aerosol therapy in patients receiving noninvasive positive pressure ventilation. J. Aerosol Med. Pulm. Drug Deliv. 2012; 25: 63–78. doi: 10.1089/jamp.2011.0929

[53] Willis LD, Berlinski A. Survey of aerosol delivery techniques to spontaneously breathing tracheostomized children. Respir. Care. 2012; 57: 1234–1241. doi: 10.4187/respcare.01518

7

Smart Drug Delivery Strategies Based on Porous Nanostructure Materials

Qun Wang, Jianying Huang and Yuekun Lai

Abstract

The control of drug delivery can have a great effect on its efficacy. An optimum concentration range of drugs can play a significant role in the human body, and it can cause harm to humans when it exceeds the range of the drug concentration. Recently, a variety of drug deliveries and their targeted systems have been studied to minimize drug loss and maximize the amount of drug accumulated in the required area, thus increasing drug bioavailability. In addition, we should especially consider the prevention of its harmful side-effects in the human body. Innovative drug delivery systems based on biodegradable, natural or synthetic polymers, micro- or nano-particles, lipoproteins, micelles, TiO_2 nanotube arrays (TNTs), nanoporous anodic aluminum oxide (AAO), and so on were developed, which combined magnetic targeting and stimulus-responsive in drug delivery systems. The composition of delivery carriers and the stimulus-responsive elements proved stimulus-responsive drug release as a smart drug delivery system.

Keywords: Drug delivery system, carriers, stimulus-responsive, TiO_2

1. Introduction

In recent years, nanomaterials and nanotechnology have been applied in the medical field such as in disease diagnosis and therapy. Research about drug delivery and targeting systems based on nanomaterials is carried out in nanomedicine to establish systems of drug delivery [1]. Based on the systems, it is easy to find disease tissues and implement the therapy in the required location.

Drug carriers included micro- or nano-particles made of biodegradable, natural or synthetic polymers, microcapsules, lipoproteins, micelles, TNTs, nanoporous aluminum oxide, and so on. Due to its controlled size, morphology and release, and excellent biocompatibility, biodegradable organic/inorganic micro/nano-particles have been studied extensively [2–5]. In fact, stimuli-responsive systems could facilitate drug release to reach a target environment. Stimuli-responsive elements have a functionality that sustains an energetic change in response to pH, temperature, magnetism, sound, and light [6–18].

Preparing particles from stimulus-responsive polymers can respond to certain pH value and temperature and so on to controllably release. The pH-responsive polymer was studied as a delivery system for therapeutic drugs [19–20] and was verified to prolong drug release circulation in vivo. Due to their special magnetic and optical properties, magnetic nanoparticles have played a great potential in drug release [21] and it has been used in disease diagnosis and therapy. Therefore, targeting drug delivery systems was built with the help of magnetic targeting. In addition, micellar solutions, vesicle and liquid crystal dispersions show great potentials as well as nanoparticle dispersions [22–23]. The drug delivery systems based on colloidal drug carriers can realize the target by obtaining systems of drug loading and release, low toxicity, and so on.

Recent progress in controlling drug release from nanotube and nanopore materials include TNT arrays, anodic aluminum oxide nanoporous, and so on [24–26]. TNT arrays have been applied in drug releases of therapies based on drug delivery because of its excellent properties, and it has been confirmed that TNT arrays change localized drug delivery therapies thoroughly. Furthermore, the method of preparing TNT arrays breaks a new nano-engineering path to propose the limitations of drug administration systems. Nanoporous materials with ordered pore structures were studied to avoid limitations of conventional drug therapies, especially for implantable drug delivery systems. In addition, porous AAOs are able to imitate dimensions of the natural bone and AAO films can be seen as promising coatings for the medical industry. Therefore, AAO has been used for new nano-platform for drug releases.

2. Energetic transitions of materials for drug delivery

As is known to us, it is necessary that the chemical functionalities exhibit stimuli-responsive behavior. In some cases, the triggering stimuli are in the proximity of the internal physiological environment of the drug delivery system [27]. It is also imagined that multiple stimuli-responsive systems operating in tandem assemble into a drug delivery system [28]. For example, a temperature change in a thermo-responsive system may be induced by a magnetic system.

2.1. pH-sensitive drug delivery

Polymer materials own structures with ionizable functionalities that become ionized at a specific pH where they acquire a positive or negative charge [29]. The transition of the functional group from one of water insolubility to one of water solubility under the effect of the ionization is called polyelectrolytes because of the presence of electrostatic charges in the water-soluble polymer structure.

There is a significant difference in the behavior of polymeric-charged functionalities and their uncharged counterparts in terms of their intermolecular effects on the surrounding environment and intramolecular effects within their own polymer molecules. The two types of interaction can be segregated into a polyelectrolyte and a solvent [29], and those between a polyelectrolyte and a surface [30]. In terms of the interaction between a polyelectrolyte and a solvent, there is a transition of the Gibbs free energy of mixing shifts from negative ($-\Delta G$) in solubility to positive ($+\Delta G$), where it is insoluble because the transition from an intermolecular hydrogen-bonded species to an intramolecular hydrogen-bonded species causes poor entropy of mixing [31]. The function is easily seen in the change in the secondary structure of polypeptides or proteins where there is a transition from an α-helical to a random coil secondary structure as a result of deprotonation or protonation, as is shown in Fig. 1 [32].

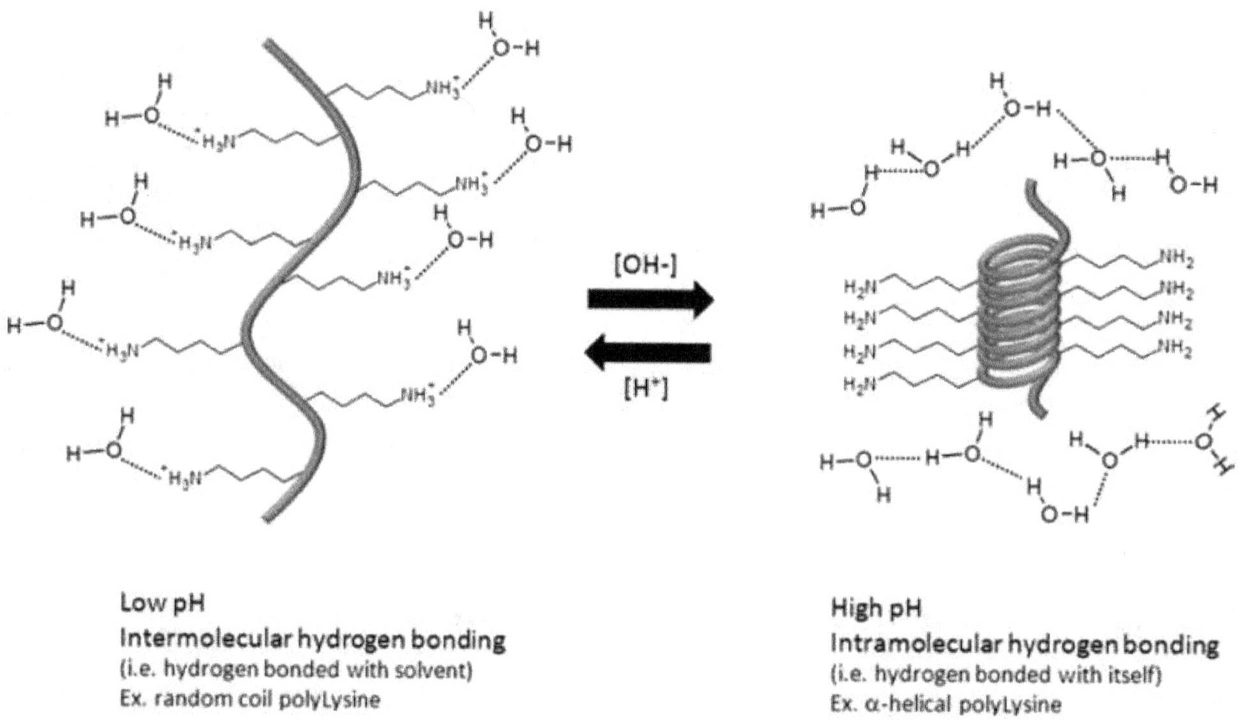

Figure 1. Diagram of the intramolecular versus intermolecular hydrogen bonding through the protonation–deprotonation of the pendant groups on the polymer chain [32].

In addition, several characteristic interactions between the polyelectrolyte and the surface can be seen. If a surface owns an oppositely charged energy, the polyelectrolyte is proposed to interact in a number of different ways. If there is a long-range of electrostatic interaction, it is possible that the rearrangement of the polyelectrolyte chain expresses charged functionalities at the surface [33]. This rearrangement would change based on the pH, the charge density, the composition and distribution of charges along the polymer chain and the ionic strength of the solvent and so on. For the purposes of our discussion in this section, we focus on the pH and ionic strength.

We know that the introduction of salt will screen the electrostatic forces between the polyelectrolyte and the surface, as well as reduce both the intermolecular and intramolecular electrostatic repulsions. There is also a non-electrostatic affinity under certain conditions in the case of interactions between polyelectrolytes and charged surfaces [34]. Any increase in the ionic strength under the presence of salts would decrease the electrostatic affinity of the polyelectrolyte to the charged surface when the adsorption of polyelectrolyte on a charged surface is driven by only electrostatic forces, and the adsorption increases to an upper limit when the non-electrostatic affinity is high enough.

The responsiveness of a molecule to pH presents an interesting target for stimulated drug delivery. As we know, when an encapsulated drug species is internalized by a cell, it will enter the lysosome at some point within the process. The lysosome cell has a pH of 4.5–5.0 [35], which is exclusively different from other intracellular vesicle species. Therefore, a collapse or dissociation of the self-assembled species is triggered by pH and will result in the release of the encapsulant.

We know the role of the hydrophobic domain in the self-assembly of micellar systems is to minimize the interfacial free energy between incompatible phases. The hydrophobicity could be adjusted by increasing the molecular weight into the entanglement regime, which more effectively stabilizes both the hydrophobic domain and the self-assembled species. If we begin to change the composition of the hydrophobic domain, it will destabilize the condensed, self-assembled structure [36].

The pH-responsive vesicle or micellar systems would not be orally relevant if the stimuli range is ~5 since the premature release of drug cargo would occur in the acidic environment of the stomach (pH 1–3) [37]. The hydrogel particles are designed such that the cross-linked domains are a combination of covalent bonds and the collapse of multiple hydrophobic domains. In these cases, a change in the pH of the environment surrounding leads to a nonpolar, collapsed hydrophobic species to turn into a charged species. The change to charged groups also leads to the electrostatic repulsion of polyelectrolyte chains within close proximity to one another, which further drives the expansion of the gel network pore structure [38]. The design is typically used in drug applications where the drug needs to be delivered within the immediate proximity of a desired cell and does not require the system to facilitate the cellular internalization response. In either of these cases, systems can be designed with negative charges as well, which shifts the operable pH range to more basic stimuli. One can envision tuning their respective systems by compositionally shifting their ratios of cationic to anionic stimuli-responsive groups to allow for a specific release window (Fig. 2) [38].

2.2. Temperature-sensitive drug delivery

The combination of a polymer with a solvent in a binary mixture involves a series of phases of varying degrees of stability primarily in relation to its composition and temperature. Within some compositional range, a material can reach a minimum energy equilibrium state known as the binodal curve that describes a critical limit at which two phases can be either stable on one side or unstable on the other side, representing the limits of solvent interaction between two phases [39]. Plus, a curve known as the spinodal curve describes the limit of absolute

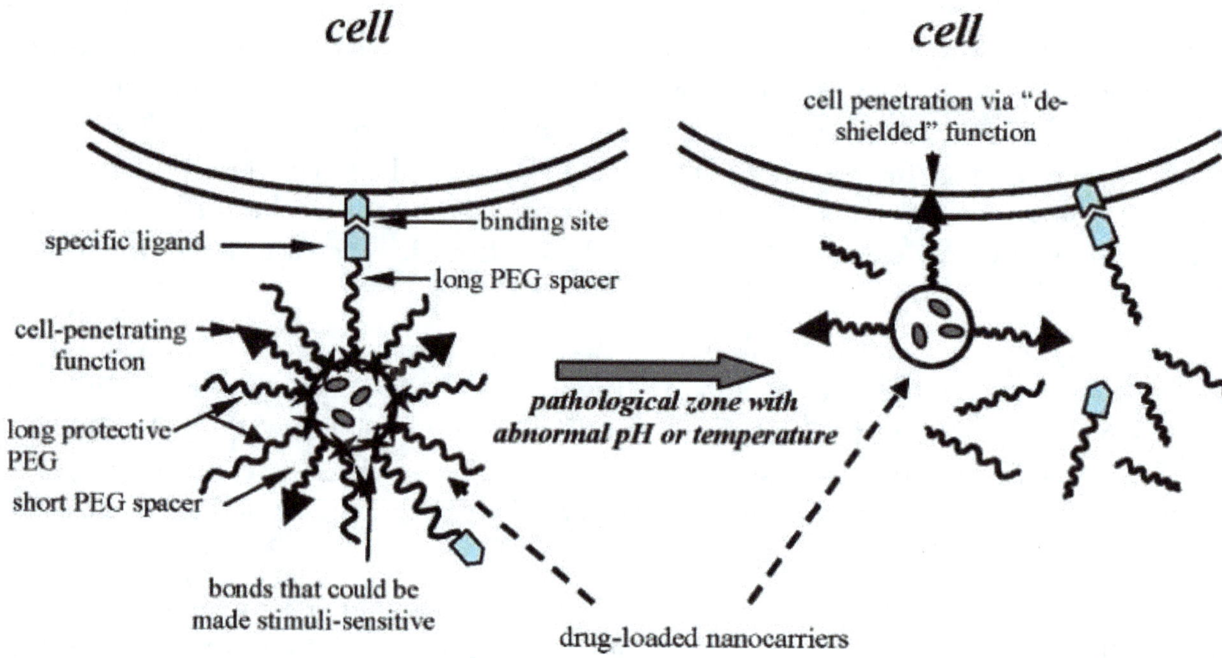

Figure 2. Interaction of the multifunctional pH-responsive pharmaceutical nano-carrier with the target cell. Local stimuli-dependent removal of protecting PEG chains or mAb-PEG moieties allows for the direct interaction of the CPP moiety with the cell membrane [38].

instability between phases. A complete decomposition of the system is produced when it is changed to composition within the spinodal curve [40].

The point at which the spinodal and binodal curves meet is known as the lower critical solution temperature (LCST) [41]. The LCST represents a point below which the material becomes miscible, where the Gibbs free energy of mixing is negative ($-\Delta G$) and above which it is completely immiscible, and where the Gibbs free energy of mixing is positive ($+\Delta G$) due to poor entropy of mixing [42]. The degree of polymerization and the polydispersity of the polymer chains can be a strong influence on the energetics of mixing and therefore can shift the values for the LCST. Typically, polymer chains with higher degrees of polymerization lead to higher values for the LCST. Polymers that exhibit an LCST behavior can have their solubility tuned based on temperature change.

We have known that the self-assembly of vesicle and micellar species is controlled by several factors, such as chemical composition, shape, charge, and so on, and species with specific size, shape, stability, and delivery efficiency are assembled under the effect of these factors [43]. For a vesicle species comprised of amphiphilic copolymers, there is much focus about their design. The chemical functionality tells us the rigidity of the system and the way hydrophobic or hydrophilic are, as well as whether a charged species is present [44].

The bond rotation of rigid species require a higher number of polymer repeats, and there are limitations in the modes of bending, so higher molecular weights is required in order to reach the entanglement regime for the more rigid systems. The closer the molecular weight is to the entanglement molecular weight, the more stable the assembled species [45]. The chemical composition will tell us the ratio of the hydrophilic and hydrophobic components, as well as the degree of polymerization of the collapsed hydrophobic domain.

Yatvin and Weinstein pioneered the concept of temperature-triggered local drug delivery using temperature-sensitive liposomes (TSLs) [46–47]. Here, a chemotherapeutic drug is encapsulated in a heat-sensitive nanovesicle that prevents extravasation of the drug into healthy tissues at physiological temperature. The experiment about temperature-induced drug delivery was performed in small rodents with a subcutaneous tumor on the hind limb where hyperthermia was realized through putting the leg into a water bath [48]. Both tumor tissue and the whole hind limb were found with temperature-induced drug delivery phenomenon. The control of the temperature remained demanding when temperatures were monitored with thermocouples inserted into the tumor. The concept of temperature-triggered drug delivery has been extended to magnetic resonance (MR) image-guided drug delivery by the co-encapsulation of a paramagnetic magnetic resonance imaging (MRI) contrast agent in the lumen of TSLs (Fig. 3) [49].

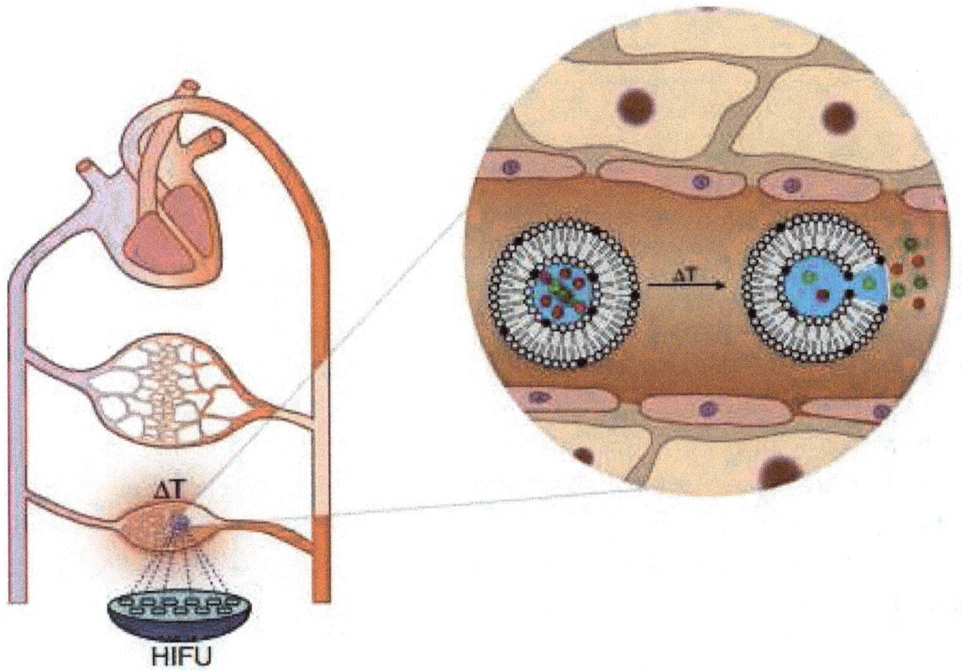

Figure 3. MR image-guided drug delivery illustration of the release of temperature-triggered drug using temperature-sensitive liposomes and HIFU. The co-release of MRI contrast agents from the liposome loaded with temperature-sensitive drug allows to non-invasively visualize and quantify the drug release process [49].

It has been revealed that the external aqueous medium was separated from the liposomal aqueous lumen by a single continuous bilayer of phospholipids that is from the self-assembly of phospholipids into liposomes [50]. These self-assembled structures have been investigated as molecular MRI contrast agents for drug delivery systems. Temperature-sensitive liposomes release encapsulated drugs at the melting phase transition temperature (Tm) of the lipid bilayer (Fig. 3). Structural changes in the lipid membrane occur as it transfers from a gel to the liquid-crystalline phase at transition temperature [51]. In comparison to the liquid-crystalline phase, liposomal membranes in the gel phase are less permeable to water and drugs.

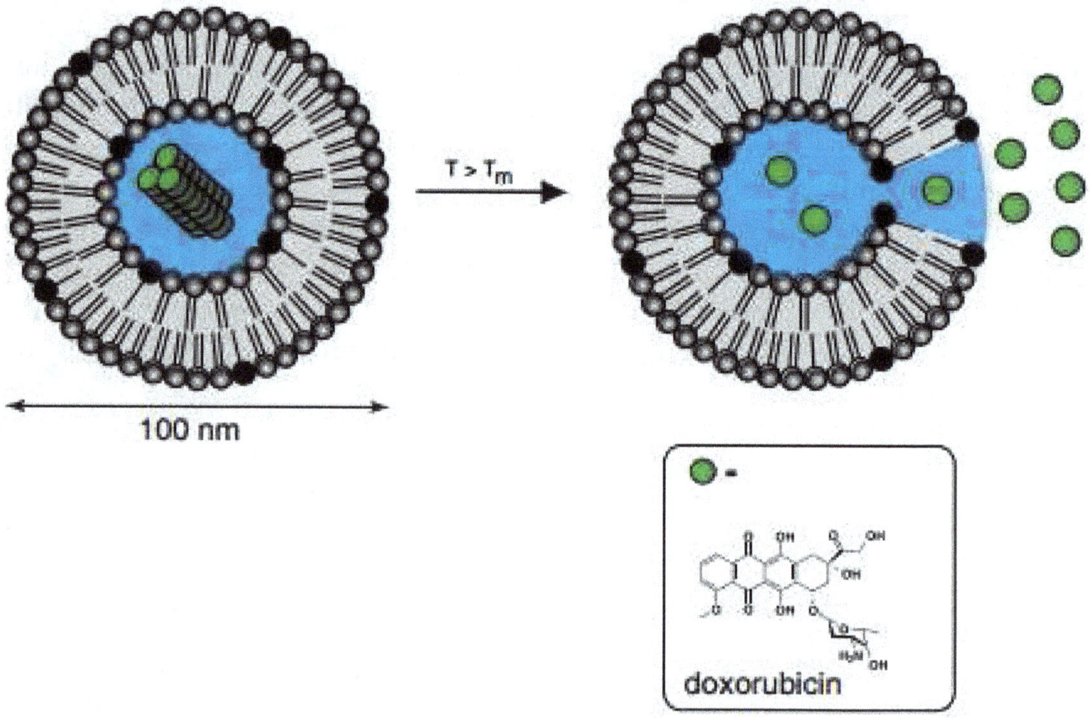

Figure 4. Schematic representation of heat-triggered dox release from TSLs [49].

There are several other thermo-responsive functionalities that can be incorporated within the polymer domain in order to stimulate porosity or swelling of a system in addition to NIPAAm, and each system has a different LCST, or in some cases a tunable LCST [52]. Appropriate selection of the thermo-responsive functionality for eliciting the desired behavior is critical. It is also important to keep in mind that the selection of the responsive functionality should reflect the rationalization that the system should be at the very least bioinert in order to be a candidate for a drug delivery system.

2.3. Magnetic-sensitive drug delivery

The stimuli-responsive behavior is dependent on the local physiological environment, such as in both cases of pH and temperature. We could direct the stimuli toward the targeted area of delivery instead of the stimuli-responsive behavior depending on a localized environment. We will adjust the chemical functionality to allow for a relevant response if there is fine control over sources that induce a direct movement including a magnetic field, light, and sound. The response is an attractive or repulsive force relative to the field direction in the case of magnetic materials. Both the material chemical functionality and the viscosity properties of the particle within a physiological system are critical in determining the extent of the response to a magnetic field (Fig. 5) [53–54]. Magnetic particles are typically divided based on size into single-domain and multi-domain particles [55]. The single-domain particles fall in a small size regime, where decreases in size correspond to an increase in coercivity to a peak level before dropping to zero. The zero point identifies a superparamagnetic material, which is one whose magnetic moment is induced in the direction of the applied magnetic field and in the absence of a magnetic field returns to an unaligned state [56].

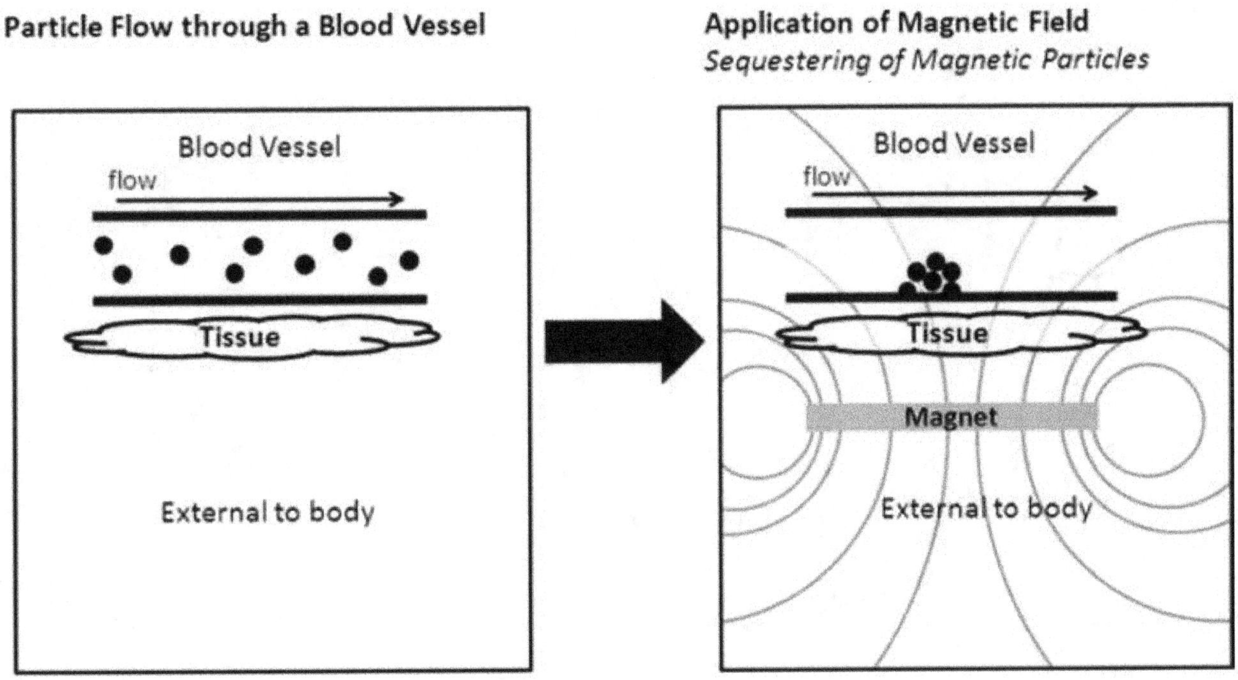

Figure 5. Diagram of the basic forces involved in the sequestration of magnetic nanoparticles in the bloodstream [53].

As was the case of thermo-responsive and pH-responsive systems, magneto-responsive materials represent systems that interact with an applied stimulus as opposed to an encountered stimulus. Light and sound are also suitable for responsive materials as an applied stimulus [57]. The stimulus is an externally applied magnetic field that can immobilize a particle under flow in terms of magnetic materials [58]. The design of magnetic materials involves several factors including particle size, stabilizing material, atomic identity, and so on [59]. In terms of the size of the magnetic particle, paying attention to the larger the magnetic particle size, the more susceptible it will be toward manipulation by a magnetic field. The stabilizing functionality is that the particle surface is necessary to allow for the particle to effectively function as a physiological system. The atomic identity refers to the metal atoms used in the particle composition.

In the application of a magnetic field, we should pay attention to a single-domain magnetic particle strategy for the immobilization of drug species [60]. The system depends on a small particle system in order to fall within the superparamagnetic regime. For example, systems of iron oxide (Fe_3O_4) are used where drug species are conjugated to the surface. A larger silica particle system is used as matrix by these ferromagnetic particles, which is then surface-functionalized with chemically inert groups [60]. Fig. 6 displays the schematic illustration of the synthesis process of the drug-loading magnetic and fluorescent chitosan nanoparticles [61]. Amino groups of chitosan consisted of cationic linear polysaccharide molecules keep positively charged under weakly acidic conditions, result in the form of a long and intertwined chain with positive charges along its backbone. The aqueous negatively charged QDs, Fe_3O_4 nanoparticles, and the ionized COO^- of cefradine (pKa = 2.5 and 7.3) along the positive backbone are electrostatically attracted in weakly acidic conditions are electrostatically attracted [61].

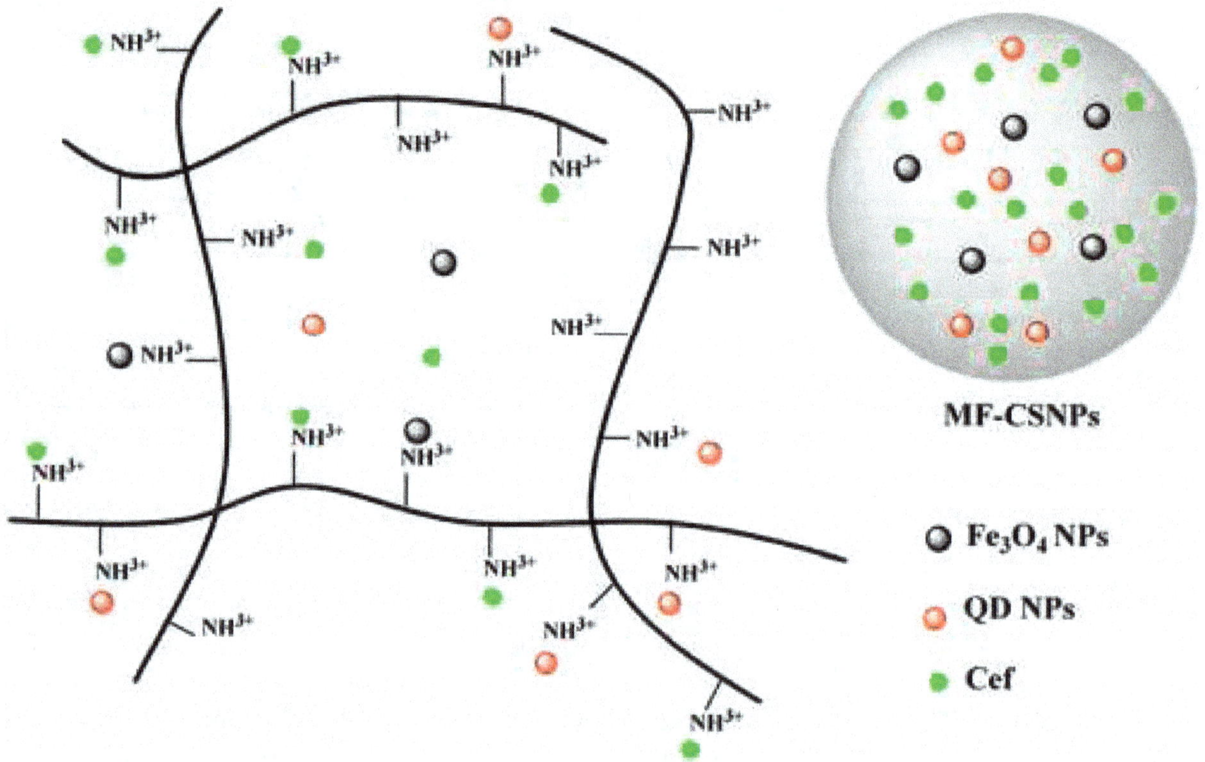

Figure 6. Schematic representation of the fabrication process of the drug-loading magnetic and fluorescent chitosan nanoparticles [61].

The introduction of surface-modifying groups for biocompatibility and the magnitude of the magnetic moment at the surface of the particle are reduced, which may limit its physiological application. Therefore, the design of these immobilized magnetic systems involves three basic factors: particle size (<10 nm), bioinert surface functionalities, and mode of drug incorporation (conjugated or dispersed within matrix) [62]. Magnetic drug delivery systems formed using this design strategy have shown promise for clinical evaluation and treatment of brain tumor patients using a tandem approach involving acoustic and magnetic targeting of tissue across the blood–brain barrier.

The domain choices allow tunable size and magnetic susceptibility for the drug delivery system. This degree of versatility allows for a multitude of surface functionalizations in order to present a drug delivery system that is physiologically bioinert.

2.4. Ultrasound-sensitive drug delivery

A self-assembled species can be induced by the use of ultrasound technology to act as a nucleation site for pore formation in a membrane barrier to enhance delivery [63]. A process of acoustic droplet vaporization pushes a superheated droplet through a phase transition to yield gas micro-bubbles, which leads to membrane pore formation by a process of sonoporation [64]. For transdermal drug delivery, the permeabilizing effects of ultrasound have been applied to a number of treatments, such as for diabetes [65]. Ultrasound has been employed for targeted disruption of drug carrier vessels such as contrast or acoustically active liposomes, releasing their therapeutic payload for uptake by the target cells (Fig. 7) [66]. In addition, sonoporation has been associated with gene therapy for the introduction of nonviral plasmid DNA into target cells.

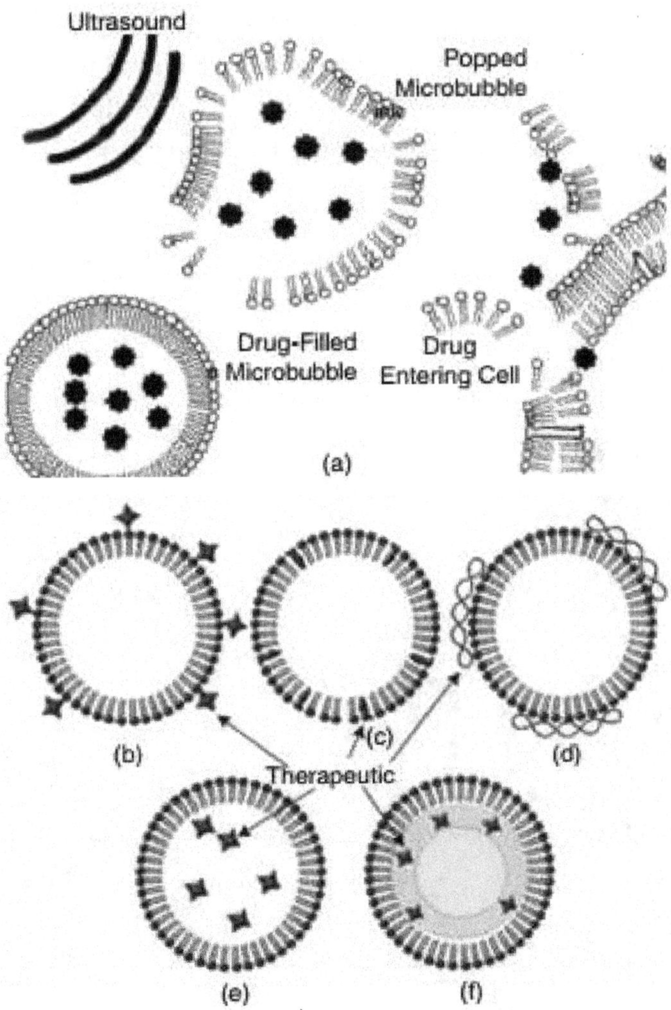

Figure 7. Various drug delivery strategies with micro-bubble carriers. (a) Schematic representation of drug delivery via targeted micro-bubble destruction with ultrasound. Models of different therapeutic agents loading styles, such as the (b) attaching to the micro-bubble membrane, (c) imbedding in the membrane, (d) bonding noncovalently to the micro-bubble surface, (e) packing in the interior of the micro-bubble, and (f) incorporating into an oily film surrounding the micro-bubble [66].

In the case of ultrasound responsive systems, it is required for the stabilization of acoustic cavitation's gas–liquid interface and the compatibility with liquid interface to generate gas bubbles. The primary requirements of the stabilized system are extended circulation lifetime, effective size range, and efficient stimulated release of encapsulated drug via the application of ultrasound [67–68].

The circulation lifetime of the gas microbubbles is associated with the amphiphilic component that stabilizes the interface. We have known that lipid bilayer systems have a significantly short thickness, which offers little stability of microbubbles in vivo in the case of gas–liquid interfaces. Amphiphilic copolymer systems offer a significant improvement to the interfacial membrane stability, while maintaining tunability to drive membrane curvature [69].

It is known that the targeted size of allowing for tumor membrane permeability and gas microbubble stabilization is less than 750 nm. The curvature can be further tuned to form nanobubbles as a preform to merge into microbubble systems at the cell membrane interface. It is an example of improving the stability of the microbubble with no discernible effect to the biological delivery. The energy of the applied ultrasound stimulus can adjust the size regimes and stabilize the desired interfacial curvature effectively (Fig. 8) [70].

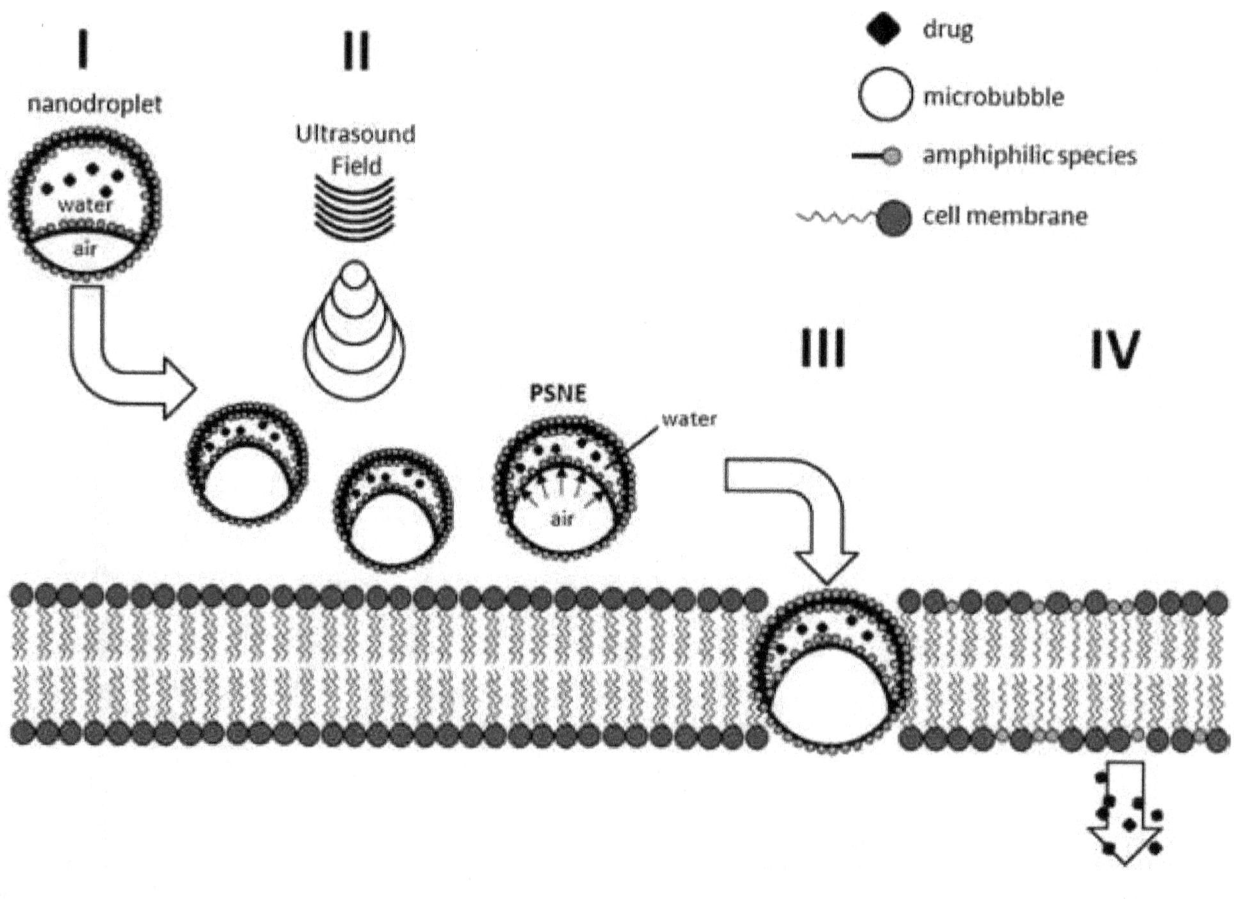

Figure 8. Diagram of the cavitation of PSNE (Phase-Shift Nanoemulsion) nanodroplets from ultrasound [70].

The effective delivery of the adhered drug is relevant to the echogenicity or the ability to bounce a signal base on oscillation, growth, and collapse of the microbubble system [71]. The echogenicity is affected by the choice of component mixtures such as water and PFP, the surfactant, and the size of the microbubble system. The trend appears to be that the maximization of the impedance between components and the stabilization of high-curvature systems can improve drug release profiles in vivo [72].

2.5. Light-sensitive drug delivery

The materials species is influenced by the presence of a specific energy wavelength of light as well as the particle species is influenced by the direction of the magnetic field in magnetic systems. The chemical structure of the drug delivery system destabilizes or changes conformation in response to the absorbed energy input when visible, ultraviolet (UV), or infrared (IR) light is directed at a desired target region. TiO_2 photocatalysts have been mostly used for the purification of air and water by UV light irradiation. However, the limited photocatalytic activity of TiO_2 within the UV range presents difficulties in biomedical and tissue engineering applications owing to the potential harmful effects of UV light. In this part, we focused on the extension of the photocatalytic activity of TiO_2 to the visible light region by doping nitrogen into the TiO_2 crystal structure, which would allow remote control of antibiotic elution by visible light irradiation [73].

A new delivery system that affords control of the time of drug elution and accurate dosing of antibiotics to the target area is required. TiO_2 nanotubes have been studied predominantly in the field of photocatalysis [74–76], solar cells [77], and biomedical engineering [78–80], because of their excellent photocatalytic activity and biocompatibility. In addition, the high surface area and unique shape of TiO_2 nanotubes make them a promising option for application in drug delivery systems. TiO_2 nanotubes arrays fabricated by electrochemical anodization can be described as a layer of tightly packed, vertically aligned and ordered nanotube structures with hexagonal arrangement, which grow perpendicularly to the Ti surface [81]. Fig. 9A and 9B show illustrations of the chemical cell and the fabrication process of TNTs by electrochemical anodization of Ti. Typical scanning electron microscopy images of prepared TNTs are shown in Fig. 9c, with the top and the cross-sectional views showing nanotubes separated into individual entities featuring closed ends at the bottom side [82].

Kyung-Suk Moon et al. [83] immobilized Gold nanorods (GNR) at the surface of TiO_2 nanotubes via a grafting technique and investigated on-off drug release triggered by near-IR laser irradiation. In addition, antimicrobial activity was monitored to assess the effectiveness of GNR-grafted TiO_2 nanotubes in allowing remotely controlled drug release by IR laser irradiation. The elution concentrations of tetracycline loaded at the surface of GNR-grafted TiO_2 nanotubes were evaluated after 30 s of IR light irradiation with a near-IR laser. The release concentrations of tetracycline from GNR-grafted TiO_2 nanotubes with IR light irradiation (674.52 ± 169.58 μ μg/mL) were significantly higher than those from other experimental conditions, such as TiO_2 nanotubes with or without IR light irradiation and GNR-grafted TiO_2 nanotubes without IR laser irradiation (Fig. 10) [83].

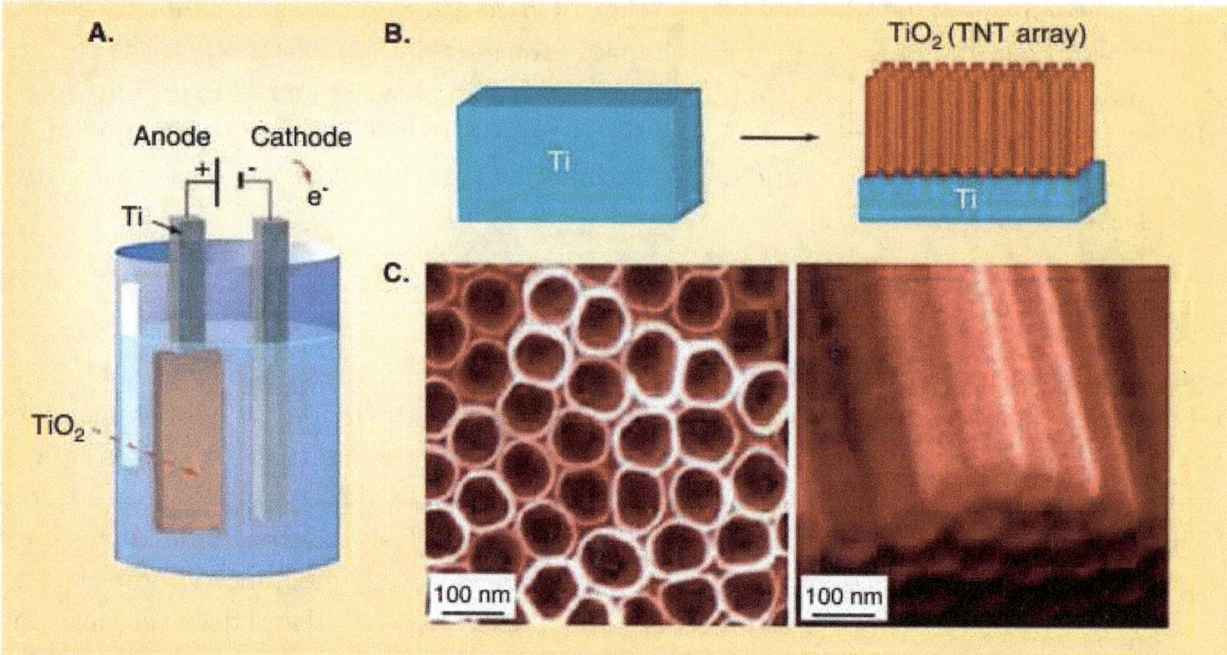

Figure 9. Schematic illustration of TNTs synthesis process and corresponding SEM images of typical morphology and structure. (a) Preparation of TNTs layer by electrochemical cell and anodization process. (b) Formation of self-organized and vertically aligned TNTs on Ti substrate. (c) SEM images of the typical morphology of TNT structures [82].

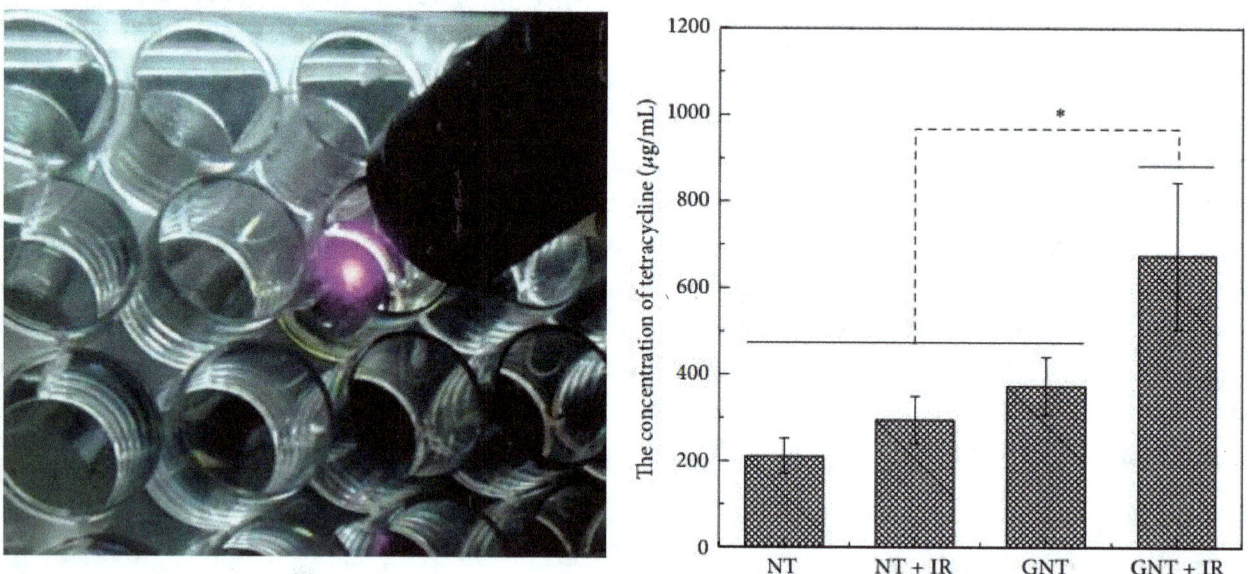

Figure 10. a) Near-IR laser and IR light irradiation and (b) the concentration of tetracycline released by IR light irradiation (NT, NT + IR, GNT, and GNT + IR in the graph designate TiO_2 nanotubes only, near-IR laser irradiated TiO_2 nanotubes, GNR-grafted TiO_2 nanotubes, and near-IR laser irradiated GNR grafted TiO_2 nanotubes, resp.) [83].

For photo-responsive materials, light can either induce the formation of an isomer or degrade a self-assembled component [84–85]. The photoisomerization strategy relies on the effective destabilization of a liquid crystal phase within the hydrophobic domain of micelle or vesicle species that are formed from amphiphilic molecules or macromolecules. The aggregated region will be highly rigid and densely packed in the trans state if the hydrophobic domain consists of liquid crystal groups [86]. The visible light or heat is used to return the structure to its native initial state in photo-isomerization-induced systems that involve highly stable vesicle or micellar self-assembled systems that rapidly reform their densely packed domains.

2.6. Nanoporous engineered drug delivery

Recently, nanoporous anodic alumina (NAA) has become one of the most popular self-ordered periodic, porous templates. In general the highly developed, superior ordering of nanopores in NAA templates is obtained by using a two-step anodization process. NAA has been of great interest due to its outstanding material properties, including electrical insulation, optical transparency, and chemical stability, and most recently, because of its biologically inert and biologically compatibility properties [87]. The use of NAA as a drug delivery platform has been explored in several fields, such as biomedical devices for dental and bone implants, vectors, or carriers for cells transplantion. The suitability of NAA loaded with catalase, endostatin, and vitamin C as sustainable, quasi-linear drug-releasing platform for ophthalmic applications has been demonstrated by Orosz et al. [88].

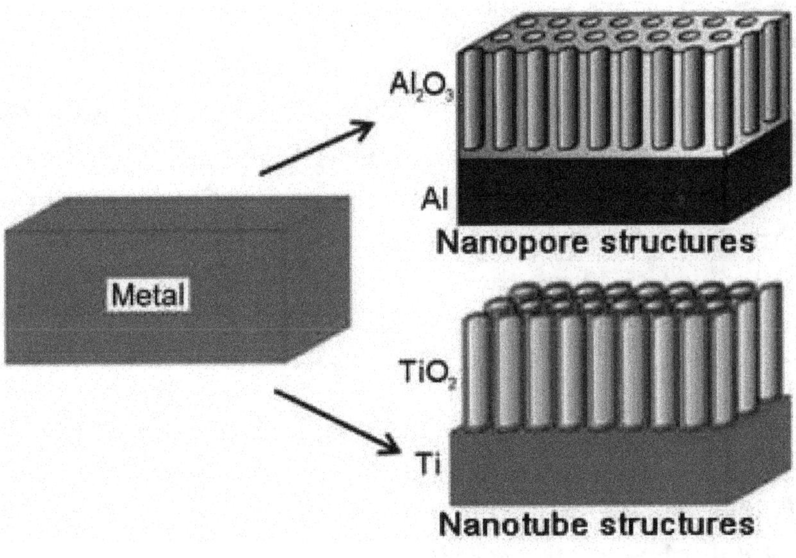

Figure 11. Schematic diagram showing the self-ordering anodization on selected metals (Al and Ti) to produce nanoporous and nanotube metal oxides (Al_2O_3 and TiO_2) with highly-ordered and self-aligning uniform structures. These two materials were explored as non-eroding drug-releasing implants for LDD applications [89].

Depending on the metal type, electrolyte, current, and voltage, two different oxide growth morphologies, such as nanoporous aluminum oxide (Al_2O_3) and nanotube titanium dioxide (TiO_2), can be obtained by a self-ordering electrochemical anodization process as shown in Fig. 11 [89]. The structural features of NAA can be controlled by the anodization parameters, so the functionalities of NAA in terms of pore geometry is an advantage for developing drug-releasing implants as the diffusion of molecules from the nanopores can be tuned by geometry

[90]. Jeonet et al. [91] developed a sophisticated system by combining NAA chips with electrically responsive polymers, in which the pore mouths of NAA were modified with polypyrrole doped with dodecylbenzenesulfonate anion (PPy/dB) by electro-polymerization on the upper surface of NAA platforms. The large volume change of that polymeric blend was used to achieve pore mouth actuation by an external electrical stimulus (Fig. 12) [90].

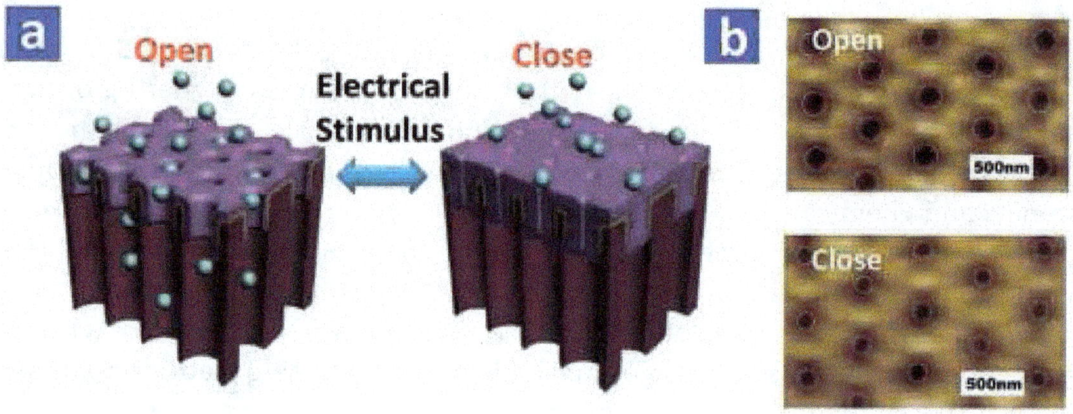

Figure 12. Electrically responsive drug-releasing NAA chip. (a) The mechanism of an electrically responsive drug-releasing chip based on NAA and PPy-DBS (reversible cycle). (b) AFM images of NAA chips before and after the application of electrical stimulus (pore mouth reduction) [90].

Titania nanotubes (TNTs) can be produced by anodizing metallic titanium (Ti) in different acid electrolytes as well as NAA; TNTs feature a nanotube structure during the anodization process (Fig. 13A and B) [92]. Different electrochemical approaches have made it possible to engineer the nanoporous structure of TNTs. TNT-based implants are recognized as one of the most promising nanomaterials to address the inherent drawbacks of conventional systemic drug administration due to their capability to localize the release of drugs over affected bones sites in a controllable manner [91].

In terms of the drug loading and release properties and capabilities of TNTs layers, the drug release from nanotubes is governed by a diffusion process when TNTs come into contact with the physiological milieu inside the host body, as schematically presented in Fig. 14 [90]. The release process is established by the mass transfer of drug molecules from the nanotubes, considering that the drug is completely soluble in the physiological solution without precipitation at particular concentrations. This diffusion-controlled process can be described by Fick's first law, which is governed by a number of factors such as the molecular size and charge of drugs, the diameter and length of nanotubes, their charge and surface chemistry, interfacial interaction between drug molecules and nanotube surface, dissolution rate of drugs, diffusion coefficient, pH, and so on [82].

In addition, the surface charges of TNTs can be rendered hydrophobic or hydrophilic to accommodate a variety of drug molecules should be mentioned. In vitro drug release with the aid of polymeric micelles as drug nano-carriers [93–94] and targeted drug release by means of

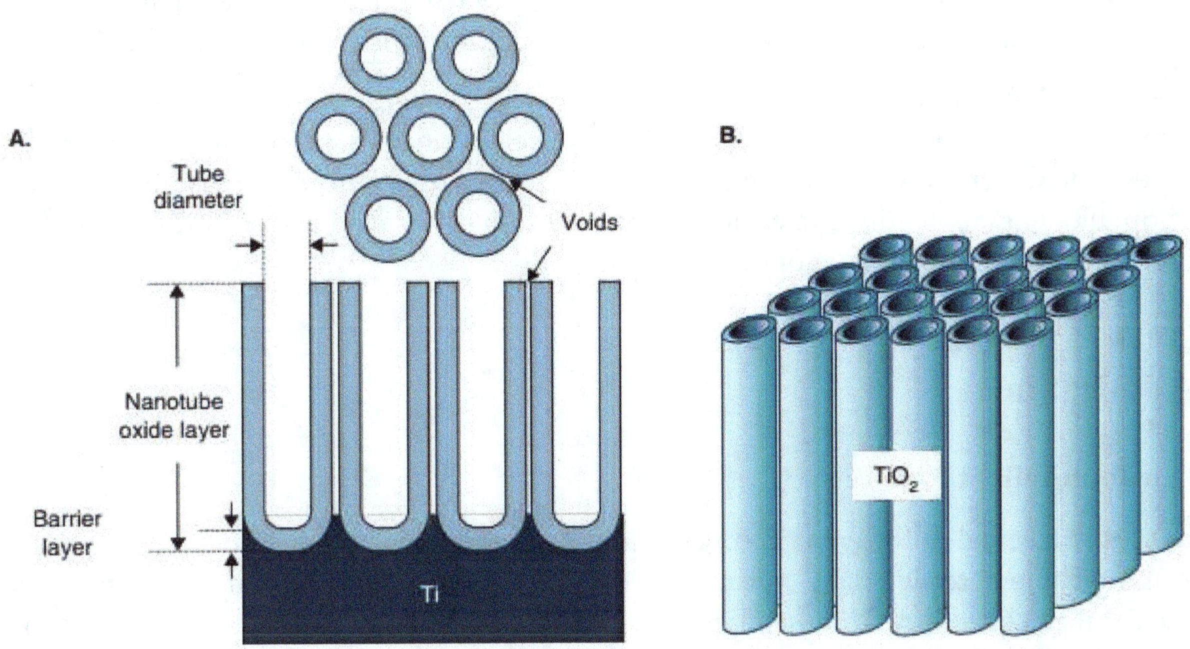

Figure 13. (a) Typical structures of nanotube titania fabricated by electrochemical anodization of titanium, (b) TiO_2 nanotube structures fabricated by electrochemical anodization in NH_4F/ethylene glycol electrolyte showing the cross-sectional image of self-supporting TiO_2 nanotube layer and the entire structure (nanotube film) not detached from Ti substrate (inset) [92].

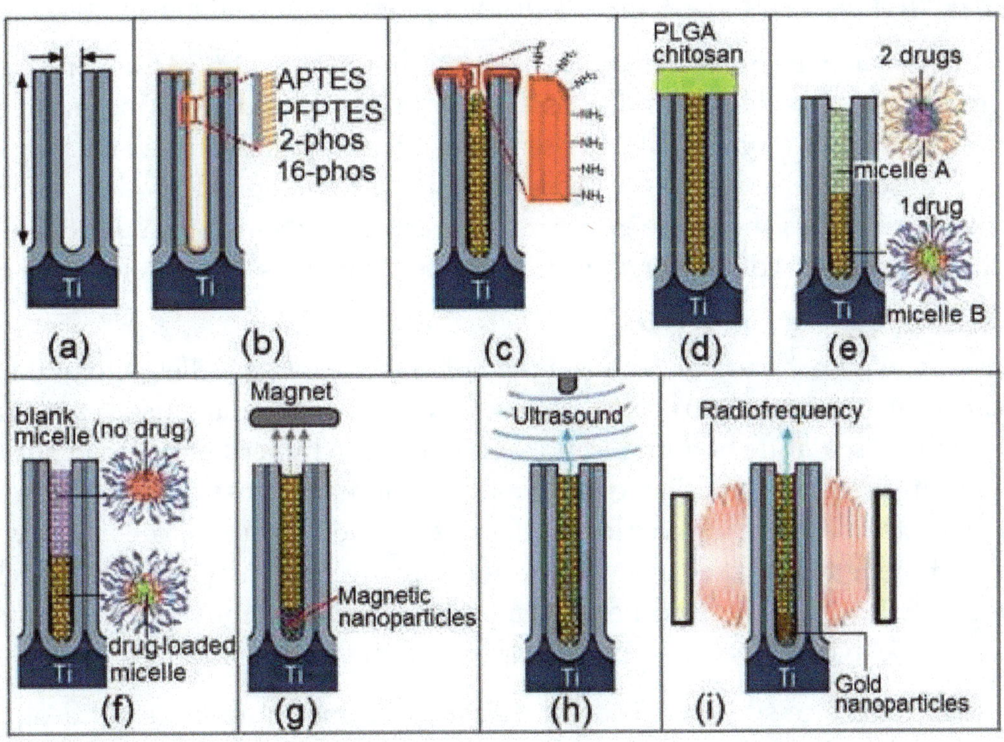

Figure 14. Schematic diagram showing different strategies developed by our group for controlling drug release from drug-releasing implants based on TNTs [90].

gold nanoparticles stimulated by radiofrequency field [95] and magnetic nanoparticles under the influence of a magnetic nanoparticles that are under the influence of a magnetic field [96].

Properties of NAA and TNTs that can control drug release but non-degrade in vivo are not suitable for some specific applications, such as drug-releasing implants for treating eye-related diseases [90]. Other nanostructure materials including porous silicon can also be applied to develop biodegradable drug-releasing implants with improved capabilities for definite requirement of clinical applications [91].

3. Applications

3.1. Smart micelles for cancer

The ways of leveraging the enhanced permeability, ligand attachment, and specific receptor-ligand attachment could make micelles target to tumors. It is essential to increase drug bioavailability and the desired cytotoxic effect for the released drug from micelles carriers when micelles reach the tumor site. In order to realize the drug release triggered specifically at the tumor site, micelle structures should be designed as environmentally responsive systems, and such functionality is typically incorporated into micelles by introducing temperature/thermo-sensitive, pH sensitive, or ultrasound-activated polymers. As "smart micelles", it is known that micelles can dynamically change their physical properties in response to environmental triggers such as pH, temperature, and chemical species.

The micelle copolymer incorporates an ionizable component and a pH-dependent stability results from the pH sensitivity to micelles. The drug is released from the micelle when it encounters an acidic environment. The pH-sensitive micelles demonstrated the long residence time and improved half-life typical of micellar nanoparticles in animal models. Comparing to non-pH-sensitive micelles, the pH-sensitive micelles achieved a satisfying effect in tumors [97]. It reveals that the potential of pH-sensitive micelles could increase drug delivery to cancerous tumors.

An alternative way of constructing environmentally responsive micelles is to build temperature sensitivity into the micelle structure. The localized hyperthermia is used clinically to treat tumors, since the vasculature of tumor is more vulnerable to hyperthermia than normal tissue [98]. Temperature-sensitive micelles could be a part of a synergistic regimen, therefore, in which the raised temperature induces local drug release and kills tumor cells directly. It is also a common technique that makes use of a thermo-sensitive polymer with LCST behavior to design temperature-responsive micelles. A temperature increase above the LCST induces the entire system to be hydrophobic and precipitate out of the solution.

An important strategy for site-specific drug release from smart micelles is ultrasound activation. A number of mechanisms could promote the drug delivery, for example, a local temperature increase in tissues, the production of highly reactive free radical species that can accelerate polymer degradation, and the cavitation that increase the permeability of cell membranes [99]. Ultrasound was used to improve the antitumor efficacy of both free doxorubicin and micelle-encapsulated doxorubicin in which micelles with ultrasound broke tumor growth an additional several days over micelles without ultrasound. Bio-distribution studies revealed that ultrasound not only increased the level of drug accumulation in the tumor, but also lowered the level of drug accumulation in the kidneys and heart [100–101]. Overall, ultrasound-sensitive micelles may have the capacity to both decrease side effects and increase chemotherapeutic effectiveness during tumor treatment.

In conclusion, micelles can be triggered by modulating temperature, pH, ultrasound, and light application. Well-designed micellar biomaterials for drug delivery could decrease mortality from cancers.

3.2. Ultrasound-sensitive drug delivery for theranostics

For smart therapies, ultrasound is a highly useful method that is already widely used clinically. In addition, ultrasound-triggered drug delivery vehicles can be combined with ultrasound contrast agents or microbubbles to create "theranostics" that incorporate both diagnostics via imaging and therapy via drug delivery [102]. Ultrasound-activated theranostics can improve the detection and treatment of cancerous tumors and cardiovascular pathologies such as atherosclerotic plaque [102].

It is demonstrated that ultrasound-triggered theranostics is a way of cancer treatment. For example, the mixtures of doxorubicin-loaded micelles with doxorubicin-loaded microbubbles were injected intravenously into mice bearing breast cancer tumors, and the agents were visualized at the tumor target site using ultrasound and were then degraded through ultrasound to release the doxorubicin at the tumor site. Ultrasound enhanced the intracellular uptake of doxorubicin by tumor cells and resulted in breast tumor regression in the mouse model. These results could have a significant impact on the treatment of other cancerous tumors via ultrasound-mediated visualization and drug delivery.

Ultrasound-triggered drug delivery vehicles can simultaneously detect areas requiring therapy and target drug delivery to these areas. The smart materials are in the early stages of development but hold potential for enabling rational treatment of diseases, improving clinical outcomes, and promoting a better quality of life for patients with complex chronic diseases.

3.3. Nanoporous implants for local drug delivery

TNTs are an alternative technology that can address some of the problems in dentistry as this is an economically affordable technology that can be easily implemented into dental implants [82]. In addition, the scope of TNT-based delivery systems can be extended to regenerative medicine and dentistry along with preventive therapy. An overview of several aspects relevant to TNT applications in dentistry, including studies of osteoblast adhesion to TNTs surfaces and its biocompatibility, release of specific drugs and silver nanoparticles and periodontium regeneration by the delivery of multiple growth factors inducing osteogenesis (Fig. 15) [82]. TNTs can also serve as a gene and DD carrier such as growth factors and stem cells, which can further enhance osseointegration and bone regeneration relevant to tooth implants [103].

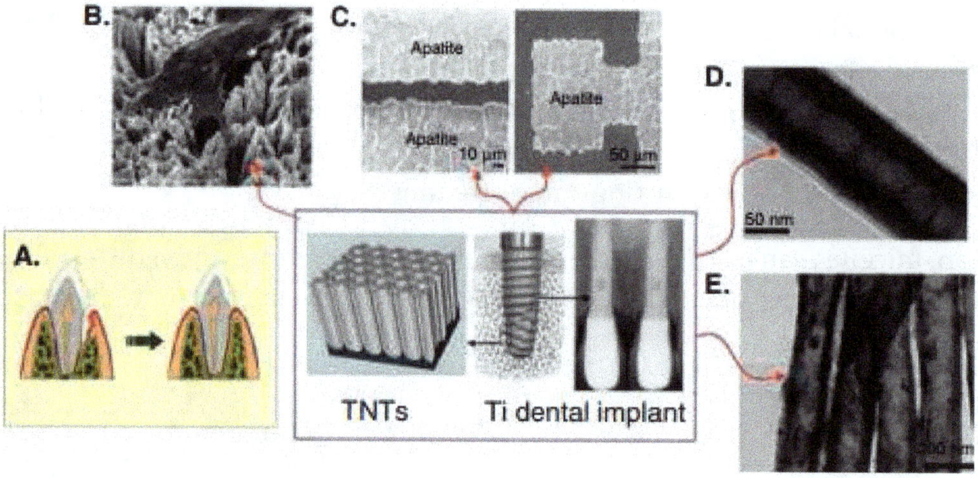

Figure 15. Schematic diagram summarizing the applications of TNTs in dentistry. (a) Periodontium problem and proposed regeneration by delivery of multiple growth factors inducing osteogenesis, (b) the adhesion of osteoblast cells to TNTs surface, (c) the growth of hydroxyapatite on TNTs, (d) the cross-sectional view of a single TNT revealing the drug sodium naproxen on the inside, and (e) anti-bacterial silver nanoparticles incorporated within TNT [82].

The encapsulation of sensitive drugs in nano-carriers such as polymer micelles were loaded in TNTs. Aw et al. put forward a prospective solution to both protect sensitive drugs and proteins from degradation and design TNT-based drug-releasing systems with an extended release capability [93]. Furthermore, based on the implementation of multi-drug payloads, polymeric micelles loaded with different drugs were loaded in the TNTs that are based on the formation of two or more immiscible layers of drug carriers that have opposite interfacial properties with hydrophobic and hydrophilic, which are used to generate a series of sequential release in a time controlled form [104].

Studies mentioned above in the discussion confirmed that NAAs and TNTs can be used for loading and releasing of wide range of therapeutics, with the ability to tune their drug releasing characteristics and provide multi-drug release of different drugs in different fashions. These approaches are aimed at achieving optimized drug dosage, release rate, and time needed for a broad range of specific therapies. The design of triggered drug-release from NAAs and TNTs using various external signaling sources (thermal, magnetic, electro-magnetic, ultrasonic, or mechanical activation) is an outstanding feature offering great perspectives and opportunities for combining NAAs and TNTs with sensing functions. NAAs and TNTs are shown to be very versatile in terms of their biomedical applications and can be applied as a new generation of smart implants and drug-delivery devices.

4. Summary

It is a highly desirable approach for effective therapeutic treatment to use smart materials to release drugs to a specific physiological environment. We have discussed the fundamental behavior and materials design associated with five stimuli-responsive systems based on pH, temperature, magnetism, sound, and light. The stimuli-responsive systems are classified as "smart" materials, and each system includes two major strategies for the material design.

Based on our previous knowledge of degradation, release, and self-assembly, we introduce new concepts of excitation, cavitation, and magnetophoresis for strategies for materials design. A cooperative strategy of magnetophoresis, thermal phase change, and selected concept strategies of light excitation were stated in the chapter. A variety of smart material systems are currently in various stages of clinical development, such as ultrasound and magnetic hyperthermia systems, for treating cancer. It has been proven that drug-releasing systems provide better capabilities and performances than conventional therapies, offering alternative ways to deliver therapeutics effectively over different parts of the host body and reducing the side effects associated with excessive dosages of highly toxic drugs. Despite the successes described above, more exhaustive research must be carried out in order to make drug-releasing implants feasible for clinical applications.

Finally, it is worth stressing that the combination localized drug-releasing systems with other traditional treatments such as surgery, radiation, and systemic chemotherapy could provide more efficient clinical therapies for treating the most challenging and resilient diseases, such as cancer, with minimal drawbacks. What's more, it is expected that the integration of TNT implants with sensors, microchips, and development of advanced triggered drug release can come true in the future. In conclusion, it is right that smart materials were used to study the drug delivery system, and materials design involved with several stimuli-responsive systems such as pH, temperature, magnetism, light, and sound. In addition, smart material systems are currently in various stages of clinical development based on ultrasound and magnetic hyperthermia systems for treating cancer.

Acknowledgements

The authors thank the National Natural Science Foundation of China (21501127; 51502185), Natural Science Foundation of Jiangsu Province of China (BK20130313; BK20140400), and Priority Academic Program Development of Jiangsu Higher Education Institutions (PAPD) for financial support of this work.

Author details

Qun Wang, Jianying Huang and Yuekun Lai*

*Address all correspondence to: yklai@suda.edu.cn

National Engineering Laboratory for Modern Silk, College of Textile and Clothing Engineering, Soochow University, Suzhou, China

References

[1] L. Li, D. Chen, Y. Zhang, Z. Deng, X. Ren, X. Meng, F. Tang, J. Ren, L. Zhang, Magnetic and fluorescent multifunctional chitosan nanoparticles as a smart drug delivery system, Nanotechnology, 2007, 18(40): 405012.

[2] N. Doshi, S. Mitragotri, Designer biomaterials for nanomedicine, Advanced Functional Materials, 2009, 19(24): 3843–3854.

[3] V. Thiviyanathan, A. D. Somasunderam, D. G. Gorenstein, Combinatorial selection and delivery of thioaptamers, Biochemical Society Transactions, 2007, 35(1): 50–52.

[4] Y. Y. Song, F. Schmidt-Stein, S. Bauer, P. Schmuki, Amphiphilic TiO2 nanotube arrays: An actively controllable drug delivery system, Journal of the American Chemical Society, 131(12): 4230–4232.

[5] S. Ghosh, C. Yang, T. Cai, Z. Hu, A. Neogi, Oscillating magnetic field-actuated microvalves for micro- and nanofluidics, Journal of Physics D: Applied Physics, 2009, 42(13): 135501.

[6] M. Hrubý, C. Konák, K. Ulbrich, Polymeric micellar pH-sensitive drug delivery system for doxorubicin, Journal of Controlled Release, 2005, 103(1): 137–148.

[7] A. Yudina, M. de Smet, M. Lepetit-Coiffé, S. Langereis, L. Van Ruijssevelt, P. Smirnov, V. Bouchaud, P. Voisin, H. Grüll, C. T. Moonen, Ultrasound-mediated intracellular drug delivery using microbubbles and temperature-sensitive liposomes, Journal of Controlled Release, 2011, 155(3): 442–448.

[8] X. Y. Li, X. L. Zheng, X. W. Wei, G. Guo, M. L. Gou, C. Y. Gong, X. Huo, D. M. Wang, L. J. Chen, Y. Q. Wei, Z. Y. Qian, A novel composite drug delivery system: Honokiol nanoparticles in thermosensitive hydrogel based on chitosan, Journal of Nanoscience and Nanotechnology, 2009, 9(7): 4586–4592.

[9] J. L. Zhang, R. S. Srivastava, R. D. K. Misra, Core-shell magnetite nanoparticles surface encapsulated with smart stimuli-responsive polymer: Synthesis, characterization, and LCST of viable drug-targeting delivery system, Langmuir, 2007, 23(11): 6342–6351.

[10] A. Ito, M. Shinkai, H. Honda, T. Kobayashi, Medical application of functionalized magnetic nanoparticles, Journal of Fermentation Technology, 2005, 100(1): 1–11.

[11] M. Shinkai, Functional magnetic particles for medical application, Journal of Bioscience and Bioengineering, 2002, 94: 600–613.

[12] A. K. Gupta, M. Gupta, Synthesis and surface engineering of iron oxide nanoparticles for biomedical applications, Biomaterials, 2005, 26(18): 3995–4021.

[13] S. Mornet, S. Vasseur, F. Grasset, P. Veverka, G. Goglio, A. Demourgues, J. Portier, E. Pollert, E. Duguet, Magnetic nanoparticle design for medical applications, Progress in Solid State Chemistry, 2006, 34(2–4): 237–247.

[14] J. Zhang, R. D. K. Misra, Magnetic drug-targeting carrier encapsulated with thermosensitive smart polymer: Core-shell nanoparticle carrier and drug release response, Acta Biomaterialia, 2007, 3(6): 838–850.

[15] S. Mornet, S. Vasseur, F. Grasset, E. Duguet, Magnetic nanoparticle design for medical diagnosis and therapy, Journal of Materials Chemistry, 2004, 14(14): 2161–2175.

[16] K. D. Harris, R. Cuypers, P. Scheibe, C. L. van Oosten, C. W. M. Bastiaansen, J. Lub, D. J. Broer, Large amplitude light-induced motion in high elastic modulus polymer actuators, Journal of Materials Chemistry, 2005, 15(47): 5043–5048.

[17] S. Juodkazis, N. Mukai, R. Wakaki, A. Yamaguchi, S. Matsuo, H. Misawa, Reversible phase transitions in polymer gels induced by radiation forces, Nature, 2000, 408(6809): 178–181.

[18] C. S. Kwok, P. D. Mourad, L. A. Crum, B. D. Ratner, Self-assembled molecular structures as ultrasonically-responsive barrier membranes for pulsatile drug delivery, Journal of Biomedical Materials Research, 2001, 57(2): 151–164.

[19] R. Fernández-Urrusuno, P. Calvo, C. Remuñán-López, J. L. Vila-Jato, M. J. Alonso, Enhancement of nasal absorption of insulin using chitosan nanoparticles, Pharmaceutical Research, 1999, 16(10): 1576–1581.

[20] O. Kayser, A. Lemke, N. Hernandez-Trejo, The impact of nanobiotechnology on the development of new drug delivery systems, Current Pharmaceutical Biotechnology, 2005, 6(1): 3–5.

[21] V. L. Colvin, M. C. Schlamp, A. P. Alivisatos, Light-emitting diodes made from cadmium selenide nanocrystals and a semiconducting polymer, Nature, 1994, 370(6488): 354–357.

[22] C. C. Müller-Goymann, Physicochemical characterization of colloidal drug delivery systems such as reverse micelles, vesicles, liquid crystals and nanoparticles for topical administration, European Journal of Pharmaceutics & Biopharmaceutics, 2004, 58(2): 343–356.

[23] R. Haag, Supramolecular drug-delivery systems based on polymeric core-shell architectures, Angewandte Chemie International Edition, 2004, 43(3): 278–282.

[24] D. Losic, S. Simovic, Self-ordered nanopore and nanotube platforms for drug delivery applications, Expert Opinion on Drug Delivery, 2009, 6(12): 1363–1381.

[25] D. Losic, M. S. Aw, A. Santos, K. Gulati, M. Bariana, Titania nanotube arrays for local drug delivery: Recent advances and perspectives, Expert Opinion on Drug Delivery, 2015, 12(1): 103–127.

[26] K. Noh, K. S. Brammer, C. Choi, S. H. Kim, C. J. Frandsen, S. Jin, A new nano-platform for drug release via nanotubular aluminum oxide, Journal of Biomaterials and Nanobiotechnology, 2011, 2(3): 226–233.

[27] K. Shimizu, H. Fujita, E. Nagamori, Oxygen plasma-treated thermoresponsive polymer surfaces for cell sheet engineering, Biotechnology and Bioengineering, 2010, 106(2): 303–310.

[28] J. F. Mano, Stimuli-responsive polymeric systems for biomedical applications, Advanced Engineering Materials, 2008, 10(6): 515–527.

[29] J. F. Joanny, L. Leibler, Weakly charged polyelectrolytes in a poor solvent, Journal de Physique, 1990, 51(6): 545–557.

[30] D. Andelman, J. F. Joanny, Polyelectrolyte adsorption, Comptes Rendus de l'Académie des Sciences-Series IV-Physics, 2000, 1(9): 1153–1162.

[31] J. L. Zhang, R. S. Srivastava, R. D. K. Misra, Core-Shell Magnetite Nanoparticles Surface Encapsulated with Smart Stimuli-Responsive Polymer: Synthesis, Characterization, and LCST of Viable Drug-Targeting Delivery System, Langmuir, 2007, 23(11): 6342–6351.

[32] Y. Goto, L. J. Calciano, A. L. Fink, Acid-induced folding of proteins, Proceedings of the National Academy of Sciences, 1990, 87(2): 573–577.

[33] M. Schmidt (Ed.), Polyelectrolytes with defined molecular architecture II (Google eBook) (p. 231), Springer: Heidelberg, 2004.

[34] M. R. Bohmer, O. A. Evers, J. M. H. M. Scheutjens, Weak polyelectrolytes between two surfaces: Adsorption and stabilization, Macromolecules, 1990, 23(8): 2288–2301.

[35] G. M. Cooper, The cell: A molecular approach (2nd ed.), Sunderland, MA: Sinauer Associates, 2000.

[36] E. G. Bellomo, M. D. Wyrsta, L. Pakstis, D. J. Pochan, T. J. Deming, Stimuli-responsive polypeptide vesicles by conformation-specific assembly, Nature Materials, 2004, 3(4): 244–248.

[37] S. K. De, N. R. Aluru, B. Johnson, W. C. Crone, D. J. Beebe, J. Moore, Equilibrium swelling and kinetics of pH-responsive hydrogels: Models, experiments, and simulations, Journal of Microelectromechanical Systems, 2002, 11(5): 544–555.

[38] R. M. Sawant, J. P. Hurley, S. Salmaso, A. Kale, E. Tolcheva, T. S. Levchenko, V. P. Torchilin, "SMART" drug delivery systems: Double-targeted pH-responsive pharmaceutical nanocarriers, Bioconjugate Chemistry, 2006, 17(4): 943–949.

[39] R. H. Kaul (Ed.), Aqueous two-phase systems: Methods and protocols, New York: Humana Press, 2000.

[40] J. W. Cahn, On spinodal decomposition, Acta Metallurgica, 1961, 9(9): 795–801.

[41] G. Charlet, G. Delmas, Thermodynamic properties of polyolefin solutions at high temperature: 1. Lower critical solubility temperatures of polyethylene, polypropylene and ethylene-propylene copolymers in hydrocarbon solvents, Polymer, 1981, 22(9): 1181–1189.

[42] N. T. Southall, K. A. Dill, A. D. J. Haymet, A view of the hydrophobic effect, The Journal of Physical Chemistry B, 2002, 106(3): 521–533.

[43] K. Kita-Tokarczyk, J. Grumelard, T. Haefele, W. Meier, Block copolymer Vesicles-Using concepts from polymer chemistry to mimic biomembranes, Polymer, 2005, 46(11): 3540–3563.

[44] A. Shavit, R. A. Riggleman, Influence of backbone rigidity on nanoscale confinement effects in model glass-forming polymers, Macromolecules, 2013, 46(12): 5044–5052.

[45] H. Aranda-Espinoza, H. Bermudez, F. S. Bates, D. E. Discher, Electromechanical limits of polymersomes, Physical Review Letters, 2001, 87(20): 208301.

[46] M. B. Yatvin, J. N. Weinstein, W. H. Dennis, R. Blumenthal, Design of liposomes for enhanced local release of drugs by hyperthermia, Science, 1978, 202(4374): 1290–1293.

[47] J. N. Weinstein, R. L. Magin, M. B. Yatvin, D. S. Zaharko, Liposomes and local hyperthermia-selective delivery of methotrexate to heated tumors, Science, 1979, 204(4389): 188–191.

[48] G. Kong, G. Anyarambhatla, W.P. Petros, R.D. Braun, O.M. Colvin, D. Needham, M.W. Dewhirst, Efficacy of liposomes and hyperthermia in a human tumor xenograft model: Importance of triggered drug release, Cancer Research, 2000, 60(24): 6950–6957.

[49] M. de Smet, E. Heijman, S. Langereis, N. M. Hijnen, H. Grüll, Magnetic resonance imaging of high intensity focused ultrasound mediated drug delivery from temperature-sensitive liposomes: An in vivo proof-of-concept study, Journal of Controlled Release, 2011, 150(1): 102–110.

[50] A. D. Bangham, R. W. Horne, Negative staining of phospholipids and their structural modifications by surface active agents as observed in electron microscope, Journal of Molecular Biology, 1964, 8(5): 660–668.

[51] E. Evans, D. Needham, Physical-properties of surfactant bilayer-membranes-thermal transitions, elasticity, rigidity, cohesion, and colloidal interactions, Journal of Physical Chemistry B, 1987, 91(16): 4219–4228.

[52] M. A. Ward, T. K. Georgiou, Thermoresponsive polymers for biomedical applications, Polymers, 2011, 3(3): 1215–1242.

[53] Y. Zhang, N. Kohler, M. Zhang, Surface modification of superparamagnetic magnetite nanoparticles and their intracellular uptake, Biomaterials, 2002, 23(7): 1553–1561.

[54] P. A. Voltairas, D. I. Fotiadis, L. K. Michalis, Hydrodynamics of magnetic drug targeting, Journal of Biomechanics, 2002, 35(6): 813–821.

[55] J. Gittleman, B. Abeles, S. Bozowski, Superparamagnetism and relaxation effects in granular Ni-SiO_2 and Ni-Al_2O_3 films, Physical Review B, 1974, 9(9): 3891–3897.

[56] A. Aharoni, Introduction to the theory of ferromagnetism, Oxford: Oxford University Press, 2000.

[57] K. Kataoka, C. Scholz, N. Rapoport, Physical stimuli-responsive polymeric micelles for anti-cancer drug delivery, Progress in Polymer Science, 2007, 32(8): 962–990.

[58] A. Senyei, K. Widder, G. Czerlinski, Magnetic guidance of drug-carrying microspheres, Journal of Applied Physics, 1978, 49(6): 3578-3583.

[59] G. P. Hatch, R. E. Stelter, Magnetic design considerations for devices and particles used for biological high-gradient magnetic separation (HGMS) systems, Journal of Magnetism and Magnetic Materials, 2001, 225(1): 262–276.

[60] S. Gómez-Lopera, R. Plaza, A. Delgado, Synthesis and characterization of spherical magnetite/biodegradable polymer composite particles, Journal of Colloid and Interface Science, 2001, 240(1): 40–47.

[61] L. Li, D. Chen, Y. Zhang, Z. Deng, X. Ren, X. Meng, F. Tang, J. Ren, L. Zhang, Magnetic and fluorescent multifunctional chitosan nanoparticles as a smart drug delivery system, Nanotechnology, 2007, 18(40): 405102.

[62] M. Mitsumori, M. Hiraoka, T. Shibata, Y. Okuno, Y. Nagata, Y. Nishimura, Targeted hyperthermia using dextran magnetite complex: A new treatment modality for liver tumors, Hepato-gastroenterology, 1996, 43(12): 1431–1437.

[63] C. X. Deng, F. Sieling, H. Pan, J. Cui, Ultrasound-induced cell membrane porosity, Ultrasound in Medicine & Biology, 2004, 30(4): 519–526.

[64] H. Pan, Y. Zhou, F. Sieling, J. Shi, J. Cui, C. Deng, Sonoporation of cells for drug and gene delivery, In Proceedings of the Annual International Conference of the IEEE Engineering in Medicine and Biology Society. 2004, 5: 3531–3534.

[65] P. Zhang, T. Porter, An in vitro study of a phase-shift nanoemulsion: A potential nucleation agent for bubble-enhanced HIFU tumor ablation, Ultrasound in Medicine & Biology, 2010, 36 (11): 1856–1866.

[66] E. C. Pua, P. Zhong, Ultrasound-mediated drug delivery, IEEE Engineering in Medicine and Biology, 2009, 28(1): 64–75.

[67] J. Du, R. K. O'Reilly, Advances and challenges in smart and functional polymer vesicles, Soft Matter, 2009, 5 (19): 3544–3550.

[68] G. Bajic, L. Yatime, R. B. Sim, T. Vorup-Jensen, G. R. Andersen, Structural insight on the recognition of surface-bound opsonins by the integrin I domain of complement

receptor 3, Proceedings of the National Academy of Sciences of the United States of America, 2013, 110(41): 16426-16431.

[69] S. R. Sirsi, M. A. Borden, Microbubble compositions, properties and biomedical applications, Bubble Science Engineering and Technology, 2012, 1(1–2): 3–17.

[70] E. Y. Lukianova-Hleb, X. Ren, J. A. Zasadzinski, X. Wu, D. O. Lapotko, Plasmonic nanobubbles enhance efficacy and selectivity of chemotherapy against drugresistant cancer cells, Advanced Materials, 2012, 24(28): 3831–3837.

[71] S. D. Tiukinhoy-Laing, S. Huang, M. Klegerman, C. K. Holland, D. D. McPherson, Ultrasound-facilitated thrombolysis using tissue-plasminogen activator-loaded echogenic liposomes, Thrombosis Research, 2007, 119(6): 777–784.

[72] A. Mueller, B. Bondurant, D. F. O'Brien, Visible-light-stimulated destabilization of PEG-liposomes, Macromolecules, 2000, 33(13): 4799–4804.

[73] S. Oh, K. S. Moon, J. H. Moon, J. M. Bae, S. Jin, Visible light irradiation-mediated drug elution activity of nitrogen-doped TiO_2 nanotubes, Journal of Nanomaterials, 2013, 2013: 802318.

[74] H. F. Zhuang, C. J. Lin, Y. K. Lai, L. Sun., J. Li, Some critical structure factors of titanium oxide nanotube array in its photocatalytic activity, Environmental Science & Technology, 2007, 41(13): 4735–4740.

[75] M. Paulose, K. Shankar, S. Yoriya, H. E. Prakasam, O. K. Varghese, G. K. Mor, T. A. Latempa, A. Fitzgerald, C. A. Grimes, Anodic growth of highly ordered TiO2 nanotube arrays to 134μm in length, Journal of Physical Chemistry B, 2006, 110(33): 16179-16184.

[76] Y. K. Lai, J. Y. Huang, H. F. Zhang, V. P. Subramaniam, Y. X. Tang, D. G. Gong, L. Sundar, L. Sun., Z. Chen, C. J. Lin, Nitrogen-doped TiO2 nanotube array films with enhanced photocatalytic activity under various light sources, Journal of Hazardous Materials, 2010, 184(1–3): 855–863.

[77] M. D. Ye, J. J. Gong, Y. K. Lai, C. J. Lin, Z. Q. Lin, High-Efficiency Photoelectrocatalytic Hydrogen Generation Enabled by Palladium Quantum Dots-Sensitized TiO2 Nanotube Arrays, Journal of the American Chemical Society, 2012, 134(38): 15720-15723.

[78] M. Bigerelle, K. Anselme, B. Noel, I. Ruderman, P. Hardouin, A. Iost, Improvement in the morphology of Ti-based surfaces: A new process to increase in vitro human osteoblast response, Biomaterials, 2002, 23(7): 1563–1577.

[79] Y. K. Lai, L. X. Lin, F. Pan, J. Y. Huang, R. Song, Y. X. Huang, C. J. Lin, H. Fuchs, L. F. Chi, Bioinspired Patterning with Extreme Wettability Contrast on TiO2 Nanotube Array Surface: A Versatile Platform for Biomedical Applications, Small, 2013, 9(17): 2945–2953.

[80] C. G. Galbraith, M. P. Sheetz, Forces on adhesive contacts affect cell function, Current Opinion in Cell Biology, 1998, 10(5): 566–571.

[81] A. Ghicov, P. Schmuki, Self-ordering electrochemistry: A review on growth and functionality of TiO2 nanotubes and other self-aligned MOx structures, Chemical Communication, 2009, 20(32): 2791–2808.

[82] D. Losic, M. S. Aw, A. Santos, K. Gulati, M. Bariana, Titania nanotube arrays for local drug delivery: Recent advances and perspectives, Expert Opinion on Drug Delivery, 2015, 12(1): 103–127.

[83] K. S. Moon, J. M. Bae, S. Jin, S. Oh. Infrared-Mediated Drug Elution Activity of Gold Nanorod-Grafted TiO2 Nanotubes, Journal of Nanomaterials, 2014, 2014: 750813.

[84] W. Brown, Thermal fluctuations of a single-domain particle. Physical Review, 1963, 130(5): 1677–1686.

[85] P. Shum, J. M. Kim, D. H. Thompson, Phototriggering of liposomal drug delivery systems. Advanced Drug Delivery Reviews, 2001, 53(3): 273–284.

[86] K. A. K. Musa, L. A. Eriksson, Photodegradation mechanism of the common nonsteroid anti-inflammatory drug diclofenac and its carbazole photoproduct. Physical Chemistry Chemical Physics, 2009, 11(22): 4601–4610.

[87] E. Gultepe, D. Nagesha, S. Sridhar, M. Amiji, Nanoporous inorganic membranes or coatings for sustained drug delivery in implantable devices, Advanced Drug Delivery, 2010, 62(3): 305–315.

[88] K. E. Orosz, S. Gupta, M. Hassink, M. Abdel-Rahman, L. Moldovan, F. H. Davidorf, N. I. Moldovan, Delivery of antiangiogenic and antioxidant drugs of ophthalmic interest through a nanoporous inorganic filter, Molecule Vision, 2004, 10(68): 555–565.

[89] M. S. Aw, M. Kurian, D. Losic, Non-eroding drug-releasing implants with ordered nanoporous and nanotubular structures: Concepts for controlling drug release, Biomaterials Science, 2014, 2: 10–34.

[90] A. Santos, M. S. Aw, M. Bariana, T. Kumeria, Y. Wang, D. Losic. Drug-releasing implants: Current progress, challenges and perspectives, Journal of Materials Chemistry B, 2014, 2: 6157–6182.

[91] G. Jeon, S. Y. Yang, J. Byun, J. K. Kim, Electrically actuatable smart nanoporous membrane for pulsatile drug release, Nano Letter, 2011, 11(3): 1284–1288.

[92] D. Losic, S. Simovic, Self-ordered nanopore and nanotube platforms for drug delivery applications, Expert Opinion on Drug Delivery, 2009, 6(12):1363–1381.

[93] M. S. Aw, S. Simovic, J. Addai-Mensah, D. Losic, Polymeric micelles in porous and nanotubular implants as a new system for extended delivery of poorly soluble drugs, Journal of Materials Chemistry, 2011, 21 (20): 7082–7089.

[94] M. S. Aw, K. Gulati, D. Losic, Controlling drug release from titania nanotube arrays using polymer nanocarriers and biopolymer coating, Journal of Biomaterials & Nanobiotechnology, 2011, 2(5): 477–484.

[95] M. Bariana, M. S. Aw, E. Moore, N. H. Voelcker and D. Losic, Radiofrequency-triggered release for on-demand delivery of therapeutics from titania nanotube drug-eluting implants, Nanomedicine, 2014, 9(8): 1263–1275.

[96] M. S. Aw, J. Addai-Mensah and D. Losic, Magnetic-responsive delivery of drug-carriers using titania nanotube arrays, Journal of Materials Chemistry, 2012, 22(14): 6561–6563.

[97] D. Shenoy, S. Little, R. Langer, M. Amiji, Poly(ethylene oxide)-modified poly(betaamino ester) nanoparticles as a pH-sensitive system for tumor-targeted delivery of hydrophobic drugs: Part 2. In vivo distribution and tumor localization studies. Pharmaceutical Research, 2005, 22(12): 2107–2114.

[98] J. van der Zee, Heating the patient: A promising approach? Annals of Oncology, 2002, 13(8): 1173–1184.

[99] S. Mitragotri, Healing sound: The use of ultrasound in drug delivery and other therapeutic applications, Nature Reviews Drug Discovery, 2005, 4(3): 255–260.

[100] A. V. Kabanov, E. V. Batrakova, V. Y. Alakhov, Pluronic block copolymers for overcoming drug resistance in cancer, Advanced Drug Delivery Reviews, 2002, 54(5): 759–779.

[101] Z. G. Gao, H. D. Fain, N. Rapoport, Controlled and targeted tumor chemotherapy by micellar-encapsulated drug and ultrasound. Journal of Controlled Release, 2005, 102(1): 203–222.

[102] A. T. Nguyen, S. P. Wrenn, Acoustically active liposome-nanobubble complexes for enhanced ultrasonic imaging and ultrasound-triggered drug delivery. Wiley Interdisciplinary Reviews in Nanomedicine and Nanobiotechnology, 2014, 6(3): 316–325.

[103] Y. H. Lee, G. Bhattarai, I. S. Park, G. R. Kim, G. E. Kim, M. H. Lee, H. K. Yi, Bone regeneration around N-acetyl cysteine-loaded nanotube titanium dental implant in rat mandible, Biomaterials, 2013, 34(38): 10199–10208.

[104] M. S. Aw, J. Addai-Mensah, D. Losic, A multi-drug delivery system with sequential release using titania nanotube arrays, Chemical Communications, 2012, 48(27): 3348–3350.

8

Enhancement of Percutaneous Absorption on Skin by Plasma Drug Delivery Method

Kazuo Shimizu and Jaroslav Krištof

Abstract

Transdermal drug delivery (TDD) is a painless method of low-dose drug delivery. The advantages and disadvantages of transdermal drug delivery methods are named and basic methods such as using chemical enhancers, iontophoresis and electrophoresis are introduced. One of the promising methods make use of plasma which is generated in atmospheric pressure mostly in volume or on surface dielectric barrier discharge (DBD) or in plasma jet. As the plasma produces various particles according to the used gas, UV radiation and heat, their effects on skin and barrier function are described. Improvement of transdermal drug delivery of hydrophilic drug galantamine hydrobromide (GaHBr) using microplasma electrode is introduced.

Keywords: microplasma, plasma jet, plasma drug delivery, skin, stratum corneum

1. Introduction of atmospheric plasma for medical application

Medical applications of atmospheric plasma have been intensively studied [1]. These studies have reported numerous applications, such as for sterilization [2, 3], decomposition of harmful substances [4] and surface treatments [5–7]. In recent years, this area of research has been focused on the practical utilization of atmospheric plasma in the medical filed, such as for blood coagulation [8, 9], wound healing [10–12] and cancer treatment [13–15]. On the other hand, dermatology is one area of medicine where atmospheric plasma applications are currently used in practice [16], such as in a device to treat acne or wrinkles [17] and to treat stretch marks in combination with ultrasonic waves [18, 19]. As explained above, various research and development efforts have been conducted in the application of plasma medicine; however, we do not yet know whether plasma irradiation can be used to treat various symptoms. Though, the basic mechanisms of cell response [13–15] and the bacterial sterilization process [2, 3] have been studied intensively, effectiveness of plasma medicine in treating depression, which is a social problem in contemporary countries such as Japan, and Alzheimer's disease, which is an increasing problem in aging societies, has not still been investigated. The use of plasma medicine to treat various other diseases, such as cerebral infarction and high blood pressure, also requires additional investigation. Reactive oxygen species (ROSs) and reactive nitrogen species (RNSs) could play important roles in the beneficial effects of plasma medicine. Mechanisms underlying these effects could be quite complicated because of the physiological activation in the body by ROS signalling [20]. Fundamental research to elucidate the cellular response is currently under investigation. In contrast, reactive species generated in plasma or exposed liquid medium have demonstrated efficacy for treating various cancers, but not for the previously mentioned mental disorders, other associated symptoms or diseases such as diabetes, cerebral infarction and high blood pressure [21]. Fortunately, mechanisms of depression and Alzheimer's disease have been revealed in detail. The inhibited production of neurotransmitters (serotonin, noradrenalin and dopamine) causes depression, and Alzheimer's disease occurs because of the deposition of a peptide called amyloid-ß on the cerebral cortex. Research and development of effective drugs for treating mental disorders are proceeding [22]. These drugs are administrated orally; however, the effects of many of these drugs are delayed because of absorption in the small intestine. Moreover, as is the case with oral administration, absorption of drugs in additional locations is different for each person. Thus, administration by injection is used if a precise or high dose of drugs is needed [23, 24]. Administration of poorly absorbed drugs is also the same. However, frequent injections are not desirable in the view of a patient's quality of life (QOL). We can point out the following questions to guide the future of plasma medicine and develop it into a strong tool for the treatment of various symptoms:

1. Is plasma medicine an effective method for treating various symptoms?
2. If not, what combination of drugs in addition to plasma irradiation will be required?
3. Can plasma irradiation be an effective method for drug administration?

As mentioned in many of the references, recent studies of plasma medicine are mostly focused on direct or indirect actions of the active species. Hence, clinical cases, such as Alzheimer's disease, diabetes, cerebral infarction and high blood pressure, have not yet been investigated to determine whether reactive species and plasma medicine could be an effective treatment. Applying plasma medicine for treatment of various symptoms, we have been considering plasma irradiation as a method to deliver appropriate drugs [25]. One instance of this use is the enhancement of percutaneous absorption by atmospheric microplasma irradiation. Percutaneous absorption is a drug administration method in which drugs are absorbed into the skin or body. In this sense, this method is similar to an injection; however, there is no need for a needle in plasma irradiation. Administering drugs in ways that do not require needles could increase patient QOL and reduce the rate of infections. In addition, percutaneous absorption has several advantages, such as preventing metabolism of the drug [24] and stabilizing the concentration of drug in the blood [26]. However, it has disadvantages as well, such as the limitation of the molecular weight of the drug [27] and the need for moderate solubility of the drug in lipids [28]. The stratum corneum layer inhibits drug penetration because the skin acts as a barrier to guard our body from foreign substances.

2. Advantages and disadvantages of TDD

Transdermal drug delivery (TDD) is an alternative to oral and parenteral routes of administration. It can offer some advantages over other methods of drug delivery [29, 30]:

1. Reduction of dosing frequency, due to longer duration of delivery.
2. Lower dosing of drugs.
3. Circumvention of first-pass inactivation by liver that can metabolize drugs.
4. Reduction of gastrointestinal irritation.
5. Lower probability of over or under dosing.
6. No pain.
7. No risk of infection by a contaminated needle or via wounds caused by a needle.
8. Suitable for patients with problems of swallowing.

Disadvantages of TTDS:

1. Only some drugs are permeable through the skin.
2. Limited to drugs with a daily dose 10 mg and less.
3. Slow drug delivery.
4. Possible skin irritation.

3. Stratum corneum structure

Stratum corneum, an upper layer of the skin, is a lipid-rich matrix with embedded corneocyte cells, which are dead keratinocytes. Corneocytes are tied together by a protein called corneodesmosome (**Figure 1**). Renewal of stratum corneum occurs every 14 days [31]. This layer is the first barrier for transdermal drug delivery. Lipid-rich matrix is used for transdermal drug delivery (TDD)—intercellular pathway. The lipid-rich matrix is composed of hydrophilic domain—head of ceramides and lipophilic domain—tails (**Figure 1**). The lipids in stratum corneum include mostly ceramides (41%), cholesterol (27%), cholesteryl esters (10%) and fatty acids (9%) with a small fraction of cholesterol sulphate (2%) [32]. The presence of ceramides indicates that lipids will be structured [31].

The permeability of stratum corneum lipid membranes depends strongly on the ceramide composition of these membranes. Molecular dynamics simulations show that ceramides with shorter (four- to eight-carbon acyl chains) fatty acid chains increase skin permeability, whereas further shortening of the chain leads to increased resistance to penetration almost as good as that of ceramides from healthy skin (24 carbons long on average) [33]. In order to enhance skin permeability, mechanisms like alternation of lipids of stratum corneum and its fluidity or creation of the disordering effect between alkyl chains of lipids of stratum corneum have been proposed [34].

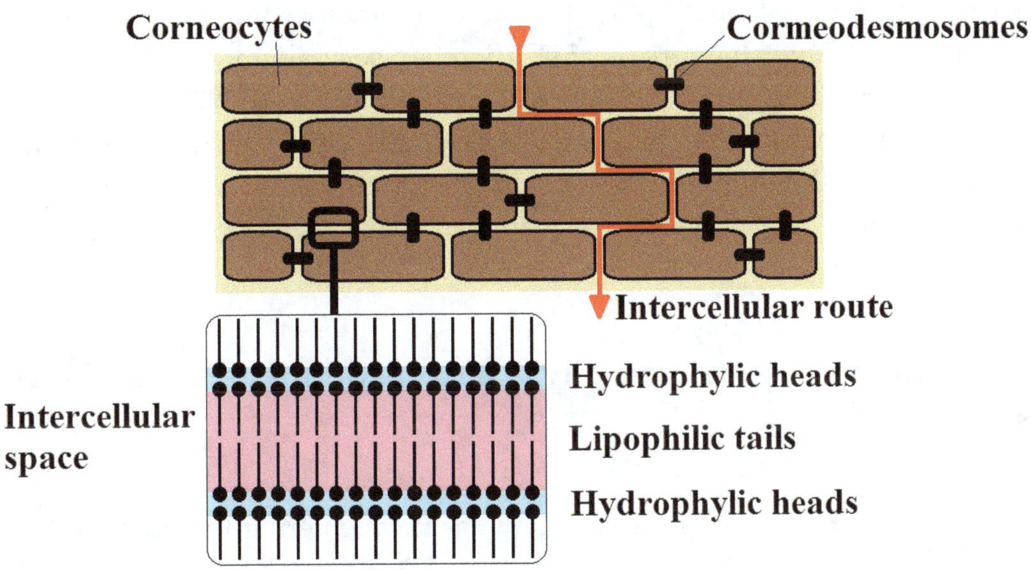

Figure 1. Stratum corneum layer with intercellular space [31].

4. Diagnostics of barrier properties of the skin—TEWL (transepidermal water loss), TST (tape stripping test), ATR-FTIR (attenuated total reflection-Fourier transform infrared spectroscopy)

There are wide varieties of methods available for analysing skin structure and other properties including its barrier function, such as Raman spectroscopy [35], X-ray diffraction [36], electron diffraction [37] and transmission electron microscopy [38]. Barrier properties of the stratum corneum can be confirmed by the transepidermal water loss (TEWL) test, which indicates water evaporation from the inner body through skin [21]. This test expresses the amount of water in grams evaporated per square metre in 1 h. Stratum corneum is a barrier against water diffusion and some other chemicals. The better the barrier function of the skin, the higher the water content and the lower the TEWL value. The tape striping test was described for the first time by Pinkus [39] in 1951. This method is based on removing of stratum corneum layers of the skin. The amount of removed stratum corneum is not constant and it depends on many parameters such as cohesion between cells, hydration or body sites [40]. This technique has been used for evaluation of the barrier function of skin, i.e. for investigating the depth of penetration of drugs [41], the influence of drug enhancers on stratum corneum [42], pH profiles [43] and many others. The tape stripping test (TST) is a representative method for estimating the barrier performance of skin and other properties of the stratum corneum [44]. When the

Scotch tape is placed on skin and peeled off, stratum corneum layer is stuck to the surface of the tape. Therefore, the barrier performance is decreased. Attenuated total reflection-Fourier transform infrared spectroscopy (ATR-FTIR) is an effective method when a material which is not well transmissive is measured, and the method can be used for liquid or solid samples. The information tells us about several micrometres of surface; thus, it is also a useful method for analysing skin [45, 46]. ATR-FTIR spectra can give us information about hydration of skin [47], structure of proteins [48] and lipids [49] and about their changes during skin treatment by chemical or other drug enhancers [50, 51]. There are several vibrational bands associated with chemical functional groups. Vibrational bands at 2850 and 2920 cm^{-1} belong to CH_2 symmetric and asymmetric stretching modes, respectively [52]. The absorbance of the spectrum decreases as the thickness of the skin decreases and the wavenumber indicates a change in chain conformation, especially a change in peak shape [49].

5. Introduction to chemical and physical transdermal drug delivery methods

The stratum corneum provides a barrier to any chemical entering the body and only small molecules having a molecular weight of less than 500 Da (Daltons) can passively diffuse through the skin at rates resulting in therapeutic effects. There are several methods for overcoming this barrier such as using chemical enhancers or physical ways using electric current or plasma discharge.

5.1. Chemical enhancers in transdermal drug delivery

Chemical enhancers are substances that change properties of skin for better penetration of drugs. The most well-known chemical enhancers are alcohols, fatty acids, terpenes and azone. An increase in permeability is very often caused by fluidising the lipids in stratum corneum. However, it is not valid for high concentration of short chain alcohols (like ethanol), where there was observed only a decrease of the absorbance of CH_2 stretching bands and no shift of their position; thus, there is only the extraction of lipids [53]. Many enhancers have long hydrocarbon chains, and it was found out that for fatty acids and fatty alcohols, enhancement is related to the length of the hydrophobic group chain [32]. Enhancer can interact with polar head or with hydrophobic tails of lipid bilayer or with proteins. Water increases fluidity of stratum corneum by insertion of water molecules between polar head groups. Dimethylsulfoxide (DMSO) interacts with intercellular lipids and keratin. Azone disrupts lipid structure, and oleic acid increases fluidity of intercellular lipids. The most effective enhancers are those which interact with lipids and also with proteins of stratum corneum [54]. Combinations of chemical enhancers have been used to maximize the effect of the permeability of drugs, and chemical enhancers are also combined with physical enhancing methods such as iontophoresis [55].

5.2. Iontophoresis in transdermal drug delivery

Iontophoresis (**Figure 2**) is a class of noninvasive methods to increase penetrations of ions through the skin by applying electric current using low voltages of up to 10 V (**Figure 2**).

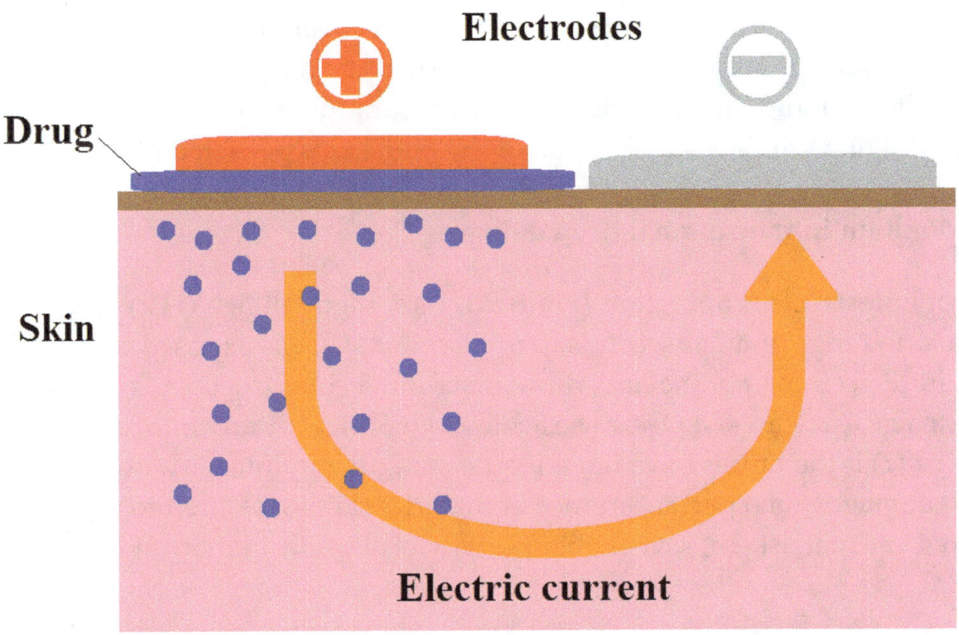

Figure 2. Application of iontophoresis to skin.

Various waveforms of applied current have been investigated [56], and it has been shown that various waveforms have various effectivities for skin permeability [57]. Iontophoresis enhances transdermal drug delivery by three mechanisms:

1. Ion-electric field interaction causing moving of drug (ions) away from the electrode through the skin.
2. Flow of electric current increases skin permeability.
3. Electro-osmosis caused by solvent flow from the anode to cathode because of negatively charged skin due to amino acids in cell membranes.

Iontophoresis is used for ionisable drugs, and it is most effective for molecules with weight of up to 7 kDa [58] or 10–15 kDa according to Kalluri and Banga [59]. The disadvantages of iontophoresis are: difficulties with stabilizing the therapeutic agent in the application vehicle, complexity of the drug release system and prolonged skin exposure to an electric current [60]. The main changes on skin after iontophoresis are an increase of the hydration of stratum corneum and a decrease of electrical resistance of the skin [61]. Analysis of asymmetric CH_2 peak, in ATR-FTIR spectra, did not show lipid alkyl chain disorders characterised by band shift or band broadening even at high current densities in some previous works [61–64]. On the other hand, in the recent work of Prasad et al. [65], they observed a shift of asymmetric CH_2 band with increasing of current density that achieved 8 cm^{-1} at 0.2 mA/cm^2. Also decreasing of lipid and protein bands intensity indicates lipid and protein extraction. The spectra also demonstrated a split in amide II band into 1553 and 1541 cm^{-1}. The split could be due to the disruption in hydrogen bonding associated with the head of ceramides, breaking interlamellar hydrogen bonding of the lipid bilayer and disrupting the barrier property of stratum corneum, resulting in loosening of lipid-protein domains, thus allowing higher flux as compared to the passive treatment [65]. Reversibility studies were conducted *in vivo* after 24 and 48 h of the application of iontophoresis. It was observed that the recovery process had started in 24 h and almost total recovery of epidermal as well as dermal changes was found in 48 h with low current density DC iontophoresis. However, with iontophoresis using 0.5 mA/cm^2 current density, edema along with focal disruption of the epidermis persisted [65].

5.3. Electroporation in transdermal drug delivery

Unlike iontophoresis, electroporation (**Figure 3**) uses high voltage (HV) (over 100 V) pulses for short time (in range of microseconds to milliseconds). Cells exposed to an electrical pulse open pores in the cell membrane and allow macromolecules to enter. It was confirmed that delivery of drugs of at least 40 kDa can be achieved [66]. The disadvantages of electroporation are as follows: (1) if the pulses have not adequate length and intensity, pores can be too large or cause cell damage, non-specific amount of material can be released to the cell [67]. (2) The created pores can persist for several hours, which allow a higher amount of drug to be delivered [30].

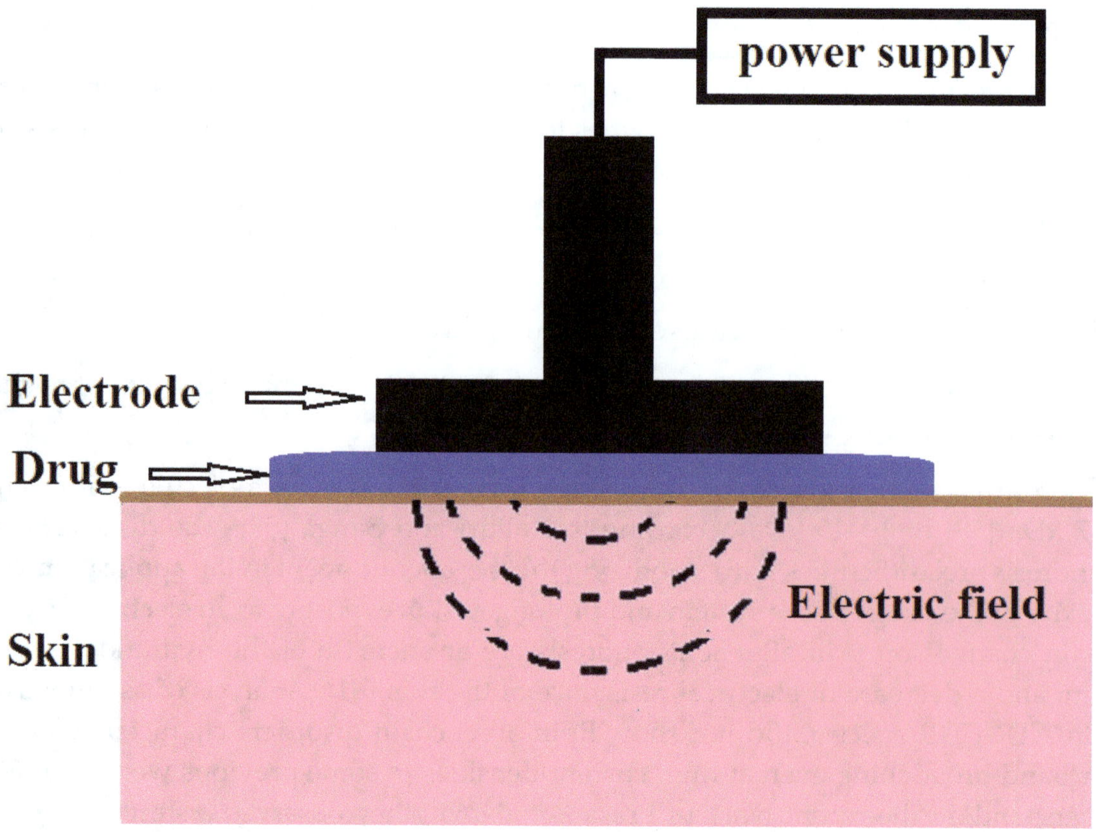

Figure 3. Application of electroporation application.

6. Plasma sources used for skin treatment

Several kinds of plasma sources were used for investigation of transdermal drug delivery so far, such as volume dielectric barrier discharge (DBD), surface DBD and plasma jet.

6.1. Volume DBD

Volume DBD (**Figure 4**) with one isolated electrode has been used in the study of Kalghatgi et al. [68]. Plasma can be with direct contact with a treated object (placed between electrodes) but with increasing distance of electrodes, ignition voltage also increases, too. This means that very high voltages need to be used in real applications. Kalghatgi et al. used pulsed discharge with a pulse duration of 1–10 μs. They applied 10 kV in the frequency range of 50–3.5 kHz to HV electrode isolated by quartz glass. The skin was treated from 15 to 120 s.

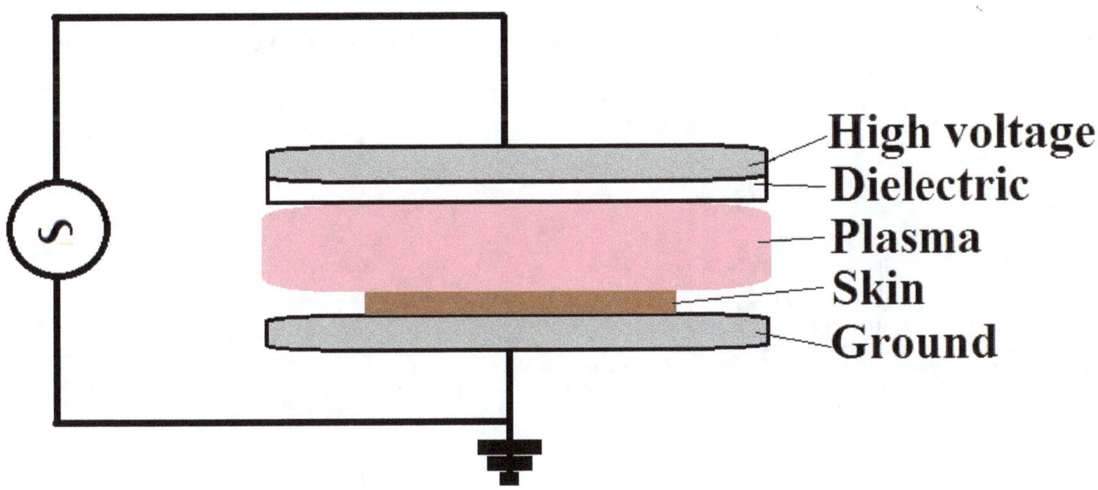

Figure 4. Volume dielectric barrier discharge.

6.2. Surface DBD

Another version of DBD is surface DBD used in Shimizu et al. [23, 69]. Both electrodes were in contact with isolator layer. Each electrode had a thickness in micrometre dimensions. These low dimensions allowed the decrease of ignition voltage to hundreds of volts. During treatment of skin, electrodes were powered by 600 V with an AC frequency of 27 kHz. Electrodes are created by two copper grids each with a thickness of 18 μm with insulation layer between them with thickness of 100 μm. The high-voltage electrode was covered with an insulation layer and the grounded electrode faced the skin samples at a distance of approximately 1.5 mm (**Figure 5**). Thus, there was no risk of electric shock to users, even when touching the surface of the film electrode. The waveform of the applied voltage and corresponding discharge current are shown in **Figure 5**. Holes between electrode lines allowed gas to pass towards the sample (**Figures 5** and **6**). Argon gas was supplied to the microplasma electrode systems with a flow rate of 5 L/min through the tube that was connected to the electrode. The exposure time was usually between 1 and 5 min (**Figure 7**).

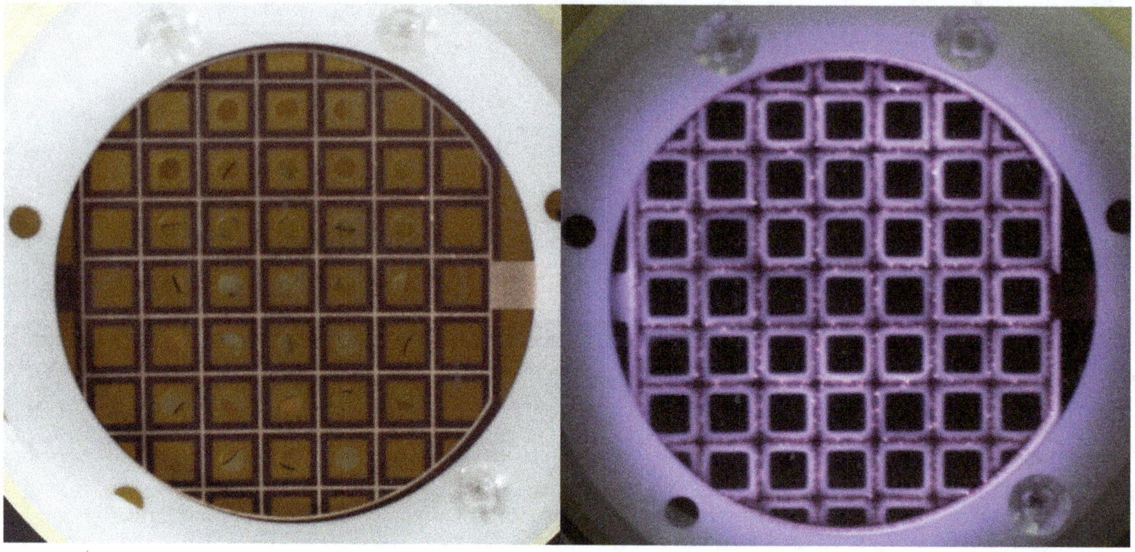

Figure 5. Top view of microplasma electrode, before discharge (left), discharge with Ar gas – 600 V (right) [69].

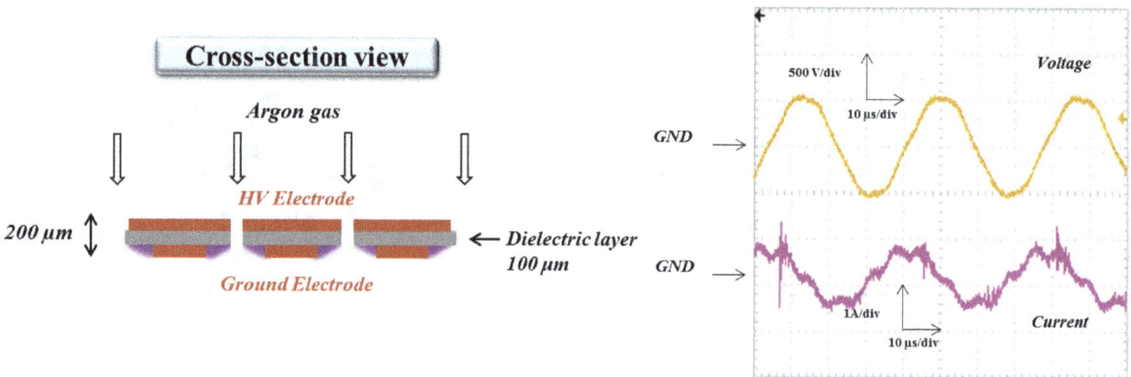

Figure 6. Cross section of microplasma electrode (left); waveforms of microplasma discharge (right) [69].

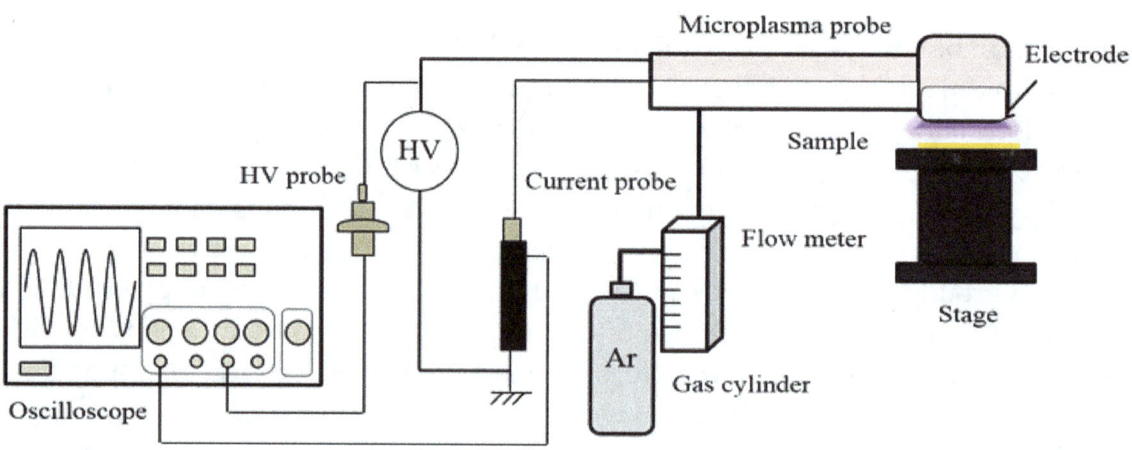

Figure 7. Experimental set-up with microplasma electrode [23].

6.3. Plasma jet

Plasma jets consist usually from a gas nozzle with one, two or three electrodes [70, 71]. The plasma jet can be realised by two ways—active plasma jets (expanding plasma contains free and high energetic electrons) and remote plasma jets (plasma is potential free and consists of relaxing and recombining active species from inside the nozzle) [70]. The plasma jet in **Figure 8** consists of a Pyrex tube and a central tungsten high voltage (HV) electrode. The grounded electrode is an aluminium ring located at the end of the outer surface of the Pyrex tube. The distance between the skin sample and the outlet of the plasma jet was set to 2 mm. The sample was isolated from the holder by a 30-mm thick PVC isolator or without isolator to compare the effect of the conductive layer under the skin surface as the human body is not isolator. The treatment time of the sample was set from several seconds to 1 min. Argon, nitrogen or argon-water vapour gases were introduced into the plasma jet. The waveform of the voltage and current of argon plasma jet is depicted in **Figure 8** [72].

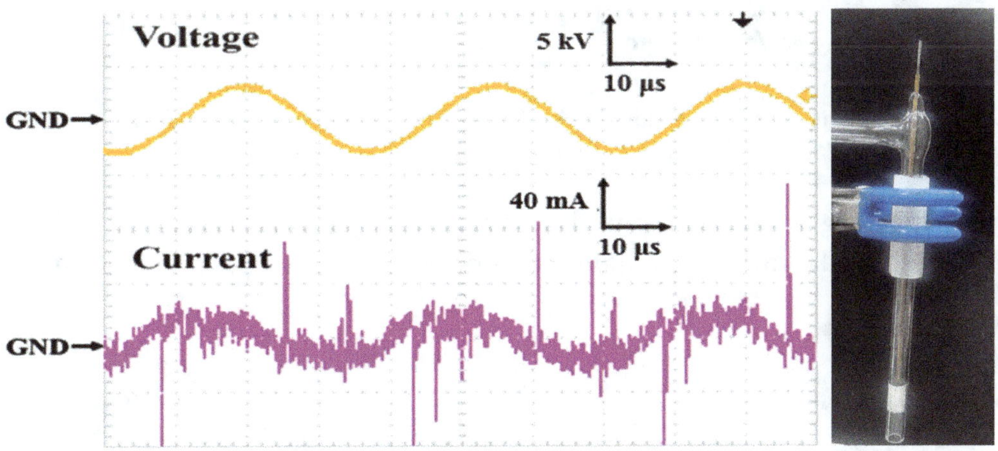

Figure 8. Waveform of plasma jet discharge (left) [72] and plasma jet electrode (right).

7. Plasma effects on skin barrier and transdermal drug delivery

7.1. Chemical reactions plasma particles with the skin

If argon plasma is used for skin treatment, the plasma produces electrons, argon ions, metastable and excited states. These particles can react with the skin directly. But, if argon or nitrogen plasma is working in atmospheric air, it makes the situation more complex because molecules of air (O_2, N_2, CO_2 and H_2O) can enter the volume of the plasma jet [73, 74]. In this case, argon can react with skin also indirectly through the excitation or dissociation or ionization process with air molecules. The reaction results in the creation of a number of species. It is difficult to find the molecule causing changes in skin. Pig skins treated by argon, nitrogen and argon/water plasma were compared by measuring ATR-FTIR spectra and monitoring of the shift of asymmetric stretching CH_2 band near 2920 cm^{-1}. A comparison of argon and nitrogen plasma jets has shown that argon can play a role in reactions with molecules of stratum corneum, but a similar effect can be achieved by nitrogen plasma itself as similar shift can be observed. A significantly higher value of shift was observed when argon with water vapours was used. The asymmetric stretching band was shifted 3.5 cm^{-1} (**Figure 9**). This result indicates that the stratum corneum became the most permeable after treatment of Ar plasma with water vapours. On the other hand, we observed low wavenumber shifts of the maxima of amide I and amide II (**Figure 9**).

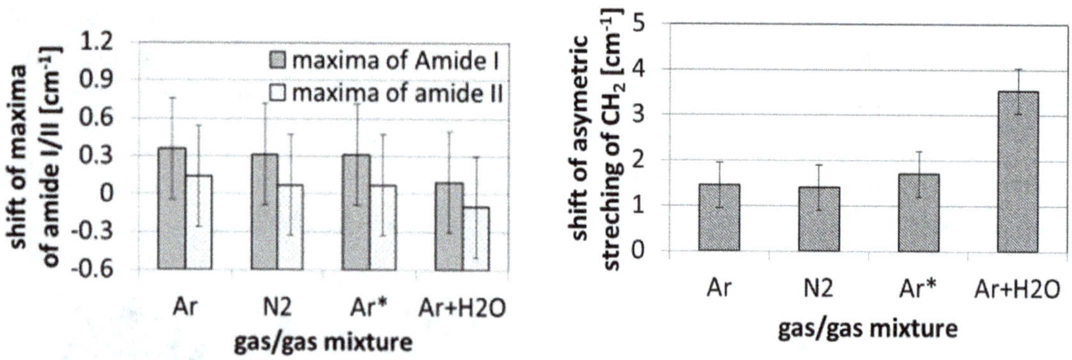

Figure 9. Shift of asymmetric stretching band of CH_2 to higher wavenumbers for the gases used in plasma jet discharge. Flow 10 L/min = (Ar*; N_2), 3 L/min = (Ar; Ar+H_2O).

Pig skin treated by argon microplasma shows shift of asymmetric stretching CH_2 band near 2920 cm^{-1} after 1, 3 and 5 min of irradiation comparable with the plasma jet (**Figure 10**).

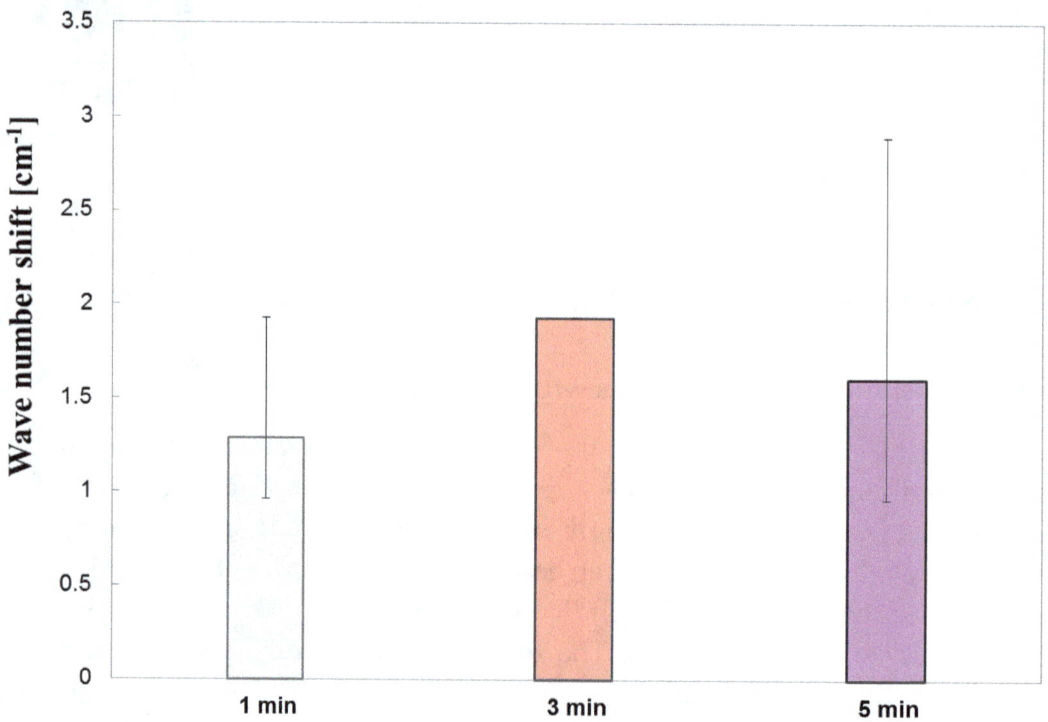

Figure 10. Shift of asymmetric stretching band of CH_2 to higher wavenumbers for Ar gas after microplasma irradiation [69].

When argon flew through the water reservoir, the argon ensured a higher concentration of water vapours in the discharge. The high shift of the asymmetric stretching band of CH_2 indicates that H_2O and the created OH molecules can play important roles in increasing the shift of the asymmetric stretching band of CH_2 in stratum corneum. OH could be created mainly by two channels [75]:

$$Ar_m + H_2O \rightarrow OH + H + Ar \tag{1}$$

$$H_2O + e \rightarrow OH + H + e \tag{2}$$

Simulation of the interaction of O and OH radicals with α-linolenic acid as a representative of fatty acid [76] showed that OH radicals most typically abstract an H atom from the fatty acids, which can lead to the creation of a double bond and also to the incorporation of alcohols or aldehyde groups, increasing hydrophilic properties of fatty acids and changing the lipid composition of the skin, causing an increase of skin permeability. Creation of these groups increases the hydrophilic character of the lipid layer. Incorporation of oxygen to stratum corneum lipids was also confirmed by increasing of C–O and C=O bonds after treatment of skin layer by atmospheric plasma [77]. Also, micropores (10 nm–1 μm in size) were observed in an artificial cell membrane system consisting of supported lipid bilayers after DBD plasma irradiation [78]. Later, it was found out that these micropores are induced transient species such as OH and OOH formed by plasma and they caused lipid peroxidation leading to truncated lipid chains, which induced pore formation [79]. These temporal pores were observed in skin after DBD plasma treatment and it was allowed to penetrate large molecules through the skin in several minutes. These pores had lifetimes of less than 5 min after treatment [68].

7.2. Effect of heating on skin barrier

Heating of the skin can increase permeability of stratum corneum [80]. Reasons of improving of transdermal delivery through the skin by increasing temperature are structural changes of stratum corneum lipids. Plasma can raise skin temperature from 30°C to more than 100°C which depends on the irradiated time, power of plasma source or used gas. Structural changes of stratum corneum lipids occur between 20 and 40°C, from orthorhombic to hexagonal ordered lipids. These changes can be indicated by CH_2 symmetric stretching frequency with an increase of 0.5 cm^{-1} in ATR-FTIR spectra or it is possible to observe by CH_2 scissoring mode where transition is revealed by splitting of the scissoring modes to produce a doublet with components at 1473 and 1463 cm^{-1}. Ordered lipid chains change to disordered chains at around 80–90°C. But some scientific groups identified more transitions in lipid structure [52]. For example, four phase transitions in temperature ranges 35–42°C, 65–75°C, 78–86°C and 90–115°C, respectively. Transitions below 75°C are reversible [81]. Between 35°C and 42°C two transitions can occur belonging to solid fluid transition and disruption of lipids covalently linked to corneocites at 37 and at 40°C to 'orthorhombic to hexagonal' change in structure. But too high a temperature can cause damage to the skin. Thermal conditions that cause burns of the skin are functions of the time and method of how the skin is exposed to the heat. Longer exposure of skin to a temperature higher than 43°C can lead to the formation of blisters [82]. It was found out that fast heating of skin can increase skin permeability without damaging deeper tissues. Investigation of high temperatures of up to 315°C applied to skin for 100 ms, 1 s and 5 s showed small variations between drug deliveries of calcein [82]. Exposure for 1 s or 5 s should be sufficient to equalize temperature in the full thickness of skin, but the 100 ms exposure should have influence only on stratum corneum. Between 100 and 150°C, permeability of skin was increased a few fold. This increase was attributed to lipid melting in the stratum corneum. In the range of 150–250°C, transdermal flux increased by two orders, attributable to disruption of stratum corneum keratin network structure. Above 300°C, transdermal flux increased by three orders, attributable to decomposition and vaporization of the stratum corneum [83].

7.3. Effect of UV radiation on skin barrier

The wavelength range of 100–400 nm is called UV light and is usually divided into three ranges: UVA (320–400 nm), UVB (280–320 nm) and UVC (100–280 nm). UV light can cause damage to skin. It is well-known that atmospheric plasma can generate wide range of UV light dependent on the used gas [84, 85]. UVC radiation can reach only stratum corneum and it consists of emission of excited NO molecule (200–280 nm—NO-gama system) or nitrogen molecule (120–200 nm—LBH system) in plasma discharges. The source of UVB radiation is emission of OH and nitrogen (second positive system of nitrogen). UVA is composed mostly of second positive system of nitrogen. UVA and UVB can reach deeper layers of skin like epidermis and UVA also dermis. UV radiation can cause formation of hydroxides and epoxides, hydrogenation of double bonds and breaking of carbon chains. The effect of UV on lipids depends on their structure, and only double bonds of fatty acids are sensitive to the formation of oxygenated molecules by oxygen in the air. These changes can be amplified or weakened by the surrounding atmosphere around the treated skin. When lipids of stratum corneum like cholesterol, cholesterol sulphate, ceramide III, linolenic acid and dipalmitoylphosphatidylcholine were irradiated by UV light up to 240 min, peroxidative changes occurred only in lipids with double bonds such as cholesterol and linolenic acid [86]. But the changes are not permanent and the order of stratum corneum lipids and water-loss protection can recover after 3 days and it returns to its initial state, thanks to repair processes in the skin [87]. Reactive oxygen species like superoxide anion radicals, singlet oxygen, hydrogen peroxide and hydroxyl radical can be created by UV light. For example, superoxide anion radicals are precursors to other oxygen reactive species, and it was found that there exists a correlation between the superoxide anion radical's concentration and degree of oxidation of lipids [88]. UV light is also used for treatment of some skin diseases but delivered doses have to be controlled and maintained in safety level to not penetrate to deeper layers of skin [89].

7.4. Acidifying effect of plasma on skin

Acidifying effect was observed after applying plasma to stripped lipids from stratum corneum. A higher decrease of pH was observed in discharges, which produced a higher amount of NO_x species. The same effect was observed on human skin, but after 30 min after plasma treatment, the pH of skin return to initial value [90]. The decrease of pH depends on parameters of the plasma discharge and the treatment time. Previous work has attributed the pH shift of water on plasma-treated lipids to the interaction of reactive species with the surface. Nitrates formed in water droplets could form nitric acid. NOx species could adhere on lipid surface or deposited nitric acid on the film surfaces by gaseous HNO_3 [91]. The recovery of pH in the post-plasma phase was attributed to the decrease of acidifying agents on the substrate surfaces by both diffusion and desorption processes.

7.5. Skin etching and skin damage by plasma

The etching effect of plasma is demonstrated in **Figure 11** by a cross section of the skin. The stratum corneum layer (the white part in (a) control sample) was removed after 20 tape stripping cycles, as shown in (b). After 30 s of atmospheric plasma jet irradiation, most of the stratum corneum layer was removed, as shown in (c). In the microplasma case, even after 5 min irradiation (d), the stratum corneum layer remained similar to the control sample, as shown in (a) [23]. Little difference in physical appearance was observed between the control pig skin sample and after microplasma irradiation. For the tape stripping test, surface asperity was decreased and after 10 s of atmospheric plasma jet irradiation, small pores (ranging from 40 to 100 μm) were observed. Physical damages on skin could be considered to arise from the electric field or an etching effect from bombardment with charged particles [92].

Surface potential can lead to a strong electric field across the skin and finally penetrate the skin to form holes. Holes were confirmed after longer operation (3–5 min) of atmospheric plasma irradiation. Pores and holes are shown in **Figure 12** after 10 and 30 s of operation of the plasma jet.

This physical damage could affect the barrier function of skin samples. When the effect of plasma jet was tested on PEN film, after 10 s of plasma jet irradiation, the surface potential increased to about 10% of the driven voltage. After long-term operation, it reached almost the same value as the driven voltage [23]. A similar problem could happen in electroporation but it uses very short operation times in the range of microseconds or milliseconds. High surface potential can induce current flow through the skin and it will increase the skin temperature and might affect cells of skin and cause thermal damage of skin [93]. On the contrary, the surface potential remained low in the microplasma case. The thickness of stratum corneum after 30 s of treatment of plasma jet is equivalent to 20 times of striping by tape. This is also confirmed by TEWL (**Figure 13**), which also shows the same values. On the other hand, TEWL after 5 min of microplasma irradiation of the pig skin sample, TEWL increased to almost double its original value, suggesting that the barrier properties were decreased through atmospheric microplasma irradiation but it is less effective than plasma jet [23].

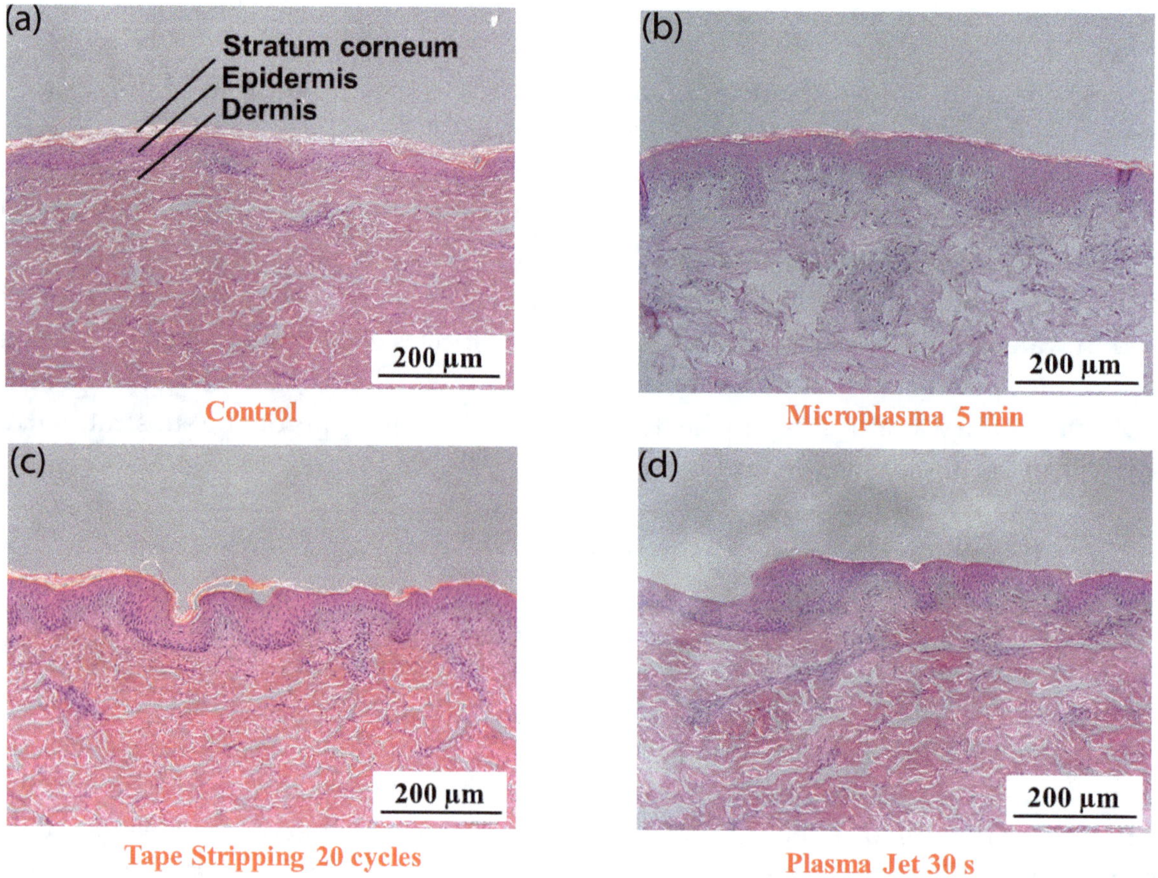

Figure 11. Cross section of pig skin after atmospheric plasma irradiation, and tape stripping test. (a) Control sample, stratum corneum thickness: 18.09 ± 1.64 µm; (b) tape stripping test — 20 times, stratum corneum thickness: 5.99 ± 1.24; (c) plasma jet — 30 s, stratum corneum thickness: 3.49 ± 0.61; (d) microplasma — 5 min, stratum corneum thickness: 13.40 ± 1.46 [72].

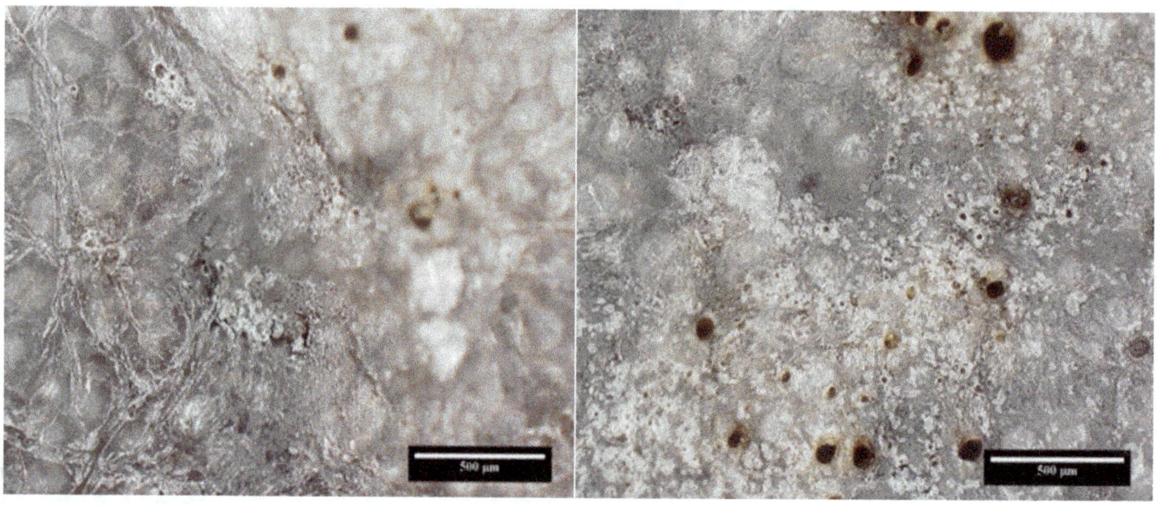

Figure 12. Left: 10 s of treatment by plasma jet; Right: 30 s of treatment by plasma jet [72].

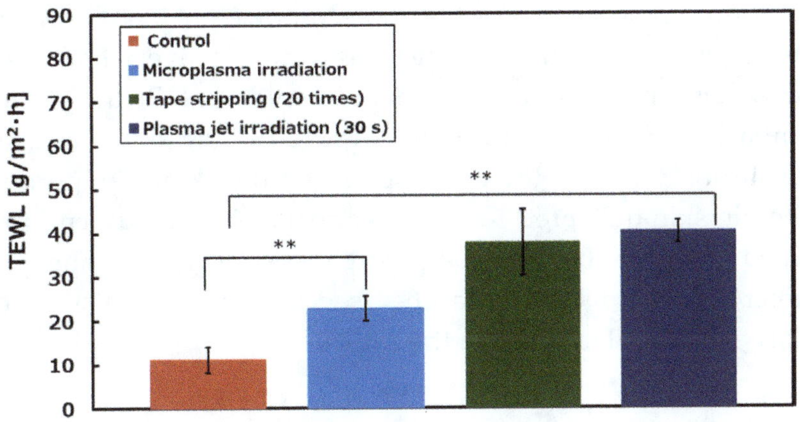

Figure 13. Variations of TEWL values before and after microplasma irradiation, tape striping test and plasma jet irradiation [72].

8. Improvement of galantamine hydrobromide (GaHBr) permeation by plasma irradiation

Galantamine hydrobromide (GaHBr) (**Figure 14**) is an alkaloid, isolated from plant species such as Narcissus and Lycoris species [93]. Treatment of Alzheimer's disease occurs by inhibition of acetylcholinesterase enzyme. The chemical structure of galantamine hydrobromide is shown in **Figure 14**.

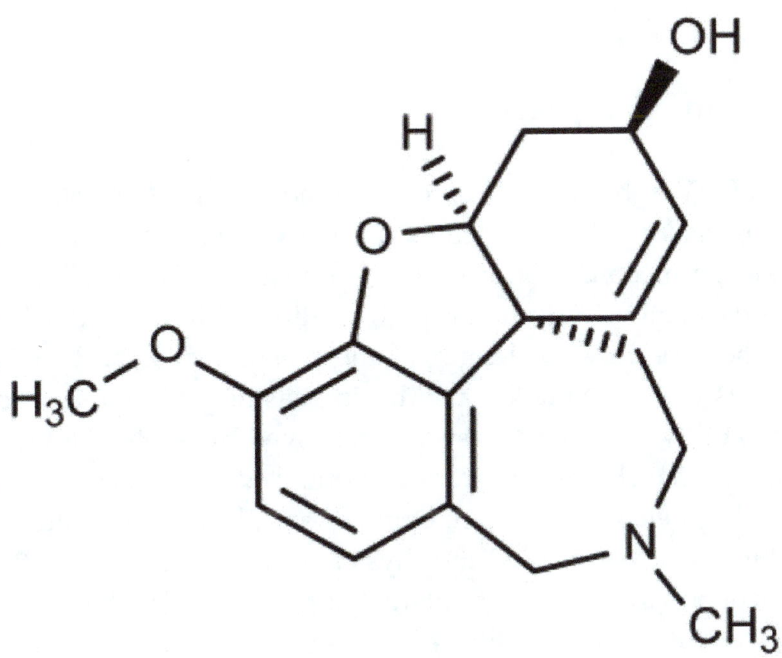

Figure 14. Chemical structure of galantamine hydrobromide.

As GaHBr is a hydrophilic molecule with a low molecular weight (368 Da), usually transdermal patches with chemical enhancers are used for transdermal delivery [94]. Using microplasma for the first time for enhancement of transdermal delivery of GaHBr, a slight improvement was observed with comparison of passive diffusion (**Figure 15**). Pig skin was irradiated for 3 min and then a water solution with GaHBr was applied on the skin. The permeation profiles of GaHBr through the pig skin delivered 5.35 ± 2.34 and 11.53 ± 2.89 μg/cm² for the control and the plasma-irradiated sample 24 h post-experiment, respectively [69]. These results lead to the expectation that microplasma discharge can be used to enhance the skin delivery of hydrophilic drugs and larger molecular drugs in the future.

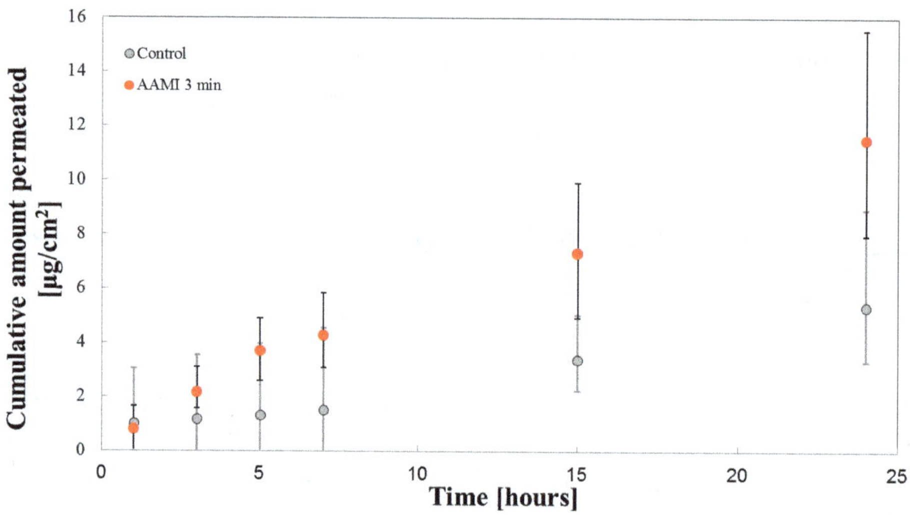

Figure 15. Amount of penetrated GaHBr—passive diffusion and after microplasma irradiation (red circles) [69].

9. Outlook of plasma drug delivery

Plasma as a source of UV light, heat, ions, reactive radicals and metastable states could be a successful tool for transdermal drug delivery. Each of these parameters can be used for improvement of skin permeability. Stratum corneum can be altered by chemical reaction of reactive oxygen species or by UV causing peroxidation of intercellular lipids. Undesirable heating effects can be tuned by the length of the plasma pulse and then a change of the conformation of lipids can be achieved also by increasing gas temperature in plasma. Improvement of permeability of skin by plasma was proved by ATR-FTIR and TEWL methods. A plasma jet is effective in etching of stratum corneum but can cause damage to skin because of the presence of a high electric field. We believe that plasma jet could be considered as a trade-off relationship, i.e. accompanied by physical damage or pain on the skin, similar to needles and creation of pores can cause risk of infection. On the other hand, microplasma seems to be more suitable for future drug delivery because it caused lower damage of skin. Transdermal drug delivery of galantamine hydrobromide by microplasma showed slight improvement in comparison with passive diffusion but further investigation is needed for drug testing or improvement in plasma properties in the future. We suggest that the use of a transdermal drug delivery with plasma irradiation is feasible, and thus, could be combined with appropriate drugs to target various symptoms such as Alzheimer's disease, diabetes and other symptoms that cannot be cured by applying plasma irradiation alone. This novel method will reveal new directions for the future of plasma medicine. Our aim is to combine a safe transdermal drug delivery method with a transdermal agent such as a peptide vaccine without requiring an injection needle and causing physical damage to the skin. Safety of patients, without causing harmful damage or physical damage to the skin, is critical for enabling this novel technology.

Acknowledgements

We would like to thank to Professor Akira Yamamoto and Dr. Kosuke Kusamori of Kyoto Pharmaceutical University, Professor Damon M. Chandler, Ms. An N. Tran and Dr. Marius G. Blajan of Shizuoka University, for fruitful discussion. This work was supported by JSPS KAKENHI Grant Number JP16H04085.

Author details

Kazuo Shimizu* and Jaroslav Krištof

*Address all correspondence to: shimizu@cjr.shizuoka.ac.jp

Shizuoka University, Hamamatsu, Japan

References

[1] Fridman G, Friedman G, Gutsol A, Shekhter A B, Vasilets V N and Fridman A. Applied plasma medicine. Plasma Process. Polym. 2008;5:503–533. DOI: 10.1002/ppap.200700154

[2] Shimizu K, Blajan M and Tatematsu S. Basic study of remote disinfection and sterilization effect by using atmospheric microplasma. IEEE Trans. Indust. Appl. 2012; 48:1182–1188. DOI: 10.1109/TIA.2012.2199953

[3] Kim J E, Lee D U and Min S C. Microbial decontamination of red pepper powder by cold plasma. Food Microbiol. 2014;38:128–136. DOI: 10.1016/j.fm.2013.08.019

[4] Shimizu K, Blajan M and Kuwabara T. Removal of indoor air contaminant by atmospheric microplasma. IEEE Trans. Ind. 2011;47:2351–2358. DOI: 10.1109/TIA.2011.2168509

[5] Pankaj S K, Ferrer C B, Misra N N, O'Neill L, Jimenez A, Bourke P and Cullen P J. Characterization of polylactic acid films for food packaging as affected by dielectric barrier discharge atmospheric plasma. Innov. Food Sci. Emerg. Technol. 2014;21:107–113. DOI: 10.1016/j.ifset.2013.10.007

[6] Kostov K G, Nishime T M C, Castro A H R, Toth A and Hein L R O. Obtaining, structural, magnetic and corrosive properties of Nd–Fe–B alloy thin films on glass. Appl. Surf. Sci. 2014;314:30–39. DOI: 10.1016/j.apsusc.2014.06.143

[7] Shimizu K, Fukunaga H, Tatematsu S and Blajan M. Atmospheric microplasma application for surface modification of biomaterials. Japan. J. Appl. Phys. 2012; 51:11PJ01. DOI: 10.1143/JJAP.51.11PJ01

[8] Ponsky T A, Gasior A C, Parry J, Sharp S W, Boulanger S, Parry R, Ostlie D J and Peter S D S. Need for subsequent fundoplication after gastrostomy based on patient characteristics. J. Surg. Res. 2013;179:1–4. DOI: 10.1016/j.jss.2012.03.064

[9] Haertel B, Woedtke T V, Weltmann K D and Lindequist U. Non-thermal atmospheric-pressure plasma possible application in wound healing. Biomol. Ther. 2014;22:477–490. DOI: 10.4062/biomolther.2014.105

[10] Ishaq M, Evans M M and Ostrikov K K. Effect of atmospheric gas plasmas on cancer cell signaling. Int. J. Cancer. 2014;134:1517–1528. DOI: 10.1002/ijc.28323

[11] Ahn H J, Kim K I, Hoan N N, Kim C H, Moon E, Choi K S, Yang S S and Lee J S. Targeting cancer cells with reactive oxygen and nitrogen species generated by atmospheric-pressure air plasma. PLoS One. 2014;9:e86173. DOI: 10.1371/journal.pone.0086173

[12] Ikawa S, Kitano K and Hamaguchi S. Effects of pH on bacterial inactivation in aqueous solutions due to low-temperature atmospheric pressure plasma application. Plasma Process. Polym. 2010;7:33–42. DOI: 10.1002/ppap.200900090

[13] Tresp H, Hammer M U, Weltamn K D and Reuter S. Differential viability of eight human blood mononuclear cell subpopulations after plasma treatment. Plasma Med. 2013;3:1–13. DOI: 10.1615/PlasmaMed.2014008450

[14] Haertel B, Backer C, Schulze C, Funke A, Wurster M, Woedtke T V and Lindequist U. Plasma-based stimulation of biotechnological processes in *Ganoderma lucidum* mycelia as example for a eukaryotic organism. Plasma Med. 2014;4:17–28. DOI: 10.1615/PlasmaMed.2014011874

[15] Gaens W V and Bogaerts A. Reaction pathways of biomedically active species in an Ar plasma jet. Plasma Sources Sci. Technol. 2014;23:035015. DOI: 10.1088/0963-0252/23/3/035015

[16] Liu D X, Iza F, Wang X H, Kong M G and Rong M Z. He+O_2+H_2O plasmas as a source of reactive oxygen species. Appl. Phys. Lett. 2011;98:221501. DOI: 10.1063/1.3592775

[17] Heinlin J, Morfill G, Landthaler M, Stolz W, Isbary G, Zimmermann J L, Shimizu T and Karrer S. Plasma medicine: possible applications in dermatology. J Dtsch Dermatol Ges. 2010;8:968–976. DOI: 10.1111/j.1610-0387.2010.07495.x

[18] Bos J D and Meinardi M. The 500 Dalton rule for the skin penetration of chemical compounds and drugs. Exp. Dermatol. 2000;9:165–169. DOI: 10.1034/j.1600-0625.2000.009003165.x

[19] Flynn G L and Yalkowsky S H. Correlation and prediction of mass transport across membranes I: influence of alkyl chain length on flux-determining properties of barrier and diffusant. J. Pharm. Sci. 1972;61:838–852. DOI: 10.1002/jps.2600610603

[20] Wiechers J W. The barrier function of the skin in relation to percutaneous absorption of drugs. Pharm. Weekblad. 1989;11:185–198. DOI: 10.1007/BF01959410

[21] Ya-Xian Z, Suetake T and Tagami H. Number of cell layers of the stratum corneum in normal skin - relationship to the anatomical location on the body, age, sex and physical parameters. Arch. Dermatol. Res. 1999;291:555–559. DOI: 10.1007/s004030050453

[22] Babaeva N Y and Kushner M J. Intracellular electric fields produced by dielectric barrier discharge treatment of skin. J. Phys. D: Appl. Phys. 2010;43:185206. DOI: 10.1088/0022-3727/43/18/185206

[23] Shimizu K, Hayashida K and Blajan M. Novel method to improve transdermal drug delivery by atmospheric microplasma irradiation. Biointerphases. 2015;10:029517. DOI: 10.1116/1.4919708

[24] Zorin S, Kuylenstierna F and Thulin H. In vitro test of nicotine's permeability through human skin. Risk evaluation and safety aspects. Am. Occup. Hyg. 1999;43:405–413. DOI: 10.1093/annhyg/43.6.405

[25] Suksaeree J, Charoenchai L, Madaka F, Monton C, Sakunpak A, Charoonratana T and Pichayakorn W. Zingiber cassumunar blended patches for skin application: formulation, physicochemical properties, and in vitro studies. Asian J. Pharm. Sci. 2015;10:341–349. DOI: 10.1016/j.ajps.2015.03.001

[26] Shen S, Liu S Z, Zhang Y S, Du M B, Liang A H, Song L H and Ye Z G. Compound antimalarial ethosomal cataplasm: preparation, evaluation, and mechanism of penetration enhancement. Int. J. Nanomed. 2015;10:4239–4253. DOI: 10.2147/IJN.S83402

[27] Franken A, Eloff F C, Du Plessis J and Du Plessis J L. In vitro permeation of metals through human skin: a review and recommendations. Chem. Res. Toxicol. 2015;28:2237–2249. DOI: 10.1021/acs.chemrestox.5b00421

[28] Klimundova J, Satinsky D, Sklenarova H and Solich P. Automation of simultaneous release tests of two substances by sequential injection chromatography coupled with Franz cell. Talanta. 2006;69:730–735. DOI: 10.1016/j.talanta.2005.11.011

[29] Jhawat V C, Saini V, Kamboj S and Maggon N. Transdermal drug delivery systems: approaches and advancements in drug absorption through skin. Int. J. Pharm. Sci. Rev. Res. 2013;20(1):47–56.

[30] Prausnitz M R and Langer R. Transdermal drug delivery. Nat Biotechnol. 2008;26:1261–1268. DOI: 10.1038/nbt.1504

[31] Hadgraft J and Lane M E. Skin: the ultimate interface. Phys. Chem. Chem. Phys. 2011;13:5215–5222. DOI: 10.1039/c0cp02943b

[32] Suhonen T M, Bouwstra J A and Urtti A. Chemical enhancement of percutaneous absorption in relation to stratum corneum structural alterations. J. Controlled Release. 1999;59:149–161. DOI: 10.1016/S0168-3659(98)00187-4

[33] Paloncyova M,Vavrova K, Sovova Z, DeVane R, Otyepka M and Berka K. Structural changes in ceramide bilayers rationalize increased permeation through stratum corneum models with shorter acyl tails. J. Phys. Chem. B. 2015;119:9811–9819. DOI: 10.1021/acs.jpcb.5b05522

[34] Moghadam S H, Saliaj E, Wettig S D, Dong Ch, Ivanova M V, Huzil J T and Foldvari M. Effect of chemical permeation enhancers on stratum corneum barrier lipid organizational structure and interferon alpha permeability. Mol. Pharmaceutics. 2013;10:2248–2260. DOI: 10.1021/mp300441c

[35] Caspers P J, Lucassen G W, Wolthuis R, Bruining H A and Puppels G J. In vitro and in vivo Raman spectroscopy of human skin. Biospectroscopy. 1998;4:S31–S39. DOI: 10.1002/(SICI)1520-6343(1998)4:5+<S31::AID-BSPY4>3.0.CO;2-M

[36] Bouwstra J A, Gooris G S, Weerheim A, Kempenaar J and Ponec M. Characterization of stratum corneum structure in reconstructed epidermis by X-ray diffraction. J. Lipid Res. 1995;36:496–504.

[37] Nakazawa H, Imai T, Hatta I, Sakai S, Inoue S and Kato S. Low-flux electron diffraction study for the intercellular lipid organization on a human corneocyte. BBA-Biomembranes. 2013;1828:1424–1431. DOI: 10.1016/j.bbamem.2013.02.001

[38] Honeywell-Nguyen P L, de Graaff A M, Groenink H W and Bouwstra J A. The in vivo and in vitro interactions of elastic and rigid vesicles with human skin. Biochim Biophys Acta. 2002;1573:140–130. DOI: 10.1016/s0304-4165(02)00415-4

[39] Pinkus H. Examination of the epidermis by the strip method of removing horny layers. I. Observations on thickness of the horny layer, and on mitotic activity after stripping. J Invest Dermatol. 1951;16:383–386. DOI: 10.1038/jid.1951.45

[40] Escobar-Chávez J J, Merino-Sanjuán V, López-Cervantes M, Urban-Morlan Z, Piñón-Segundo E, Quintanar-Guerrero D and Ganem-Quintanar A. The tape-stripping technique as a method for drug quantification in skin. J Pharm Pharm Sci. 2008;11:104–130.

[41] Pardeike J, Hommoss A and Müller R H. Lipid nanoparticles (SLN, NLC) in cosmetic and pharmaceutical dermal products. Int J Pharm. 2009;366:170–184. DOI: 10.1016/j.ijpharm.2008.10.003

[42] Bommannan D, Potts R and Guy R. Examination of stratum corneum barrier function in vivo by infrared spectroscopy. J. Invest. Dermatol. 1990;95:403–408. DOI: 10.1111/1523-1747.ep12555503

[43] Wagner H, Kostka K H, Lehr C M and Schaefer U F. pH profiles in human skin: influence of two in vitro test systems for drug delivery testing. Eur. J. Pharm. Biopharm. 2003;55:57–65. DOI: 10.1016/S0939-6411(02)00125-X

[44] Lawler J C, Davis M J and Griffith E C. Electrical characteristics of the skin. J. Invest. Dermatol. 1960;34:301–308. DOI: 10.1038/jid.1960.52

[45] Kazarian S G and Chan K. Applications of ATR-FTIR spectroscopic imaging to biomedical samples. BBA-Biomembranes. 2006;1758:858–867. DOI: 10.1016/j.bbamem.2006.02.011

[46] Chan K L A and Kazarian S G. Attenuated total reflection Fourier-transform infrared (ATR-FTIR) imaging of tissues and live cells. Chem. Soc. Rev. 2016;45:1850–1864. DOI: 10.1039/C5CS00515A

[47] Lucassen G W, van Veen G N A and Jansen A J. Band analysis of hydrated human skin stratum corneum attenuated total reflectance Fourier transform infrared spectra in vivo. J. Biomed. Opt. 1998;3:267–280. DOI: 10.1117/1.429890

[48] Karande P, Jain A, Ergun K, Kispersky V and Mitragotri S. Design principles of chemical penetration enhancers for transdermal drug delivery. Proc. Natl. Acad. Sci. U S A. 2005;102:4688–4693. DOI: 10.1073/pnas.0501176102

[49] Boncheva M, Damien F and Normand V. Molecular organization of the lipid matrix in intact Stratum corneum using ATR-FTIR spectroscopy. Biochim. Biophys. Acta. 2008; 1778:1344–1355. DOI: 10.1016/j.bbamem.2008.01.022

[50] Zhang D, Wang H-J, Cui X-M and Wang C-X. Evaluations of imidazolium ionic liquids as novel skin permeation enhancers for drug transdermal delivery. Pharm. Dev. Technol. 2016;13:1–10. DOI: 10.3109/10837450.2015.1131718

[51] Balázs B, Sipos P, Danciu C, Avram S, Soica C, Dehelean C, Varju G, Erős G, Budai-Szűcs M, Berkó S and Csányi E. ATR-FTIR and Raman spectroscopic investigation of the electroporation-mediated transdermal delivery of a nanocarrier system containing an antitumour drug. Biomed. Optics Express. 2016;7:67–78. DOI: 10.1364/BOE.7.000067

[52] Mendelsohn R, Flach C R and Moore D J. Determination of molecular conformation and permeation in skin via IR spectroscopy, microscopy, and imaging. BBA-Biomembranes. 2006;1758:923–933. DOI: 10.1016/j.bbamem.2006.04.009

[53] Levang A K, Zhao K and Singh J. Effect of ethanol/propylene glycol on the in vitro percutaneous absorption of aspirin, biophysical changes and macroscopic barrier properties of the skin. Intl. J. Pharmaceut. 1999;181:255–263. DOI: 10.1016/S0378-5173(99)00055-1

[54] Barry B W. Penetration enhancers. Mode of action in human skin. J. Control. Release. 1987;6:85–97. DOI: 10.1016/0168-3659(87)90066-6

[55] Prasad R, Anand S, Khar R K, Dinda A K and Koul V. Studies on in vitro and in vivo transdermal flux enhancement of methotrexate by a combinational approach in comparison to oral delivery. Drug Dev. Ind. Pharm. 2009;35:1281–1292. DOI: 10.3109/03639040902882322

[56] Coston A F and Li J K-J. Iontophoresis: modeling, methodology, and evaluation. Cardiovasc. Eng. 2001;1:127–136. DOI: 10.1023/A:1014042109687

[57] Prasad R, Koul V, Anand S and Khar R K. Effect of DC/mDC iontophoresis and terpenes on transdermal permeation of methotrexate: In vitro study. Int. J. Pharm. 2007;333:70–78. DOI: 10.1016/j.ijpharm.2006.09.058

[58] Turner N G, Ferry L, Price M, Cullander C and Guy R H. Iontophoresis of poly-L-lysines: the role of molecular weight?. Pharm. Res. 1997;14:1322–1331 . DOI: 10.1023/A:1012100100865

[59] Kalluri H and Banga A K. Transdermal delivery of proteins. AAPS PharmSciTech. 2011;12:431–441. DOI: 10.1208/s12249-011-9601-6

[60] Krueger E, Junior J L C, Scheeren E M, Neves E B, Mulinari E and Nohama P. Iontophoresis: principles and applications. Fisioter Mov. 2014;27:469–481. DOI: 10.1590/0103-5150.027.003.AR02

[61] Jadoul A, Bouwstra J and Preat V. Effects of iontophoresis and electroporation on the stratum corneum: review of the biophysical studies. Adv. Drug Delivery Rev. 1999;35:89–105. DOI: 10.1016/S0169-409X(98)00065-9

[62] Thysman S, Van Neste D and Preat V. Noninvasive investigation of human skin after in vivo iontophoresis. Skin Pharmacol. 1995;8:229–236. DOI: 10.1159/000211352

[63] Jadoul A, Doucet J, Durand D and Preat V. Modifications induced on stratum corneum after in vitro iontophoresis: ATR-FTIR and X-ray scattering studies. J. Control. Release. 1996;42:165–173. DOI: 10.1016/0168-3659(96)01452-6

[64] Van der Geest R, Elshove D A R, Danhof M, Lavrijsen A P M and Bodde H E. Noninvasive assessment of skin barrier integrity and skin irritation following iontophoretic current application in humans. J. Control. Release. 1996;41:205–213. DOI: 10.1016/0168-3659(96)01329-6

[65] Prasad R, Anand S and Koul V. Biophysical assessment of DC iontophoresis and current density on transdermal permeation of methotrexate. Int. J. Pharm. Investig. 2011;1:234–237. DOI: 10.4103/2230-973X.93011

[66] Lombry C, Dujardin N and Preat V. Transdermal delivery of macromolecules using skin electroporation. Pharmaceut. Res. 2000;7:32–37. DOI: 10.1023/A:1007510323344

[67] Weaver J C and Chizmadzhev Y A. Theory of electroporation: a review. Biochem. Bioenerget. 1996;41:135–160. DOI: 10.1016/S0302-4598(96)05062-3

[68] Kalghatgi S, Tsai C, Gray R and Pappas D. Transdermal drug delivery using cold plasmas . In: 22nd Int'l Symposium on Plasma Chemistry; 5–10 July; Antwerp, Belgium. 2015. pp. O-22-6.

[69] Shimizu K, Tran A N, Kristof J and Blajan M G. Investigation of atmospheric microplasma for improving skin permeability. In: Proceedings of the 2016 Electrostatics Joint Conference; 13–18 June; Lafayette, USA. 2016. p. I4.

[70] Weltmann K D, Kindel E, von Woedtke T, Hähnel M, Stieber M and Brandenburg R. Atmospheric-pressure plasma sources: prospective tools for plasma medicine. Pure Appl. Chem. 2010;82:1223–1237. DOI: 10.1351/PAC-CON-09-10-35

[71] Stoffels E, Flikweert A J, Stoffels W W and Kroesen G M W. Plasma needle: a non-destructive atmospheric plasma source for fine surface treatment of (bio)materials. Plasma Sources Sci. Technol. 2002;11:383–388. DOI: 10.1088/0963-0252/11/4/304

[72] Shimizu K, Tran N A, Hayashida K and Blajan M. Comparison of atmospheric microplasma and plasma jet irradiation for increasing of skin permeability. J. Phys. D: Appl. Phys. 2016;49:315201. DOI: 10.1088/0022-3727/49/31/315201.

[73] Tsai I-H and Hsu C-C. Numerical simulation of downstream kinetics of an atmospheric pressure nitrogen plasma jet. IEEE Trans. Plasma Sci. 2010;38:3387–3392. DOI: 10.1007/s11090-013-9480-6

[74] Van Gaens W and Bogaerts A. Kinetic modelling for an atmospheric pressure argon plasma jet in humid air. J. Phys. D: Appl. Phys. 2013;46:275201. DOI: 10.1088/0022-3727/46/27/275201

[75] Bruggeman P and Schram D C. On OH production in water containing atmospheric pressure plasmas. Plasma Sources Sci. Technol. 2010;19:045025. DOI: 10.1088/0963-0252/19/4/045025

[76] Van der Paal J, Aernouts S, van Duin A C T, Neyts E C and Bogaerts A. Interaction of O and OH radicals with a simple model system for lipids in the skin barrier: a reactive molecular dynamics investigation for plasma medicine. J. Phys. D: Appl. Phys. 2013;46:395201. DOI: 10.1088/0022-3727/46/39/395201

[77] Marschewski M, Hirschberg J, Omairi T, Viol W, Emmert S and Maus-Friedrichs W. Electron spectroscopy analysis of the human skin barrier: cold atmospheric plasma-induces changes in lipid composition. Exp. Dermatol. 2012;21:921–925. DOI: 10.1111/exd.12043

[78] Tero R, Suda Y, Kato R, Tanoue H, and Takikawa H. Plasma irradiation of artificial cell membrane system at solid–liquid interface. Appl. Phys. Express. 2014;7:077001. DOI: 10.7567/APEX.7.077001

[79] Suda Y, Tero R, Yamashita R, Yusa K and Takikawa H. Reduction in lateral lipid mobility of lipid bilayer membrane by atmospheric pressure plasma irradiation. Jpn. J. Appl. Phys. 2016;55:03DF05. DOI: 10.7567/JJAP.55.03DF05

[80] Petersen K K, Rousing M L, Jensen C, Arendt-Nielsen L and Gazerani P. Effect of local controlled heat on transdermal delivery of nicotine. Int. J. Physiol. Pathophysiol. Pharmacol. 2011;3:236–242

[81] Wood D G, Brown M B and Jones S A. Understanding heat facilitated drug transport across human epidermis. Eur. J. Pharmaceut. Biopharmaceut. 2012;81:642–664. DOI: 10.1016/j.ejpb.2012.03.019

[82] Hao J, Ghosh P, Li S K, Newman B, Kasting G B and Raney S G. Heat effects on drug delivery across human skin. Expert Opin. Drug Delivery. 2016;13:755–768. DOI: 10.1517/17425247.2016.1136286

[83] Park J-H, Lee J-W, Kim Y-C and Prausnitz M R. The effect of heat on skin permeability. Int. J. Pharm. 2008;359:94–103. DOI: 10.1016/j.ijpharm.2008.03.032

[84] Yu L, Laux Ch O, Packan D M and Kruger C H. Direct-current glow discharges in atmospheric pressure air plasmas. J. Appl. Phys. 2002;91:2678–2689. DOI: 10.1063/1.1435421

[85] Sewraj N, Merbahi N, Gardou J P, Rodriguez Akerreta P and Marchal F. Electric and spectroscopic analysis of a pure nitrogen mono-filamentary dielectric barrier discharge (MF-DBD) at 760 Torr. J. Phys. D: Appl. Phys. 2011;44:145201. DOI: 10.1088/0022-3727/44/14/145201

[86] Trommer H, Plätzer M, Wolf R and Neubert R H H. Mass spectrometric examinations of stratum corneum lipid models exposed to ultraviolet irradiation. Skin Pharmacol. Appl. Skin. Physiol. 2003;16:291–304. DOI: 10.1159/000072069

[87] Merle C, Laugel C and Baillet-Guffroy A. Effect of UVA or UVB irradiation on cutaneous lipids in films or in solution. Photochem. Photobiol. 2010;86:553–562. DOI: 10.1111/j.1751-1097.2009.00690.x

[88] Kaneko T, Kaise Ch, Kimoto Y, Suzuki S, Kondo T and Yuasa M. Detection of superoxide anion radical in a stratum corneum intercellular lipid model using an electrochemical sensor. J. Oleo. Sci. 2011;60:647–654. DOI: 10.5650/jos.60.647

[89] Lademann J, Richter H, Alborova H, Humme D, Patzelt A, Kramer A, Weltmann K D, Hartmann B, Ottomann Ch, Fluhr J W, Hinz P, Hübner G and Lademann O. Risk assessment of the application of a plasma jet in dermatology. J. Biomed. Opt. 2009;14:054025. DOI: 10.1117/1.3247156

[90] Hirschberg J, Gerhard C, Braun A, Grottker S, Krupp A, Emmert S and Viöl W. Validation of the suitability of stripped lipid as a skin model in plasma medical investigations. Open J. Appl. Sci. 2015;5:40–49. DOI: 10.4236/ojapps.2015.52005

[91] Helmke A, Hoffmeister D, Mertens N, Emmert S, Schuette J and Vioel W. The acidification of lipid film surfaces by non-thermal DBD at atmospheric pressure in air. New J. Phys. 2009;11:115025. DOI: 10.1088/1367-2630/11/11/115025

[92] Babaeva N Y, Ning N, Graves D B and Kushner M J. Ion activation energy delivered to wounds by atmospheric pressure dielectric-barrier discharges: sputtering of lipid-like surfaces. J. Phys. D: Appl. Phys. 2012;45:115203. DOI: 10.1088/0022-3727/45/11/115203

[93] Martin G T, Pliquett U F and Weaver J C. Theoretical analysis of localized heating in human skin subjected to high voltage pulses. Bioelectrochemistry. 2002;57:55–64. DOI: 10.1016/S1567-5394(01)00176-1

[94] Yen W F, Basri M, Ahmad M and Ismail M. Formulation and evaluation of galantamine gel as drug reservoir in transdermal patch delivery system. Sci. World J. 2015;2015: 495271. DOI: 10.1155/2015/495271

9

Nuclear Medicine and Drug Delivery

Ana Rita Fernandes, Ana Oliveira, Jorge Pereira and Pedro Silva Coelho

Abstract

Nuclear Medicine is a molecular-imaging modality that diagnoses and treats diseases with very small amounts of radioactive materials, known as radiopharmaceuticals. Drug delivery refers to approaches, formulations, technologies, and systems for transporting a pharmaceutical compound in the body as needed to safely achieve its desired therapeutic effect. The use of nuclear medicine and radiopharmaceuticals allows studying the *in vivo* behavior of developed drug-delivery systems, and pharmacoscintigraphy is, from the beginning, one of the most promising aspects of this medical specialty. In this chapter, we review the technologies, fundaments, rationales, and strategies more frequently used and present examples of their application in the development and evaluation of drug-delivery systems.

Keywords: nuclear medicine, radiopharmaceuticals, drug delivery, *in vivo* analysis

1. Introduction

Nuclear Medicine is a medical speciality that involves the application of small amounts of radioactive materials, known as radiopharmaceuticals, for the diagnosis and treatment of disease, without causing any physiological effect.

Drug-delivery strategies have been steadily being developed in order to obtain better therapeutic results, enhance adhesion to treatment, and mitigate side effects. The ever-increasing complexity of the systems, combined with the regulatory demands by the Medicines Authorities, made the *in vivo* analysis of those systems' behavior almost compulsory.

The unique characteristics of Nuclear Medicine and Radiopharmaceuticals make dynamic, noninvasive studies and therefore are frequently used in the evaluation and development of new drug-delivery systems. This chapter aims to review the different techniques available, their rationale and applications, using, whenever possible, examples from the literature as well as from the authors' own experience.

2. Molecular imaging and Nuclear Medicine

Molecular imaging is defined as the visualization, characterization, and measurement of physiological mechanisms at the molecular and cellular levels, in living systems. Apart from Nuclear Medicine, it includes several other techniques, such as magnetic resonance imaging and spectroscopy, certain ultrasound technologies, and others [1, 2].

One of the biggest advantages of molecular imaging is the ability to characterize specific disease processes in different individuals, using noninvasive assessment and quantification; i.e., providing information that is inaccessible with any other imaging techniques or that otherwise would require more invasive procedures such as biopsy or surgery. Also, it identifies disease in its earliest phases and determines the precise location of a tumor, frequently before symptoms occur or changes can be detected at the anatomical level. Identifying small differences between patients allows the tailoring of specific treatments for each individual [1–3].

Nuclear Medicine is a molecular-imaging modality that diagnoses and treats diseases using radioactive materials, known as radiopharmaceuticals. Radiopharmaceuticals, at diagnostic levels, have the ability to portray human physiology, biochemistry, or pathology without causing any physiological effect [1, 3].

For example, it can be used to identify the presence or absence of specific receptors or molecular changes, which are crucial for the selection of patients for certain targeted therapies [1].

This step for "personalized medicine" also allows a more precise identification of research subjects, leading to more exact and cost-effective clinical trials [3].

3. Detectors and imaging systems

Diagnostic imaging refers to the techniques and processes used to create anatomical and functional images and is one of the fields in Medicine with the greater recent development [1].

The first reference to structural imaging dates to 1895, when Wilhelm Conrad Röntgen identified electromagnetic radiation in a wavelength range now known as X-rays. Functional imaging started following the discovery of the scintillation scanner by Benedict Casen (using I-131 as a radiotracer for diagnostic imaging purpose), and developed as a diagnostic specialty in 1958, when Hal Anger introduced the gamma camera (based on the principle of scintillation counting). Since then, Nuclear Medicine has considerably changed our view of looking at disease, by showing images of radiotracer distributions, providing functional images [1, 4].

A gamma camera is single-photon imaging equipment, also known as Anger camera or as scintillation camera. It contains a large radiation detector, consisting of a large thallium-activated sodium iodide crystal—the scintillator. A collimator, placed in front of the crystal, enables the γ-rays to be focused onto the detector. Coupled to the crystal are photomultiplier tubes, which detect the light pulses. The whole detection part of the equipment is shielded from undesirable radiation. An electronic system links the photomultiplier tubes to a computer and visual display unit [1, 5, 6, 7].

The basic principle of gamma cameras is that radionuclide concentrations in the body can be measured *in vivo*, by detecting the photons emitted during their radioactive decay. The first gamma cameras were only able to create two-dimensional (2D) representations. But in 1963, David Kuhl and Roy Edwards presented the first tomographic images using the Anger camera, by acquiring multiple planar images from different angles around the body and creating a three-dimensional representation. This technology, called single-photon emission computerized tomography (SPECT or SPET), is of special interest when studying complex three-dimensional anatomical structures [1, 6]. Besides static 2D and tomographic images, it is also possible to obtain dynamic, sequential images of the radiopharmaceutical's variation over time within a particular segment of the body [8].

Another indispensable nuclear-imaging method consists of positron emission tomography (PET). The distinction between SPECT and PET is based on the physical properties of the radioisotopes used for imaging. SPECT (single-photon imaging) relies on single γ-ray photon emitters. By contrast, PET uses positron emitters—radioisotopes that simultaneously emit two 511-keV photons, at approximately opposite directions. These photons are detected in the PET camera by a ring of detectors configured to detect coincidence. The registered events are then reconstructed into a three-dimensional image [5, 9].

Although PET offers some advantages over SPECT, such as improved resolution and increased quantitative capabilities, SPECT is often more practical because of its wider availability and lesser cost [3].

A typical nuclear-imaging procedure starts with the administration of the selected radiotracer, followed by image acquisition (through the detection of γ-rays, X-rays, or annihilation quanta in PET, using either a gamma camera or a PET scanner). The resulting image illustrates the tracer's location within the body [5, 10].

More recent developments in Nuclear Medicine include hybrid-imaging techniques. Hybrid imaging refers to the fusion of two (or more) imaging modalities, such as SPECT/CT, PET/CT, or PET/magnetic resonance (MR) devices. These modalities have the advantage of condensing molecular and anatomical information in a single examination, thus surpassing one major drawback of highly specific tracers: the lack of anatomical landmarks within the image [3, 4].

It should be noted that Nuclear Medicine can also operate without imagery. This can be achieved by the measurement of radioactivity in specified sites of accumulation or in biological samples following the administration of the radiopharmaceutical [1, 8].

4. Radiopharmaceuticals

The first radioactive tracer experiment was performed by George Charles de Hevesy in the 1920s. In the 1930s, Irene Curie and Frederic Joliot discovered artificial radioactivity. The discovery of the cyclotron by Ernest Lawrence opened the door for the production of radiotracers of practically every element, thus enabling investigators to design radiotracers for the study of specific biochemical processes.

The European Pharmacopoeia describes "radiopharmaceutical" as any medical product which, when ready to use, contains one or more radionuclides included for a medicinal purpose [11].

Although the field of Nuclear Medicine evolved into a more sophisticated molecular-imaging technology, the term "radiopharmaceuticals" has extended to novel radiolabeled molecular-imaging probes [1, 4].

Most radiopharmaceuticals consist of a combination of a radioactive molecule—a radionuclide —and a biologically active molecule or a drug that acts as a carrier and determines localization and biodistribution. For a few radionuclides (such as radioiodine, gallium, or thallium), the radioactive atoms themselves act as the radiopharmaceuticals [3].

The radionuclide emits radiation that is detected externally using gamma cameras or PET cameras. Certain characteristics are desirable for clinically useful radiopharmaceuticals. Radionuclide decay should result in emissions of suitable energy (100–200 keV is ideal for gamma cameras) and in sufficient abundance for external detection. Particulate radiation (e.g., beta emissions) increases the patient radiation dose, and should be reserved for therapeutic use. Effective half-life should be only long enough for the intended application (usually a few hours). The radionuclide should be carrier-free—that is, not contaminated by other stable radionuclides or other radionuclides of the same element. Technetium-99m most closely fulfills these features for the gamma camera, and fluorine-18 for PET [2, 3].

Once a decision about a suitable nuclide has been made, an appropriate agent must be selected to carry the isotope. There are many different radiopharmaceuticals available to study the different parts of the body, which can be administered by injection, ingestion, or even inhalation. They are administered in sub-pharmacological doses (<100 μg) and "trace" a particular physiological or pathological process in the body, portraying the physiology, biochemistry, or pathology, without affecting it or without causing any other physiological effect [2, 3]. Thus, with the exception of some tracers in radio-immunoscintigraphy and radiotherapy, hypersensitivity reactions against tracers are very rare, as the administered quantities are below a threshold to trigger immune response. Even in known hypersensitivity to iodinated substances (i.e., hypersensitivity against contrast media in radiology), iodine tracers can be safely used for diagnosis and therapy [1].

Understanding the mechanism and rationale for the use of each agent is critical to understanding the normal and pathological findings demonstrated scintigraphically.

5. Nuclear Medicine: its applications

Taking advantage of the combination of individual characteristics of the patient and molecular specificities of the disease, Nuclear Medicine aims to integrate patient- and disease-specific information [4, 8].

Apart from its major diagnostic and therapeutic roles, Nuclear Medicine is important in establishing prognosis, assessing disease progression, identifying recurrence, selecting the most effective therapy, monitoring therapy, and adapting treatment plans in response to changes in cellular activity [1, 4, 8].

Additionally, Nuclear Medicine is an important tool in the development of new targeted drugs and in the design and implementation of improved patient-tailored therapies [1, 4, 8].

5.1. Diagnosis

Nuclear Medicine dedicates primarily to the diagnosis of medical conditions. Depending on the type of examination, radiopharmaceuticals are administered in the most suitable way, for example, intravenously or orally. Afterwards, external detectors capture the radiation emitted by those radiopharmaceuticals and images are formed, showing the radiopharmaceutical uptake distribution and, subsequently, the targeted sites.

5.2. Targeted therapy

Drugs are designed to treat diseases, correcting abnormal cellular or molecular processes [4]. In theory, any highly specific imaging tracer can be used for therapy if labeled with the suitable radionuclide.

The term theranostics refers to substances that have both diagnostic and therapeutic roles. One classic example is radioiodine, used to diagnose and treat some thyroid pathologies. Theranostics has played a vital role in radiation-based therapies, especially when using targeted radiopharmaceuticals [9, 12].

Therapeutic procedures in Nuclear Medicine use high-dose, nonpenetrating radiation emitting, targeted radiopharmaceuticals. Most therapies use beta-emitters (I-131, Y-90, and Lu-177), but Auger-, Alpha-, or conversion electron emitters are also good candidates [3, 8]. The targeting ligands can also be radiolabeled with suitable positron emitters such as F-18 and Ga-68, for PET monitoring and evaluation purposes [9].

Theranostics agents play a major role in the development of radiopharmaceuticals, validating its target profile and early-disease diagnostics. They help choose the more adequate candidates and therefore are frequently used by the pharmaceutical industry [9].

5.3. Drug and formulation development and drug-regulatory affairs

Nuclear Medicine studies on drug delivery have been accepted by regulatory authorities as supporting evidence in product registration dossiers such as Investigational New Drug Applications or New Drug Applications [13].

Nuclear Medicine stimulates and supports drug development in a noninvasive way. With the radiolabeling of drug molecules, it is possible to monitor distribution, release, and kinetics, through the observation of its *in vivo* distribution and allowing the visualization of their metabolism in both target and nontarget sites [1, 13]. These studies can be performed in both animals and humans.

In drug approval, most studies are performed with new chemical entities (NCEs), because information on their metabolic outcome is required. Studies of biopharmaceuticals metabolism using radiotracers are less frequent, because it can be difficult to substitute a radiotracer for a naturally occurring stable isotope [6].

Regulatory drug-testing programs that employ radiotracers are generally classified into two groups: explorative and standard studies. Standard studies are habitually done for the majority of NCEs, with varying characteristics, depending on the drug class and specific circumstances. Explorative studies, although very important (even mandatory sometimes), are not usually required. More than 80% of all drug-safety-testing assessment programs (by the US safety assessment process) used radiotracers [14].

6. Drug delivery and Nuclear Medicine

Drugs are usually administered as pharmaceutical dosage forms. In the development of these dosage forms, it is fundamental to ensure they will perform correctly. Before the submission to the regulatory authority for approval of a new medicine, detailed testing is required. To improve therapeutic effects and minimize toxicity, it is crucial to deliver the therapeutic drugs to the right target, in the desired time, and in the precise concentration—a "magic bullet" [7, 9].

The controlled and targeted delivery of therapeutic drugs improves their bioavailability (either by preventing premature degradation or by improving uptake), maintains their concentrations within the therapeutic window (by adjusting the release rate), and reduces side effects (by targeting disease site/cells). The ability to deliver therapeutic drugs to the target, in a minimally invasive approach, has advanced considerably with the growth of molecular-imaging techniques [9].

When molecular-imaging radiotracers are part of the drug-delivery system, they enable monitoring of its *in vivo* behaviour: pharmacokinetics, distribution, release at the target site, and excretion. Some of these evaluations (such as *in vivo* fate or delivery efficiency) are not possible with a nonimage-guided approach. Another issue with nonimaging techniques is that much testing (bioavailability, therapeutic efficacy, and dose response) must be done in separate experiments, which makes for a rather expensive and stressful process [9].

The use of Nuclear Medicine imaging in the study of a drug-delivery process dates back to the late 1970s and is well established in pharmaceutical development. Understanding drug action and providing key information about the drug-delivery process through a variety of routes, Nuclear Medicine can be used in the various stages of studies [6, 9, 13]. Without radiotracers, the comprehension of numerous biochemical processes would have been tremendously difficult and, in some cases, maybe impossible. Its strength lies in the quantitative nature of the images. Only Nuclear Medicine techniques can determine the precise location of tablet disintegration in the gastrointestinal (GI) tract, the depth of penetration of a nebulized solution in the lungs, or for how long does the formulation stay in the cornea [6, 9, 13].

In image-guided drug delivery assessment, the image techniques are used for determining disease location, drug-targeting levels and localization, and release kinetics (before and during treatment). The type and stability of the labeling will depend upon whether the study is meant to examine release, deposition, retention/dispersion, or is being used to monitor the effects of physiological process [13, 15].

The majority of studies have evaluated gastrointestinal, pulmonary, and nasal drug delivery, but ophthalmic, buccal, rectal, vaginal, and parenteral routes have also been subject of research [6].

The required quantity of radiotracer in a drug formulation is very small and does not commit with the performance of the delivery system. Radiolabeling must reveal high *in vitro* and *in vivo* stability and can be performed in two different ways. The radiolabeled compound can be directly incorporated into the preparation, or a dosage form that contains a nonradioactive tracer can be neutron-activated. The latter is advantageous in extensive or complicated delivery systems, and also has the advantage of the dosage formulation being manufactured and produced under normal conditions [7, 9]. Still, Nuclear Medicine imaging of drug-delivery processes involves several challenges and is affected by numerous factors such as target expression, *in vivo* availability of the receptor, type of drug, enhanced permeability and retention effect, tracer protein dose, and timing of imaging [9].

Once administered, the radiolabeled compound will be monitored *in vivo* over a period of time (depending on its half-life), using appropriate image equipment: gamma-scintigraphy or PET. It is then crucial to choose the most suitable radioisotopes, with fitting half-lives to pair with the pharmacokinetics of their drug carriers, and the most adequate imaging system [6, 9, 13].

In the last decades, most studies used gamma-scintigraphy and Tc-99m-labeled radiopharmaceuticals containing chelating agents (such as diethylene-triamine-pentaacetic acid (DTPA)), colloids (such as sulfur colloid), diphosphonates (such as hydroxymethane diphosphonate (HDP)), cells and blood elements, and cellulose macromolecules [7, 13].

More recently, the use of PET is increasing, including in drug-delivery development studies. An important attribute of PET studies is that some of the radioactive atoms available include radioisotopes of carbon, nitrogen, and fluorine. This makes it possible to synthesize PET radiotracers with the same chemical structure as the unlabeled molecules, without altering their biological function [9, 13].

Unlike radiological imaging, Nuclear Medicine allows serial images to be obtained without submitting the subjects to higher radiation burdens, and radioactive concerns are neglected. Besides the reliability and reproducibility of Nuclear Medicine studies on the nature and characteristics of products, they may also be performed in the groups of patients intended to receive the dosage forms therapeutically, which is important since the presence of pathology can have significant impact on physiology [13].

It is well established that diseases alter physiological processes, and subsequently biodistribution of drug formulations. Thus, studies in humans are the most relevant and Nuclear Medicine imaging probably represents the only technique available that allows the quantification of drug release and pharmacokinetics in specific groups, namely patients with diseases [13]. This know-how has the potential for patient selection for targeted therapy and for the monitoring of therapeutic response after the drug is delivered [9].

Targeted therapy involves the integration of multidisciplinary fields such as cell and molecular biology, chemistry, physics, and so on. Significant advances in the field have been attributed to the progress in nanotechnology, with the development of nanosized, multifunctional drug-delivery platforms. For example, a single platform can be used to detect, treat, and monitor treatment response in tumors. These systems present several advantages, including minimal clearance by the immune system, prolonged circulating times, attachment to suitable vectors (peptides, proteins, antibodies, etc.) and targeting of specific receptors, and improved treatment effects by shielding entrapped drugs from degradation [9].

For example, stimulus-responsive polymeric nanomaterials can be synthesized to mimic the behavior of biological molecules, minimizing side effects and maximizing predictability. Another example, the liposomal carriers (the first and most extensive studied drug-delivery carriers), is used in the delivery of anticancer drugs, antineoplastic agents, antimicrobial compounds, immunomodulators, anti-inflammatory agents, cardiovascular drugs, and so on. Some other nanosized drug-delivery systems that have also been developed for molecular-imaging purposes are metallic nanoparticles, oxide nanoparticles, polymeric nanoparticles, and carbon nanostructures [9].

The major goal of molecular imaging is to maximize therapy effect in diseased tissues, and reduce systemic effects and toxicity as much as possible [9].

6.1. Gastrointestinal tract studies

Despite the vast diversity of new drug-delivery systems, oral administration is still preferred.

Most commonly, oral-dosage forms immediately release in the stomach, but the use of more sophisticated, modified release systems is increasing and requires new methods of evaluation. Furthermore, regulatory authorities require evaluation of the *in vivo* performance of new oral formulations.

Nuclear Medicine imaging is one of the most popular methods to investigate those GI release systems, because pharmacokinetic measurements are often unreliable. Its combination with pharmacokinetic studies provides accurate data about transit, absorption, and release performance of oral-dosage formulations [7].

Nuclear Medicine imaging provides information, from both control and patient groups, on swallowing dynamics of tablet and capsule formulations, disintegration of immediate release formulations, gastric emptying and gastroesophageal reflux, release of enteric-coated formulations, GI transit times, the effect of formulation size on GI delivery, visualization of targeted release or delivery to the colon, the effects of time of dosing on delivery, local permeability within the colon, disintegration characteristics likely to influence drug absorption, and residence time of the material within the colon [7, 9].

GI nuclear studies often require both solid- and liquid-phase markers, there being two conventional approaches for the labeling of the oral-dosage forms. One method involves incorporating a nonabsorbable chelate of the radioactive isotope (e.g., DTPA-Tc-99m). The other incorporating a radiolabeled ion-exchange resin, which has the advantage of giving information about the *in vivo* position of the radiolabeled drug, because the resin remains within the device [7].

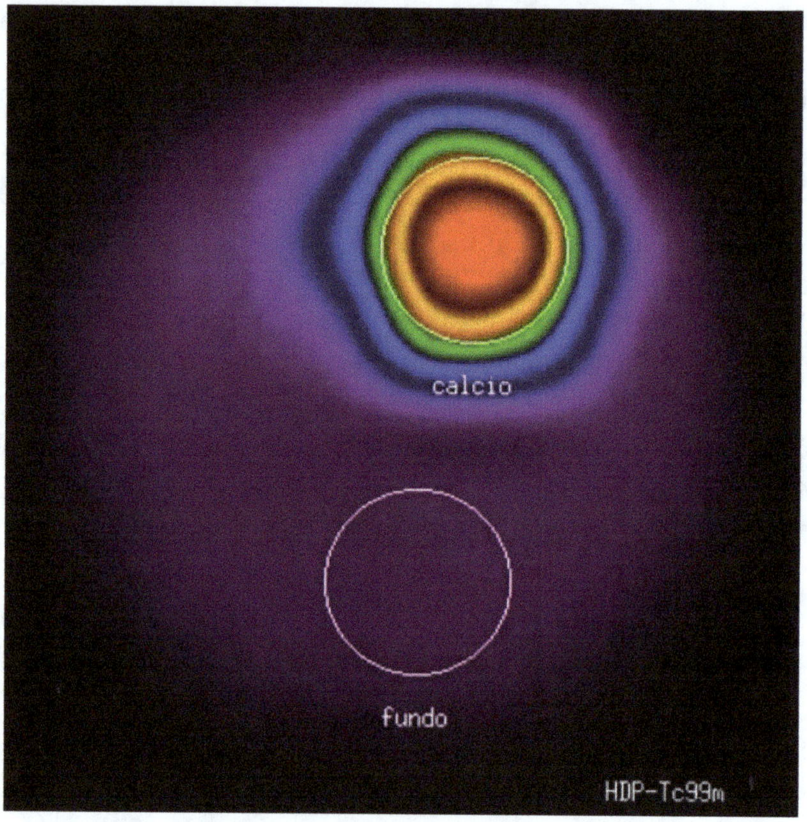

Figure 1. *In vitro* radiolabeling and evaluation of the drug-delivery system.

In two different studies aimed at evaluating the gastroretentive behavior of pharmaceutical dosage forms, Barata et al. used Tc-99m-HDP to label HMPC tablets supplemented with calcium phosphate. The radiolabeling process consisted in soaking the tablet in a Tc-99m-HDP and NaCl 0.9% solution, with activity counts of 400–600 millicuries. The addition of calcium to the systems did not affect drug release, but significantly increased the binding of the radiopharmaceutical to the dosage form. In fact, the dosage form remained integer and well radiolabeled for a period of over 4 h, which was sufficient to study the gastroretentive pattern of the produced tablets. This proved to be an easy and reproducible method of extemporaneously radiolabeling tablets produced outside Nuclear Medicine Department facilities, solving radiation-related transportation problems (see **Figure 1**).

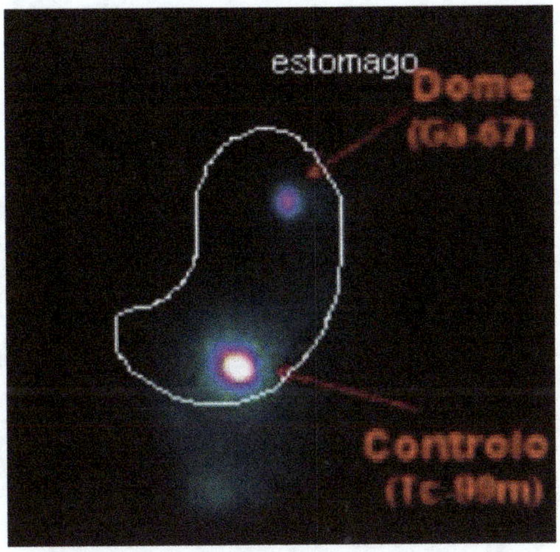

Figure 2. *In vivo* analysis of the drug-delivery system floating behavior.

For the floating-device study, a non-floating tablet was labeled with Tc-99m-HDP, while the floating pharmaceutical dosage form was labeled with Ga-68 (gallium-68), using the same soaking method. Despite not as effective as Tc-99m-HDP labeling, Ga-68 labeling was enough to allow a clear visualization of the system. The physical properties of the two radiopharmaceuticals (different energy photons) enabled the simultaneous identifying of each system over time: initially, both in the stomach (floating in the upper part of the stomach or staying in the antrum), then, the effective gastroretention of the floating device for over 4 h (see **Figure 2**).

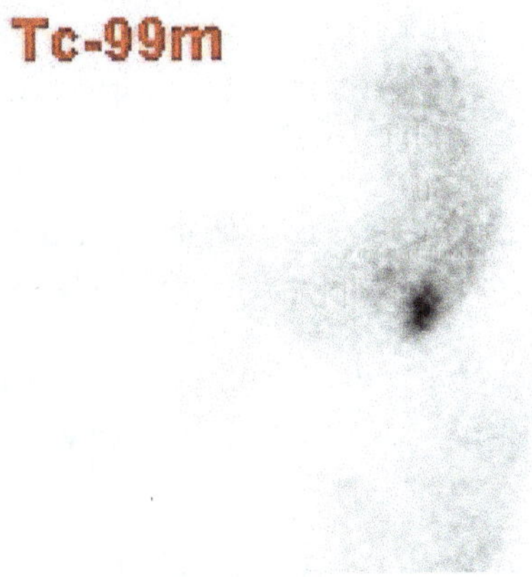

Figure 3. *In vivo* analysis of the drug-delivery system gastroretentive behavior.

In the other study, aiming to demonstrate the gastroretentive efficacy of high-density tablets, a similar process was used to radiolabel the produced tablets. Again, it was possible to see the *in vivo* positioning of the pharmaceutical dosage form and confirm that the high-density controlled release strategy is effective for delivering drugs with a narrow upper GI absorption window (see **Figure 3**).

These examples prove that incorporating gamma-emitting radionuclides into a delivery device or formulation provides an appropriate, simple method of observing the transit and residence within the GI tract—of particular interest in determining the time and site of release of delayed release formulations.

6.2. Other system studies

Both SPECT and PET imaging play an increasing role in the development of new targeted drug-delivery systems [13].

Nuclear Medicine is being used to surpass the severe systemic toxicity of anticancer drugs, which are usually more effective in high doses. Additionally, numerous conventional therapeutic agents repeatedly fail to reach their target, rendering them ineffective. The ideal drug should be specific for the cancer cell and devoid of systemic effects. For these reasons, the ideal drug-delivery system is aimed, and Nuclear Medicine, with all its already-known advantages, plays an important role in this area [9, 16].

PET image-guided drug delivery allows for the treatment of a variety of diseases with minimal systemic involvement (sparing normal cells), while monitoring its efficacy.

In cancer-targeted treatment, chemotherapeutic drugs can be loaded onto multifunctional drug carriers (such as liposomes, micelles, and nanoparticles) and coupled with several targeting ligands (such as monoclonal antibodies, peptides, and antibody fragments). Carriers are multifunctional and may also carry PET radiopharmaceuticals for diagnostic purposes. These systems are important examples of theranostics. One example is the streptavidin/biotin interaction that is used for binding numerous carriers to targeting proteins and antibodies.

In another approach, therapeutic radionuclides are conjugated with targeting ligands (by means of bifunctional-linking strategies), without any image-enabling radionuclide. PET imaging for the diagnosis or monitoring of therapeutic response is carried out separately, by conjugation of the targeting ligands with suitable PET radioisotopes [9].

Investigation-wise, PET allows the *in vivo* quantification and drug distribution, determining its extraction fraction and washout from different organs/systems.

PET imaging allows the study of the first-pass liver elimination of a drug, a fundamental knowledge, since first-pass metabolism excludes oral delivery of several drug molecules and compounds.

PET studies are also useful in the understanding of the brain and of several neurological conditions, including anxiety and depression [13]. In Parkinson's and Alzheimer's diseases, the *in vivo* study of neuroreceptors binding is fundamental for the drug-design process (ex. enzyme/prodrug-based delivery approach with 18F for Parkinson's disease) [9, 13].

7. Conclusion

Nuclear Medicine is a very promising field and will surely increase its relevance on diagnostics and therapeutics in the near future. Also within the field of drug development and drug-delivery systems research, it is expected to demonstrate an ever-increasing applicability and importance. The advent of new and more complex drugs, combined with more ingenious and technological delivery systems, will call for a more detailed and effective *in vivo* studies during the development and regulatory phases of the research and marketing authorization process. Radiopharmaceuticals and Nuclear Medicine will therefore be predictably ever more used with the purpose of obtaining better, safer, and more reliable drug-delivery systems.

Author details

Ana Rita Fernandes[1], Ana Oliveira[1], Jorge Pereira[1] and Pedro Silva Coelho[2*]

*Address all correspondence to: pbarata@ufp.edu.pt

1 Nuclear Medicine Department, São João Hospital Center, Porto, Portugal

2 Faculty of Health Sciences, University Fernando Pessoa, Porto, Portugal

References

[1] Leitha T. Nuclear Medicine: Proof of principle for targeted drugs in diagnosis and therapy. Current Pharmaceutical Design. 2009;15:173–187. DOI: 10.2174/1381612 09787002898

[2] Society of Nuclear Medicine [Internet]. Available from: http://interactive.snm.org/docs/whatisnucmed2.pdf and http://www.snmmi.org/AboutSNMMI/Content.aspx?ItemNumber=6433 [Accessed: 2016.05.23]

[3] Ziessman HA, O'Malley JP, Thrall JH. Nuclear Medicine: The Requisites. 4th ed. Philadelphia, PA: Elsevier; 2013. 466 p. DOI: 10.1148/radiol.2223012567.

[4] Clanton J, Sandler MP. Molecular imaging radiopharmaceuticals for PET and SPECT. Journal of Nuclear Medicine. 2010;51:660–661. DOI: 10.2967/jnumed.109.072645

[5] Kim EE, Lee D, Tateishi U, Baum RP. Handbook of Nuclear Medicine and Molecular Imaging—Principles and Clinical Applications. 2nd ed. World Scientific Publishing Co. Pte. Ltd., 2012. 472 p. ISBN: 9789814366236

[6] Lappin G, Temple S. Radiotracers in Drug Development. Taylor & Francis, 2006. 320 p. ISBN: 9780849333477

[7] Wilding IR, Coupe AJ, Davis SS. The role of γ-scintigraphy in oral drug delivery. Advanced Drug Delivery Reviews. 2001;46:103–124. DOI: 10.1016/S0169-409X(00)00135-6.

[8] Calahan RJ. et al. Society of nuclear medicine procedure guideline for the use of radiopharmaceuticals 4.0. Journal of Nuclear Medicine Technology. 2007;35(4) 272–275. DOI: 10.2967/jnmt.107.044156.

[9] Chakravarty R, Hong H, Cai W. Positron emission tomography image-guided drug delivery: Current status and future perspectives. Molecular Pharmaceutics. 2014; 11(11):3777–3797. DOI: 10.1021/mp500173s

[10] Baert AL, Sartor K, Schiepers C. Diagnostic Nuclear Medicine. 2nd Revised Edition. Springer-Verlag, Berlin Heidelberg, 2006. 355 p. DOI: 10.1007/3-540-30005-8

[11] European Pharmacopoeia. 8th ed. EDQM, 01/2014., 2016. ISBN-13:9789287175274

[12] MacKay JA, Li Z. Theranostic agents that co-deliver therapeutic and imaging agents? Advanced Drug Delivery Reviews. 2010;62(11):1003–1004. DOI: 10.1016/j.addr.2010.10.001

[13] Malcolm F, Alan CP. The role of gamma scintigraphy in the study of drug delivery. Correspondence Continuing Education Courses for Nuclear Pharmacists and Nuclear Medicine Professional. 2003;X(N° 3 and 4):1–76.

[14] Roberts D, Lockley R. Radiosynthesis: A vital role supporting drug development. Drug Discovery World, Fall, 2004, pp. 59–62.

[15] Hatefi A, Minko T. Advances in image-guided drug delivery. Drug Delivery and Translational Research. 2012;2:1–2. DOI: 10.1007/s13346-011-0057-8.

[16] Haley B, Frenkel E. Nanoparticles for drug delivery in cancer treatment. Urologic Oncology. 2008;26(1):57–64. DOI: 10.1016/j.urolonc.2007.03.015.

Permissions

All chapters in this book were first published in ATDT, by InTech Open; hereby published with permission under the Creative Commons Attribution License or equivalent. Every chapter published in this book has been scrutinized by our experts. Their significance has been extensively debated. The topics covered herein carry significant findings which will fuel the growth of the discipline. They may even be implemented as practical applications or may be referred to as a beginning point for another development.

The contributors of this book come from diverse backgrounds, making this book a truly international effort. This book will bring forth new frontiers with its revolutionizing research information and detailed analysis of the nascent developments around the world.

We would like to thank all the contributing authors for lending their expertise to make the book truly unique. They have played a crucial role in the development of this book. Without their invaluable contributions this book wouldn't have been possible. They have made vital efforts to compile up to date information on the varied aspects of this subject to make this book a valuable addition to the collection of many professionals and students.

This book was conceptualized with the vision of imparting up-to-date information and advanced data in this field. To ensure the same, a matchless editorial board was set up. Every individual on the board went through rigorous rounds of assessment to prove their worth. After which they invested a large part of their time researching and compiling the most relevant data for our readers.

The editorial board has been involved in producing this book since its inception. They have spent rigorous hours researching and exploring the diverse topics which have resulted in the successful publishing of this book. They have passed on their knowledge of decades through this book. To expedite this challenging task, the publisher supported the team at every step. A small team of assistant editors was also appointed to further simplify the editing procedure and attain best results for the readers.

Apart from the editorial board, the designing team has also invested a significant amount of their time in understanding the subject and creating the most relevant covers. They scrutinized every image to scout for the most suitable representation of the subject and create an appropriate cover for the book.

The publishing team has been an ardent support to the editorial, designing and production team. Their endless efforts to recruit the best for this project, has resulted in the accomplishment of this book. They are a veteran in the field of academics and their pool of knowledge is as vast as their experience in printing. Their expertise and guidance has proved useful at every step. Their uncompromising quality standards have made this book an exceptional effort. Their encouragement from time to time has been an inspiration for everyone.

The publisher and the editorial board hope that this book will prove to be a valuable piece of knowledge for researchers, students, practitioners and scholars across the globe.

List of Contributors

Asadullah Madni, Nayab Tahir, Mubashar Rehman, Ahmed Raza, Muhammad Ahmad Mahmood, Muhammad Imran Khan and Prince Muhammad Kashif
Faculty of Pharmacy and Alternative Medicine, The Islamia University of Bahawalpur, Bahawalpur, Pakistan

Lavinia Vlaia, Georgeta Coneac, Ioana Olariu and Vicențiu Vlaia
Faculty of Pharmacy, "Victor Babeş" University of Medicine and Pharmacy, Timişoara, Romania

Dumitru Lupuleasa
Faculty of Pharmacy, "Carol Davila" University of Medicine and Pharmacy, Bucureşti, Romania

Mohsin Kazi
Department of Pharmaceutics, College of Pharmacy, King Saud University, Riyadh, Kingdom of Saudi Arabia

Sukumaran Anil
Department of Periodontics and Community Dentistry, College of Dentistry, King Saud University, Riyadh, Saudi Arabia

Asala F. Al-Sulaimani
King Saud University, Riyadh, Saudi Arabia

Ansar E. Beeran and Harikrishna P.R. Varma
Biomedical Technology Wing, Sree Chitra Tirunal Institute for Medical Sciences & Technology, Poojappura, India

Elna P. Chalisserry
College of Dentistry, King Saud University, Riyadh, Saudi Arabia

Mohammad D. Al Amri
Department of Prosthetic Dental Sciences, College of Dentistry, King Saud University, Riyadh, Saudi Arabia

Sakthivel Lakshmana Prabu
Department of Pharmaceutical Technology, Bharathidasan Institute of Technology, Anna University, Tiruchirapalli, Tamil Nadu, India

Kandasamy Ruckmani
Department of Pharmaceutical Technology, Bharathidasan Institute of Technology, Anna University, Tiruchirapalli, Tamil Nadu, India
Centre for Excellence in Nanobio Translational Research (CENTRE), National Facility on Drug Design (NFDD), Professor and Head, Department of Pharmaceutical Technology, Bharathidasan Institute of Technology, Anna University, Tiruchirapalli, Tamil Nadu, India

Jinxiang Xi
School of Engineering and Technology, Central Michigan University, Mount Pleasant, MI, USA

Xiuhua April Si
Department of Mechanical Engineering, California Baptist University, Riverside, CA, USA

Qun Wang, Jianying Huang and Yuekun Lai
National Engineering Laboratory for Modern Silk, College of Textile and Clothing Engineering, Soochow University, Suzhou, China

Kazuo Shimizu and Jaroslav Krištof
Shizuoka University, Hamamatsu, Japan

Ana Rita Fernandes, Ana Oliveira and Jorge Pereira
Nuclear Medicine Department, São João Hospital Center, Porto, Portugal

Pedro Silva Coelho
Faculty of Health Sciences, University Fernando Pessoa, Porto, Portugal

Index

www.ingramcontent.com/pod-product-compliance
Lightning Source LLC
LaVergne TN
LVHW081025210926
848485LV00004B/953